TRENDS IN ALCOHOLIC LIVER DISEASE RESEARCH – CLINICAL AND SCIENTIFIC ASPECTS

Edited by **Ichiro Shimizu**

Trends in Alcoholic Liver Disease Research – Clinical and Scientific Aspects
Edited by Ichiro Shimizu

Published by InTech

Janeza Trdine 9, 51000 Rijeka, Croatia

Publishing Process Manager Adriana Pecar

Technical Editor Teodora Smiljanic

Cover Designer InTech Design Team

Additional hard copies can be obtained from orders@intechopen.com

Trends in Alcoholic Liver Disease Research – Clinical and Scientific Aspects,
Edited by Ichiro Shimizu
p. cm.
ISBN 978-953-307-985-1

For EU product safety concerns:
IN TECH d.o.o., Prolaz Marije Krucifikse Kozulić 3, 51000 Rijeka, Croatia,
info@intechopen.com or visit our website at intechopen.com.

Meet the editor

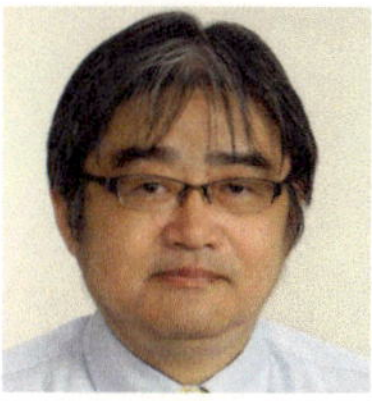

Ichiro Shimizu, MD, PhD, AGAF, is the director at Showa Clinic in Yokohama, Japan, and a former associate professor of Tokushima University School of Medicine in Japan. Dr. Shimizu has performed pioneering research on the favorable effects of estrogens on hepatic fibrogenesis and carciogenesis that are connected with the sex-associated differences of chronic liver disease. In addition, Dr. Shimizu has also identified preventive and therapeutic mechanisms for hepatic fibrosis in the Chinese herbal medicine Xiao-Chaihu-Tang (Sho-Saiko-To). Dr Shimizu published in excess of 10 books relating to hepatic fibrosis, also called "female hepatology", and Sho-Saiko-To, and was additionally awarded the Japan Society of Gastroenterology Encouragement Prize in 1998 and the Liver Forum in Kyoto Encouragement Prize in 1999.

Contents

Preface

In most Western countries, alcoholic beverages contribute significantly to a person's overall caloric intake. Of greater significance is it's status as the most widely used drug worldwide and addictive properties in addition to the damage it causes to various organs within the human body - in particular the liver. Alcoholic liver disease occurs after prolonged heavy drinking, especially among persons who are physically dependent on alcohol. Not everyone who drinks alcohol to excess develops serious forms of alcoholic liver disease. It is likely that genetic factors determine this individual susceptibility, and a family history of chronic liver disease may indicate a higher risk. Other factors include being overweight (similar to hepatitis C and non-alcoholic fatty liver disease), and iron overload. Women are more susceptible to alcoholic liver disease than men, partly because of differences in the rate of alcohol metabolism, but also for other biological reasons. Alcoholic liver disease encompasses a broad spectrum of diseases, ranging from steatosis (fatty liver), steatohepatitis, fibrosis, and cirrhosis, to hepatocellular carcinoma.

There have been major advances in our understanding of the liver, and a growing number of mechanisms underlying alcoholic liver disease continue to pose new challenges. This book presents state-of-the-art information summarizing the current understanding of a range of alcoholic liver diseases. Additionally, key cellular, biochemical, immunological and microstructural mechanisms, and diagnostic and therapeutic advances are also reviewed.

The book constitutes a collection of selected clinical and scientific topics. Some chapters treat the cellular, biochemical, immunological, and micro-structural mechanisms underlying alcoholic liver diseases. Some other chapters focus on clinical alcoholic liver disease pathophysiology, related diagnostics, and therapeutic insights. Each of the eleven chapters is followed by a detailed bibliography, enabling the reader to work in depth on specific topics. Collectively, this book represents a broad range of important updated topics.

It is hoped that the target readers, such as hepatologists, clinicians, researchers and academicians, will be afforded new ideas and exposed to subjects which extend beyond their own scientific disciplines. In addition, students and all those who wish to increase their knowledge of advances in the field of alcoholic liver disease will find this book a valuable source of information.

My thanks are extended to the authors, the publisher, and most importantly, my family.

Ichiro Shimizu, MD, AGAF
Showa Clinic, Kohoku-ku, Yokohama,
Kanagawa, Japan

1

Alcohol Drinking Patterns and Nutrition in Alcoholic Liver Disease

Sabine Wagnerberger, Giridhar Kanuri and Ina Bergheim
Universität Hohenheim
Germany

1. Introduction

In most Western countries alcoholic beverages contribute markedly to the overall caloric intake. Indeed, alcohol contributes to approximately 5% of the daily caloric intake in the American diet (Halsted, 2004). Alcohol, besides nicotine, is also the most widely used drug in our society, bearing a large potential for addiction but also organ damage and herein particularly liver damage. Chronic alcohol abuse is frequently accompanied with malnutrition with the degree of malnutrition varying not only between the type of alcohol abuse (e.g. binge drinker vs. chronic drinker) but also the degree of liver damage. For practitioners it is important to recognize the various factors contributing to the evolvement of malnutrition in alcoholic patients, as the correction of deficiencies or other strategies to improve nutritional status may have a beneficial effect in the prevention and treatment of alcoholic liver disease. The effects of alcohol ingestion on dietary pattern, nutrient intake and the intermediary metabolism have been investigated in numerous human but also animal studies. In this chapter the role of alcohol as energy source but also the effects of alcohol ingestion on energy metabolism, dietary pattern and micronutrient bioavailability as well as metabolism with special emphasize on the liver and the development of alcoholic liver disease are reviewed. Furthermore, current recommendations for treatment of malnutrition in patients with alcoholic liver disease are summarized.

2. Alcohol drinking patterns

When talking about "alcohol drinking", two main patterns have to be distinguished: acute "binge drinking" and "chronic drinking". As reviewed by Zakhari and Li (2007), the impact of the quantity and frequency of alcohol ingestion on alcoholic liver disease becomes more and more important. Indeed, the results of a Danish prospective study with a cohort of 6152 alcohol misusing men and women indicate that periodic drinking leads to a significantly lower relative risk for developing cirrhosis than daily drinking (Kamper-Jorgensen *et al.* 2004). The Italian Dionysos Study focused on drinking habits as cofactors of risk for alcohol-induced liver damage. The results of this study show that drinking without food and drinking multiple different alcoholic beverages both increase the risk of developing alcoholic liver disease (Bellentani *et al.* 1997). Furthermore, it has been shown that the metabolic effects of binge drinking and chronic drinking on the liver also markedly differ (for overview see (Zakhari and Li, 2007)). For example, binge drinking may lead to glycogen depletion, acidosis and hypoglycemia; whereas chronic drinking results in the development of alcoholic liver damages. The differences between these two alcohol drinking patterns are detailed in the following.

2.1 Binge drinking

The World Health Organization (WHO) defines binge drinking as a pattern of heavy drinking that occurs in an extended period, which is usually defined as more than one day of drinking at a time (WHO, 1994). In the United States (US), the National Institute on Alcohol Abuse and Alcoholism defined a more common definition that a "binge" is a pattern of alcohol drinking that brings blood alcohol level to 0.08 gram-percent or above. For a typical adult, the amount of alcohol that has to be ingested to reach these blood alcohol levels is on average equivalent to consuming five or more drinks (men), or four or more drinks (women), in about two hours (National Institute on Alcohol Abuse and Alcoholism, 2007). In contrast, in the United Kingdom binge drinking is defined as the consumption of more than eight drinks in men and more than six drinks in women in a single day (Institute of Alcohol Studies, 2010). In the United States, the prevalence of binge drinking among adults was 15.2% in 2009, with the prevalence being two times higher in men than in women (Kanny *et al.* 2011). This phenomenon can also be observed in most of the European countries, except for England and Ireland. In these two countries binge drinking is found to be particularly prevalent in women (Dantzer *et al.* 2006). In terms of age, the prevalence of binge drinking decreases, both in the United States and United Kingdom, with increasing age, indicating that the phenomenon "binge drinking" is as an important problem especially in young people (Institute of Alcohol Studies, 2010). In dependence on "drinking cultures" binge drinking occurs more or less in different countries. In Mediterranean culture, alcoholic beverages, especially wine, are consumed on a daily basis as part of meals and mostly in family settings. In contrast, in Northern cultures, drinking is less frequent in everyday life but heavier, typically around weekends (Institute of Alcohol Studies, 2010).

2.2 Chronic drinking

In a systemic review, the risks of moderate alcohol consumption have been weighed against its benefits. As a result of comparing the critical endpoints of alcohol intake related to morbidity and mortality, tolerable upper alcohol intake levels have been defined for the German adult population to be 20 to 24g alcohol per day for men and 10 to 12g alcohol per day for women (Burger *et al.* 2004). However, it is recommended that if this amount of alcohol is ingested, at least two days per week should be without any alcohol consumption. Exceeding this tolerable alcohol intake level alcohol consumption is classified as a risk factor for numerous organ damages (e.g. liver, pancreas, stomach, gut).

In Germany, the per-capita consumption of pure ethanol was 9.7 l in 2009. Furthermore, in 2006 3.8% of the German population met the criteria of alcohol abuse and 2.4% of alcohol dependence in 2006 (Deutsche Hauptstelle für Suchtfragen, DHS, 2006). According to the 2001-2002 National Epidemiologic Survey on Alcohol and related Conditions, 5.8% of the US adult population meet the criteria for alcohol dependence or alcoholism and 7.1% meet the criteria for alcohol abuse (for overview see Zakhari and Li, 2007). Despite intense education on the risks associated with alcohol abuse, in industrialized countries in Europe as well as in the United States, the damage of liver and other organs as a consequence of chronic alcohol consumption is still an important health problem. Especially, chronic alcohol abuse is one of the most important risk factors for liver damage (Lieber, 1994). The results of previous studies demonstrated the existence of a dose-response relation between alcohol intake and the risk of liver disease (Lelbach, 1975; Day, 1997). As a consequence of alcohol abuse different alcoholic liver disease patterns such as alcohol-caused fatty liver, alcoholic hepatitis, or alcohol-induced cirrhosis can be observed.

3. Alcohol and energy metabolism

3.1 Alcohol and its contribution to energy intake

For many people regular alcohol consumption is still a part of their daily diet. Raw alcohol and even more so alcoholic beverages are rather energy dense nutrients. Alcoholic beverages primarily consist of water, ethanol, and, depending on the beverage, variable amounts of carbohydrates as well as to a lesser extend proteins, vitamins or minerals (see Table 1).

	Energy	Protein		Fat		Carbohydrate		Ethanol	
	kcal	g	kcal	g	kcal	g	kcal	g	kcal
Whiskey	250	0.0	0.0	0.0	0.0	0.1	0.4	36	252.0
Vodka	232	0.0	0.0	0.0	0.0	0.0	0.0	33.4	233.8
Dry red wine	60	0.7	2.9	0.0	0.0	4.6	18.9	5.5	38.5
Dry white wine	42	0.5	2.1	0.0	0.0	3.1	12.7	4.0	28.0
Stout	83	0.1	0.4	0.0	0.0	3.8	15.6	19.9	139.3
Beer	67	0.1	0.4	0.0	0.0	0.2	0.8	9.5	66.5
Sweet white wine	96	0.2	0.8	0.0	0.0	5.9	24.2	10.2	71.4
Cocktail	141	0.2	0.8	0.9	8.4	9.1	37.3	13.7	95.9

Table 1. Energy and caloric content of various alcoholic beverages per 100 mL. Values were calculated with the software program EBIS pro and are based on the German food index.

Calories provided through the consumption of alcoholic beverages primarily stem from its content and metabolism of carbohydrates and ethanol. Indeed, hard spirits like whiskey, vodka and schnapps contain no sugar, whereas dry red and white wine contain 31 to 46 grams of sugar per liter. Sugar content of beer various between 2 and 38 grams per liter depending whether stout or "normal" beer is consumed. Sugar content may even be as high as 120 grams per liter in sweet white wine (on average 59 g/L) and up to 91 grams per liter in mixed cocktails (average value of several cocktails). A similarly strong variability in content is also found when ethanol contents of different alcoholic beverages are compared. For example, a liter of beer with the exception of stout on average contains 200 grams of ethanol per liter whereas wine contains 40 to 100 grams of ethanol per liter. Hard spirits may even contain up to 300 to even 500 grams of ethanol per liter. An average serving of wine (125 mL), beer (330 mL) or hard spirits (40 mL) contains 12 to 14 grams of ethanol.

3.2 Alcohol metabolism and energy yield

Using bomb calorimetry it was shown that ethanol yields 7.1 kcal (= 29.3 kJ) per gram when completely combusted (Lieber, 1991). However, as the digestibility of ethanol ranges from 98 to 100 % and approximately 5% of ethanol is also lost through respiration, faeces and urine energy provide for metabolic purposes is only approximately 6.9 kcal per gram ethanol (= 28.8 kJ per gram ethanol) (Lieber, 1991). It was further shown that even when ethanol is ingested at constant rates and high levels (e.g. up to 171 grams of ethanol per day) the loss of alcohol derived energy through the respiratory tract und urine only accounts to approximately 50 kcal per day (Reinus *et al.* 1989). Indeed, a marked loss of ethanol through urine or respiration was only observed when the amounts of ethanol ingested exceed the liver´s ethanol metabolizing capacity shown to be 105 mg/ kg body weight per h (Reinus *et al.* 1989).

Taking the caloric content of alcoholic beverages into account and the fact that only little is lost through respiration, faeces, and urine, one would expect a positive association of alcohol intake and obesity. However, results of epidemiological studies are somewhat contradictory indicating no or only a weak association of alcohol consumption and body weight in men and even an inverse association in women (Müller *et al.* 1999). The results of these studies suggest that

- ethanol either bears a negative effect on energy yield implying that ethanol is inefficiently metabolised or
- the consumption of ethanol alters dietary intake, absorption and/ or metabolism of other nutrients subsequently leading to a negative or at least diminished energy yield.

In the very early studies of Atwater and Benedict (1902), using direct calorimetry it was shown that in healthy non-alcoholic volunteers ethanol (72 grams ethanol per day) was utilized as efficiently as fat or carbohydrates as a source of energy. Furthermore, it was shown that the ingestion of 31.5 gram of ethanol per 65 kg of body weight did not increase oxygen consumption or thermogenesis in normal volunteers (Barnes *et al.* 1965). However, contrary to these early finding, in the studies of Pirola and Lieber (1972), in which it was shown in normal volunteers that the progressive substitution of carbohydrates with ethanol in an otherwise balanced, normal diet results in a decrease in body weight. In line with these findings it was further shown that the addition of 90g of ethanol to the daily diet increased the daily energy expenditure by 7% (Suter *et al.* 1992) and that lipid oxidation may be inhibited by the ingestion of additional alcohol to 50% of calories (Sonko *et al.* 1994). Furthermore, in a study in which the energy intake of middle-class patients with alcoholic liver disease ranging from non-cirrhotic to cirrhotic was compared to that of controls with the same body mass index it was shown that non-alcoholic energy intake did not differ from that of controls (Bergheim *et al.* 2003). In this study it was further shown that the average energy intake form alcoholic beverages (e.g. from beer, wine and hard spirits) accounting to ~1008 kcal/ day (= ~142 g Ethanol/ day) was added to the daily non-alcoholic energy intake without leading to the development of obesity. The results of this study are in line with other studies in which it was also shown that in middle-class alcohol consumers alcohol consumption is not associated with increased body weight compared with control subjects ingesting the same nonalcoholic energy intake, but lower total energy intake (Mezey, 1991; Rissanen *et al.* 1987). These data suggest that some of the energy ingested as alcohol is "lost" or "wasted"- that is, this energy is not available to the body for the production of energy resources that can be used to produce or maintain body mass. However, when interpreting these data, it has to be kept in mind that when assessing nutritional intake and herein especially that of alcohol underreporting may be a problem. For example, when applying the formula published by the WHO to calculate for underreporting to a study performed by Colditz *et al.* (1991) underreporting was found in ~25% of women and ~33% of men (Müller, 1999).

Several mechanisms have been proposed to be responsible for the apparent loss of alcohol-derived energy. In the following, some of the main mechanisms proposed are summarized.

Three enzyme systems are known to be able to metabolize ethanol to acetaldehyde:

- the alcohol dehydrogenase (ADH), a cytolic enzyme existing as several isoenzymes, is the major enzyme metabolizing ethanol
- the microsomal ethanol oxidizing system (MEOS), a cytochrome P450-depending enzyme system, bound to the smooth endoplasmatic reticulum
- the catalase, localized in the peroxisomes, under normal conditions plays a neglectable role and therefore shall not be discussed here (for overview also see Zakhari (2006)).

The ADH is the major enzyme metabolizing ethanol. In order to facilitate the oxidation of ethanol ADH converts its cofactor nicotinamide adenine dinucleotide (NAD^+) to NADH. The reaction mediated by the ADH are summarized as

$$\text{Ethanol} + NAD^+ \rightarrow \text{Acetaldehyde} + NADH$$

NADH is an energy rich molecule that can donate electrons to the electron transport chain in the mitochondria subsequently leading to the synthesis of adenosine triphosphate (ATP). However, as the ADH-mediated ethanol oxidation is located in the cytoplasm and NADH cannot pass the mitochondrial membrane the cellular redox potential is markedly altered when ethanol is metabolised (e.g. the NADH/ NAD^+ ratio) (van Haaren *et al.* 1999). As a consequence, ethanol derived NADH is mainly metabolized through the reduction of pyruvate to lactate and oxaloacetate to malate which in turn can then be used to utilize energy by the mitochondria (van Haaren *et al.* 1999). Acetaldehyde also produced in this reaction is rapidly metabolized, mainly by mitochondrial acetaldehyde dehydrogenase (ALDH) 2 to form acetate and NADH, which than is oxidized by the electron transport chain (for overview also see (Zakhari and Li, 2007)). The increase in mitochondrial NADH in hepatocytes resulting from the metabolism of acetaldehyde may result in a saturation of the NADH dehydrogenase and subsequently the impairment of the tricarboxylic acid (TCA) cycle as the acetyl coenzyme A (CoA) synthase 2, the mitochondrial enzyme involved in the oxidation of acetate is not found in the liver but is abundant in heart and skeletal muscles (Fujino *et al.* 2001). As a consequence, most of the acetate resulting from the breakdown of ethanol in the liver enters the circulation and is eventually metabolized to CO_2 in the TCA in tissues that possess the enzymes to convert acetate to acetyl CoA (e.g. heart and skeletal muscle).

Furthermore, ethanol is also metabolised through the MEOS. The MEOS differs from the ADH in several aspects as it has a higher Michaelis constant (K_m) (MEOS: K_m 10mM vs. ADH: K_m 1mM) (Haseba and Ohno, 2010; Lieber and DeCarli, 1970) and its activity increases when ethanol is consumed chronically (Lieber, 1997). The reaction mediated by the MEOS, which requires Nicotinamide adenine dinucleotide phosphate (NADPH) rather than NAD^+ and oxygen as a cofactor are summarized as

$$\text{Ethanol} + \text{NADPH} + \text{H}^+ + \tfrac{1}{2}\,\text{O}_2 \rightarrow \text{Acetaldehyde} + \text{NADP}^+ + 2\text{H}_2\text{O}$$

This metabolic route of ethanol was proposed as one possible explanation of the energy "waste" associated with the intake of alcohol (Lieber, 1994; Lieber, 2003). Lieber (1991) postulated that when alcohol is consumed chronically alcohol is metabolized preferentially through the MEOS implying that the production of $NADP^+$ is increased whereas the formation of NADH through the ADH is decreased. This shift between the two enzyme systems would imply a loss in the net energy gain (e.g. through MEOS "only" ~67% of the energy gain that is achieved if ethanol is metabolised through ADH). Lands and Zakhari (1991) calculated that if ethanol is readily metabolized through mitochondrial oxidation 1 Mol of ethanol can provide as much as 16 Mol of ATP. In contrast the first steps of microsomal-mediated ethanol oxidation require 1 Mol of NADPH equivalent to 3 Mol ATP. Subsequently the energy yield through this pathway is markedly lower.

In addition, it was also postulated that the metabolism of acetate may also be associated with a loss of energy. Indeed, Müller *et al.* (1995 and 1998) showed that up to 80% of the acetate derived from ethanol metabolism in the human liver was found in the liver vein. It was further shown that in fasted subjects acetate blood levels raise with 90 min after ethanol ingestion up to 900-950 Mol/L after the ingestion of 47.5 g ethanol (Frayn *et al.* 1990). At the same time, acetate uptake by muscle tissue only accounted to ~3% of the ingested ethanol. The enhanced energy use needed for the lipogenesis of acetate actually was calculated to account to ~25% of the energy content of ethanol (Müller *et al.* 1999).

3.3 Alcohol metabolism and its effect on general energy as well as fat, protein and carbohydrate metabolism

The increased ratios of NADH to NAD^+ in both mitochondria and cytosol in hepatocytes affect the "direction" of several reversible reactions resulting in alterations of hepatic lipid, carbohydrate, and protein but also lactate and uric acid metabolism. The latter are not discussed in this chapter. Most of these changes have been shown to happen as a consequence of acute excessive alcohol intake (e.g. binge drinking) and seem to be at least in part to be attenuated when alcohol is consumed chronically; however, some alterations, like the accumulation of fat in the liver are also found when alcohol is consumed chronically. Furthermore, it has been shown that acute but also chronic intake of alcohol may not only affect micronutrient uptake in the small intestine but may also disturb the absorption of macronutrients; however, most of the data summarized in the following stem from animal experiments.

3.3.1 Effect of alcohol intake on fat metabolism

Besides an altered dietary pattern (e.g. higher intake of pork and subsequently polyunsaturated fatty acids) found to be associated with an increased intake of alcohol (French, 1992) results of early animal studies suggested that the concomitant ingestion of alcohol and plant derived oils is associated with a markedly reduced absorption of these fats (Bode, 1980); however, this effect of alcohol was probably due to a slowed gastric empting resulting from the combination of the oil with a relatively high dose of alcohol. In later human and animal studies it was found that absorption of lipids decreased by the ingestion of alcohol doses of $\geq$ 1g/ kg body weight (Bode and Bode, 1992). It has further been suggested, that fat malabsorption found in patients with alcoholic hepatitis may be due to reduced bile and pancreas enzyme secretion (Soberon *et al.* 1987). Regarding the effects of alcohol metabolism on hepatic lipid metabolism it has been shown that the altered ratio of NADH/ NAD^+ results in an increase of the intermediate metabolite α-glycerophosphate, which favours the accumulation of triglycerides in hepatocytes, but also inhibits β-oxidation of fatty acids in mitochondria (for overview also see Zakhari and Li (2007); Lieber (1984)).

3.3.2 Effect of alcohol intake on protein metabolism

In Europe the average intake of proteins has been shown to be normal in patients with chronic alcohol abuse or alcoholic liver disease in the earlier stage (e.g. steatohepatitis) (Bergheim *et al.* 2003). However, results of animal but also human studies suggest that absorption of amino acids in the small intestine is markedly impaired when alcohol is consumed concomitantly. Indeed, it has been shown in animal studies that in the presence of 2-4.5% of alcohol the uptake of L-alanin, L-glycine, L-leucine, L-proline, L-methionine, L-phenylalanin, and L-valin is in the small intestine impaired by more than 20% (Abidi *et al.* 1992). Especially the decreased uptake of methionine but also the inhibition of the methionine synthase in combination with the deficiency of folic acid and pyridoxine has been shown to be a critical factor in the development and progression of alcoholic liver disease. Recent data from animal studies suggest that the shift in the NADH/ NAD^+ ratio resulting from alcohol metabolism may also affect liver methionine metabolism (Watson *et al.* 2011). Indeed, it has been shown that the supplementation of methionine but also its metabolite S-adenosyl-L-methinone may improve alcoholic liver disease (for overview also see Beier and McClain (2010)).

3.3.3 Effect of alcohol intake on hepatic glucose metabolism

In animal experiments it was shown that alcohol at concentrations found in humans after moderate drinking (e.g. 1-5% w/v) depresses glucose uptake in the brush border membrane in a dose- and time-dependent manner (Dinda and Beck, 1981). Furthermore, the increase in NADH resulting from the ADH-mediated oxidation of alcohol has been shown to prevent the conversion of pyruvate to glucose, which in turn impairs the rate limiting step of the gluconeogenesis, the pyruvate carboxylase reaction (Krebs *et al.* 1969) subsequently leading to hypoglycaemia. Fasting, sustained physical exercise and malnutrition may even increase the likelihood of hypoglycaemia.

4. Alcohol and dietary pattern

Alcohol consumption and potential alterations of dietary habits have been extensively studied in various cohort studies in various regions of the world (Thomson *et al.* 1988; Gruchow *et al.* 1985; Suter *et al.* 1997).

4.1 Binge drinking and dietary pattern

Kim *et al.* (2007) reported that both male and female binge drinkers have higher energy intake in comparison to non-binge drinkers. Among men, an inverse association between the frequency of binge drinking and the intake of polyunsaturated fatty acids (PUFA) including linoleic acid, α-linolenic acid and eicosapentaenoic acid was found; a similar association was not found in female binge drinkers (Kim *et al.* 2007). The lower intake of PUFA implies that binge drinking affects the choice of foods (e.g. intake of fish maybe lower) (Howe *et al.* 2006). Results of Toniolo *et al.* (1997) indicate that moderate drinkers (< 5 g/d) have reduced intake of milk and fresh fruits in comparison to abstainers (Toniolo *et al.* 1991). However, results of Thomson *et al.* (1988) found higher intake of fiber, cereal fiber and PUFA in moderate drinking group (0.1-9 g/day). Results of Colditz *et al.* (1991) found a strong correlation between alcohol intake and carbohydrates, and herein particularly the intake of sucrose. To further investigate this relation the study examined consumption of candy and chocolates. Results of this study are summarized in Table 2. In women the intake of only candy was negatively related with alcohol intake (Spearmann r=-0.07, p<0.0001).

	Alcohol intake		
	0g/d	0.1-4.9g/d	>50g/d
Women			
Only candy	5.67 g/d	5.39g/d	2.48g/d
Candy + chocolate	3.12 g/d	3.12 g/d	3.40g/d
Men			
Only candy	1.98 g/d	1.70 g/d	0.85g/d
Candy + chocolate	1.98 g/d	1.70 g/d	0.85g/d
Chocolate	3.69 g/d	3.69 g/d	2.27 g/d

Table 2. Intake of alcohol vs. candy and chocolate in men and women (Adapted from Colditz *et al.* 1991).

Earlier studies have repeatedly documented that consumption of alcohol is associated with losses in tissue PUFA (Salen and Olsson, 1997; Lands *et al.* 1998).

4.1.1 Chronic alcoholics, dietary pattern and nutritional intake

In Germany and in most industrialized countries chronic alcohol abuse is not only one of the most important causes of nutritional disorders but also of changes in dietary habits (Aaseth *et al.* 1986; Addolorato, 1998; Suter *et al.* 1997). For instance, studies have reported that increased alcohol consumption is positively associated with an increased consumption of coffee, cheese, eggs, fish, meat whereas negative association was found with the intake of fruits and milk consumption (Kesse *et al.* 2001). Similar results were also reported by Toniolo *et al.* (1991) in regards to intake of fruit and dairy products. As mentioned above the results of Colditz *et al.* (1991) have reported that consumption of alcohol up to 50g/d was associated with lower intake of sugar in men. Results of Nanji et al. (1985) reported that pork and alcohol consumption were significantly correlated to cirrhosis mortality (r=0.98, p<0.001). A study by Bergheim et al. (2003) performed on German male middle-class alcohol consumers found that in chronic alcohol consumption protein intake is within the recommended daily allowances. However, the intake of fat and carbohydrate was lower in alcohol consumers in comparison to controls. No significant differences were found in the intake of vitamin B1, B2, B6 and vitamin C as well as retinol in chronic alcohol consumers and controls. These results were in contrast with studies performed in the United States.

Linangpunsakul *et al.* (2010) used the Third National Health and Nutritional Examination Survey (NHANES III) to examine an association between the nutritional intake and alcohol consumption in the United States. These data reveal that in both male and female participants the energy derived from carbohydrates, proteins and fat decreased with increased alcohol consumption. The subjects consumed less fat and protein with increased consumption of alcohol. This large population study concluded that alcohol has replaced nutrients particularly in terms of energy. Furthermore, the increased consumption of alcohol has an inverse relation with macronutrient intakes. Studies have also shown that in alcohol consumers hepatic zinc and vitamin A are found to be depleted due to poor dietary intake (Leo and Lieber, 1999). Taken together, the results gathered in the United States from the above studies differ from Europe, where alcohol was added to the diet but has not substituted nutrients from food sources.

5. Alcohol and vitamins

5.1 Fat soluble vitamins

Vitamin A: Vitamin A, which is vital for bone growth and normal eye function, is found to be deficient in patients with alcoholic cirrhosis (Lieber, 2003). Indeed, it has been found in human studies that patients with severe alcoholic liver disease have reduced levels of hepatic vitamin A (Ahmed *et al.* 1994). Interestingly, in these patients ß-carotene levels in the blood were found to be normal, indicating that liver disease may modify the ability of liver to convert ß-carotene to vitamin A (Ahmed *et al.* 1994). On the other hand, results of Manari *et al.* (2003) have indicated that chronic alcohol abusers without alcoholic liver disease have lower dietary intake of vitamin A than recommended by the reference nutrient intake. However, noteworthy results of Leo and Lieber (1982) showed that chronic alcohol administration in rats fed with vitamin A supplemented diet resulted in decrease of hepatic vitamin A levels. Thus, decreased levels of vitamin A in alcohol abuse may not be linked to reduced intake or malabsorption alone, suggesting that other mechanisms might be involved. Results of animal studies suggest that chronic ethanol ingestion has increased the peripheral vitamin A status and decreased hepatic vitamin A content (Leo *et al.* 1986; Leo and Lieber, 1988).

Vitamin D: Results of several human studies have reported that chronic alcohol abuse resulted in reduction of plasma 1,25 dihydroxyvitamin D3 levels, which is an active form of vitamin D3 (Lund *et al.* 1977; Laitinen and Valimaki, 1991; Laitinen *et al.* 1990). Similar reduction of plasma 1,25 dihydroxyvitamin D3 levels were also found in animal studies after chronic ethanol exposure (Turner *et al.* 1988). Reduction of circulating vitamin D levels in alcohol abusers may lead to reduced bone mass and lower calcium levels (Sampson, 1997; Keiver and Weinberg, 2003). Vitamin D is crucial in maintaining insulin levels and deficiencies may lead to altered glucose metabolism (Clark *et al.* 1981; Gedik and Akalin, 1986).

Vitamin E: Vitamin E is a well known anti-oxidant, whose metabolism is also altered in alcohol consumption (Drevon, 1991). Results of Bergheim et al. (2003) suggest that vitamin E consumption was markedly lower in patients with different stages of alcoholic liver disease. Furthermore, several animal and human studies suggest that consumption of alcohol reduces the hepatic stores of vitamin E (Bjorneboe *et al.* 1986, 1987, 1988a, 1988b). Indeed, rats fed with ethanol have increased hepatic α-tocopherol quinine levels, a product of α-tocopherol oxidation, suggesting that ethanol promotes vitamin E degradation (Kawase *et al.* 1989).

5.2 Water soluble vitamins

Thiamine: Thiamine or vitamin B1 is essential for proper neurological and cardiovascular functioning (Wood and Breen, 1979). Thiamine is available as free thiamine (T), thiamine diphosphate ester (TDP 80%), thiamine triphosphate and thiamine monophosphate ester in the organism. Alcohol can inhibit the rate limiting mechanism of thiamine transport after its absorption from gastro-intestinal tract (Mancinelli and Ceccanti, 2009). In chronic alcohol abusers the concentrations of T and TDP were found to be reduced however, they were not related to liver injury (Mancinelli and Ceccanti, 2009). Furthermore, results of Manari *et al.* (2003) reported that 73% of the alcohol abusers have low thiamine intake in comparison to reference nutrient intake. Taken together, thiamine deficiency can be due to alcohol or malnutrition acting by itself or in combination.

Riboflavin: Riboflavin or vitamin B2 is an essential component of the cofactors flavin adenine dinucleotide and flavin mononucleotide. Riboflavin deficiency seems to be prevalent in alcoholics due to poor dietary intake (Manari *et al.* 2003). However, ethanol seems not to have an effect on riboflavin absorption (Pekkanen and Rusi, 1979).

Pyridoxine: Pyridoxine or vitamin B6 is an essential cofactor in amino acid metabolism. Studies have shown that 50% of alcohol abusers have lower circulating levels of pyridoxal-phosphate (PLP), an indicator of vitamin B6 status; this deficiency might be attributed to poor dietary intake and demolition of the vitamin by phosphotases (Lumeng and Li, 1974; Lumeng, 1978; Fonda *et al.* 1989). Acetaldehyde, a product of ethanol oxidation in chronic alcohol abusers displaces protein bound PLP and exposes PLP to destruction of phosphotases (Lumeng and Li, 1974; Lumeng, 1978). Alteration in the amino acid metabolism due to PLP deficiency might be an aspect in the development of alcoholic liver disease. Indeed, animal studies have reported that chronic PLP deficient diet leads to the development of mild fatty liver (French and Castagna, 1967).

Folic acid: Folic acid or vitamin B9 plays an important role in facilitating many body processes. Folic acid deficiency is common in chronic alcohol abuse. For instance, a British study on alcoholics has reported that most of the patients had megaloblastic anaemia in association with lower liver folate levels and lower red blood cells (Wu *et al.* 1975). The causes of the deficiency are still unclear; however, numeral mechanisms have been proposed together with lower intake of folate, reduced intestinal absorption of polyglutamyl folates, alteration in hepatic and renal folate homeostasis and augmented folate catabolism (Halsted *et al.* 1973; Tamura and Halsted, 1983; Halsted *et al.* 1971; McMartin *et al.* 1989; Shaw *et al.* 1989).

Cobalamin: Vitamin B12 deficiency in chronic alcohol abusers is rare due to large hepatic deposits (Klipstein and Lindenbaum, 1965). Results of Kanazawa and Herbert (1985) reported higher levels of plasma vitamin B12 in chronic alcohol abusers than in controls. However, analysis of the hepatic tissue confirmed that vitamin B12 concentration was significantly lower in chronic alcoholics than in controls. Therefore, it might be concluded that chronic alcohol ingestion affects hepatic cobalamin homeostasis but probably also that of other organs (Cravo and Camilo, 2000).

6. Alcohol and minerals and trace elements

Nutritional disturbances are assumed to remain among the most relevant medical problems in alcohol consumers (Aaseth *et al.* 1986; Addolorato, 1998; Suter *et al.* 1997) but it is still not clear whether chronic alcohol consumption *per se* results in malnutrition (Lieber, 2003; Leo *et al.* 1993; Leo and Lieber, 1999; Morgan and Levine, 1988). As reviewed by Lieber (2003), malnutrition and malsupplementation of certain micronutrients can be observed in alcohol abusers in the United States, whereas in another study dietary intake of German middle-class alcohol abusers with liver damage did not differ from that of control subjects consuming only very low amounts of ethanol (Bergheim *et al.* 2003). However, malsupplementation or an excessive intake of special micronutrients may contribute to the development of hepatic damage in alcoholic liver disease in single cases.

6.1 Iron

In contrast to other micronutrients iron is known to promote liver damage. Oxidative stress plays a key role in the pathogenesis of alcoholic liver diseases. By catalyzing the conversion of superoxide and hydrogen peroxide to hydroxyl radicals, iron can contribute to induce oxidative stress and, thus, induce liver cirrhosis in experimental settings in rats treated with ethanol (Tsukamoto *et al.* 1995). In other studies with rodents, iron also increased the hepatotoxicity caused by alcohol (Stal and Hultcrantz, 1993). Alcoholic liver diseases are often associated with an iron overload (Kohgo *et al.* 2008). Even mild to moderate alcohol consumption has recently been shown to increase the prevalence of iron overload (Ioannou *et al.* 2004). Iron has been shown to accumulate in Kupffer cells as well as in hepatocytes (Farinati *et al.* 1995; Ioannou *et al.* 2004). However, the mechanisms involved in the accumulation of iron in the liver when alcohol is ingested chronically are still poorly understood. Two possible mechanisms that are discussed to lead to an accumulation of iron in alcohol-inuced liver diseases are 1. an increased uptake of iron into hepatocytes, 2. an increased intestinal absorption of iron (Kohgo *et al.* 2008). In a study in Japanese patients with alcoholic liver disease it has been shown that the expression of transferrin receptor 1 was increased in hepatocytes (Suzuki *et al.* 2002) indicating that ethanol may increase iron uptake in hepatocytes. Another important factor that may be involved in iron overload found in patients with alcoholic liver disease is the systemic iron hormone hepcidin. Hepcidin plays an important role in duodenal iron absorption. In recent years it has been shown that hepcidin expression is downregulated in alcoholic liver disease (for overview see (Kohgo *et al.* 2008)).

6.2 Zinc

Zinc is an essential trace element and the daily recommended intake for adults ranges from 7 mg to 11mg. Zinc plays an essential role not only in catalytic reactions but also in the maintenance of the structural integrity of proteins by forming a "zinc finger-like" structure created by chelation centers, including cysteine and histidine residues (Klug and Schwabe, 1995) and in the regulation of gene expression. For example, metallothionein expression is regulated by a mechanism that involves the binding of zinc to the metal regulatory transcription factor 1, which in turn activates gene transcription (Cousins, 1994; Dalton *et al.* 1997). Zinc is necessary for the function of nearly 100 specific enzymes (e.g. alcohol dehydrogenase, retinol dehydrogenase) and is essential for macronutrient metabolism (e.g.

carbohydrate and protein metabolism), wound healing, the immune system, glucose control, growth, digestion, and fertility (King and Cousins, 2005; Prasad, 1995; Lipscomb and Strater, 1996). In alcoholic abusers, evidence of zinc deficiency has been reported repeatedly (Aaseth *et al.* 1986; Bjorneboe *et al.* 1988). Results of a study in German middle-class alcohol consumers indicated that zinc concentrations in plasma were significantly decreased in alcohol consumers with different stages of alcoholic liver diseases (fatty liver, hepatitis, cirrhosis), whereas urinary zinc loss was increased in this patients (Bergheim *et al.* 2003). This is in line with the findings of previous studies, which reported decreased intestinal absorption of zinc (Valberg *et al.* 1985; Dinsmore *et al.* 1985) and increased zinc excretion in urine (Sullivan, 1962) being the most important reasons for zinc deficiency caused by alcohol consumption. Indeed, zinc deficiency is one of the most commonly observed nutritional manifestations of alcoholic liver disease (McClain *et al.* 1991). It has been discussed by Kang and Zhou (2005) that a supplementation of zinc may have a high potential to be developed as an effective agent in the prevention and treatment of alcoholic liver disease.

6.3 Copper

Copper plays an essential role as component of a number of metalloenzymes acting as oxidases (e.g cytochrome c oxidase). The daily recommended intake for adults ranges from 0.9 mg to 1.5 mg. In humans, an isolated copper deficiency rarely occurs and is normally due to an insufficient intake. However, the consumption of alcohol has been shown to be associated with a significant reduction of the levels of copper in serum (Schuhmacher *et al.* 1994). Results of a study in patients with alcoholic cirrhosis indicate that liver copper contents and urinary copper excretion were higher in cirrhotic patients and were related with the severity of chronic alcoholic liver disease (Rodriguez-Moreno *et al.*, 1997). Besides zinc, copper is an essential cofactor of the copper/zinc superoxide dismutase, which is an enzyme that catalyzes the dismutation of superoxide into oxygen and hydrogen peroxide. In the liver, one of the most important antioxidants is the copper/zinc superoxide dismutase (Suter, 2005). In biopsies from patients with alcoholic liver disease it has been shown that the amount of copper/zinc superoxide dismutase reactivity was significantly lower than in control biopsies (Zhao *et al.*, 1996).

6.4 Magnesium

As a cofactor for more than 300 enzyme systems (Wacker and Parisi, 1968) magnesium plays an essential role in anaerobic and aerobic energy generation and in glycolysis, being part of the Magnesium-ATP complex or acting as an enzyme activator (Garfinkel and Garfinkel, 1985). The daily recommended intake for adults is 300-400mg. Magnesium deficiency leads to many specific and unspecific symptoms such as anxiety, insomnia, nervousness, high blood pressure, and muscle spasms. Alcohol abusers are at high risk for magnesium deficiency because alcohol dose-dependently increases urinary excretion of magnesium (Laitinen *et al.* 1992). Even in cases of moderate alcohol consumption an increased excretion of magnesium in urine can be observed (Rylander *et al.* 2001). In dependence on the severity of alcohol abuse, 30 to 60% of alcoholics and nearly 90% of patients experiencing alcohol withdrawal have low magnesium levels in serum/plasma (Flink, 1986). The increased loss of magnesium may be potentiated by an insufficient intake or by an intestinal loss (e.g. through diarrhoea and vomiting).

6.5 Selenium

Selenium plays an important role as cofactor in several enzyme systems, such as the glutathione peroxidase, which acts as a cellular protector against free radical oxidative damage (Foster and Sumar, 1997). Low levels of selenium in plasma, serum or blood have not only been reported in patients with alcohol-induced cirrhosis but also in other liver diseases (for overview see McClain *et al.* (1991)). Results of a study in German middle-class alcohol consumers indicated that selenium concentrations in plasma and in erythrocytes were significantly decreased in alcohol consumers with different stages of alcoholic liver diseases compared to healthy controls, although the dietary intake of selenium was not decreased in these patients with alcoholic liver disease (Bergheim *et al.* 2003). In contrast, in other studies depressed serum selenium concentrations correlated closely with poor nutritional status (Tanner *et al.* 1986) and with the severity of alcohol-induced liver damage (Dworkin *et al.* 1985). In patients with alcohol-induced cirrhosis an additional decreased content of selenium in the liver was observed (Dworkin *et al.* 1988).

7. Clinical manifestation, diagnosis and therapy of malnutrition

As discussed in the previous sections of this chapter, alcohol consumption and herein particularly chronic intake of alcohol but also alcohol metabolism is associated with numerous alterations such as changes in dietary pattern (e.g. elevated intake of pork), impaired intestinal absorption of micro- but also macronutrients but also metabolism in the liver. As a consequence malnutrition is frequently found in patients with alcoholic liver disease. Indeed, as reviewed by Stickel *et al.* (2003), malnutrition can be both, a primary event resulting from a poor diet and decreased caloric intake but also a secondary process resulting from malabsorption and maldigestion. The question if the progression of alcoholic liver disease can be improved by nutritional support to these patients has been addressed in several clinical trails using oral, enteral, or parenteral routs to deliver nutritional formulas (for overview also see Halsted (2004; DiCecco and Francisco-Ziller (2006)). However, many of the studies were inconclusive as in some studies control groups were inadequate or control formulas were unbalanced, duration of studies was too short or nutritional needs were not adequately assessed (Halsted, 2004). In the following, methods for the assessment of nutritional status and recommendations for nutritional support of patients with alcoholic liver disease are briefly summarized (for overview also see Halsted (2004; DiCecco and Francisco-Ziller (2006; Plauth *et al.* (2006)).

7.1 Assessment of nutritional status

Assessing the nutritional status of a patient with alcoholic liver disease may be challenging as many of the traditional tools may be affected by the disease (e.g. body weight changes may stem from fluctuation in oedema or ascites). Indeed, diminished serum levels of hepatic protein such as albumin and transferrin may rather be indication of an altered protein biosynthesis in the liver than a protein caloric malnutrition (Fuhrman *et al.* 2004). In patients without fluid overload, midarm muscle area and creatinine excretion in urine have been shown to be the most reliable measures of nutritional status, whereas in those patients with ascites and oedema creatinine height index is more reliable (Nielsen *et al.* 1993). Furthermore, serum status of vitamins such as A, D, E, and folate as well as minerals like zinc and iron as well as skin turgor, poor oral health and temporal muscle wasting or night blindness should also be assessed and may also help to identify losses of muscle mass and micronutrient deficiencies (Figueiredo *et al.* 2000). The subjective global assessment method, which combines subjective and objective measures has been found to accurately reflect the nutritional status of patients with end-stage liver disease (Hirsch *et al.* 1991, Hasse *et al.* 1993). Taken together, a detailed diet history, anthropometric measurements (e.g. triceps skinfold, arm circumference, body mass index), and measurements of handgrip strength but also measurements of vitamin and mineral status in serum are recommended when nutritionally assessing patients with alcoholic liver disease (DiCecco and Francisco-Ziller, 2006).

7.2 Oral nutritional supplementation

One of the first-line therapies to prevent and treat malnutrition in patients with alcoholic liver disease is through oral feeding including supplements. Herein, avoiding a fasting state, minimizing dietary restrictions, and offering small, frequent feedings is critical to meet the caloric and protein requirements (DiCecco and Francisco-Ziller, 2006). The benefit of oral nutritional supplementation has been assessed in many studies; however, due to poor study design or to small patients numbers included a final conclusion regarding the efficacy of this approach cannot yet be drawn. As reviewed by Stickel *et al.* (2003) and Halsted (2004) and stated in the guidelines from the European Society for Clinical Nutrition and Metabolism (ESPEN) on enteral nutrition for patients with liver disease (Plauth *et al.* 2006) oral nutritional supplements may improve nutritional status and complications of alcoholic liver disease and are recommend, although the true effect on survival is still unknown.

7.3 Enteral nutritional supplementation

Enteral tube feeding is second option to treat malnutrition in patients with alcoholic liver disease and is especially considered a save and efficient way to improve the nutritional status in those patients unable or willing to consume adequate oral nutrition. Indeed, despite the sometimes poor patient acceptance of the tube feeding it has been shown in several studies, that tube feeding may improve digestion but also has a short-term positive effect on liver function and may improve long-term survival (for overview also see Halsted, (2004; Plauth *et al.* (2006)).

7.4 Parenteral nutritional supplementation

The advantage of parenteral nutrition is the delivery of a precisely defined amount of protein, total calories, micronutrients, fluid, and electrolytes; however, clinical trails performed to evaluate the effect of parenteral nutrition in patients with alcoholic liver disease are difficult to interpret as study design was mostly inadequate (e.g. intake of controls was not adjusted, length of study, follow-up). The ESPEN guidelines advise that parental formula should provide adequate calories and protein with careful monitoring of glucose and electrolytes (Plauth *et al.* 2006).

8. Conclusion

Results of several studies suggest that quantity and frequency of alcohol consumption are important in the pathogenesis of alcoholic liver disease. Malnutrition is frequently present in patients with alcoholic liver disease and may result from an altered dietary pattern, disturbed intestinal absorption and nutrient utilization in the liver due to the concomitant alcohol metabolism and/ or alcohol-induced impairments of liver function. Nutritional support including provision of adequate calories and protein but also micronutrients avoiding extended fasting periods and restricted diets may help to improve health status of patients with alcoholic liver disease; however, more clinical trails are needed to clarify the long-term effects of nutritional treatment on liver status and survival in patients with alcoholic liver disease.

9. References

Aaseth, J., Smith-Kielland, A. & Thomassen, Y. (1986). Selenium, alcohol and liver diseases. *Ann.Clin.Res.* 18(1):43-47.

Abidi, S.A. et al. (1992). In Lieber C.S.. ed. *Medical and Nutritional Complications of Alcoholism: Mechanisms and Management.* New York: Plenum Press, pp 127-155

Addolorato, G. (1998). Chronic alcohol abuse and nutritional status: recent acquisitions. *Eur.Rev.Med.Pharmacol.Sci.* 2(5-6):165-167.

Ahmed, S., Leo, M.A. & Lieber, C.S. (1994). Interactions between alcohol and beta-carotene in patients with alcoholic liver disease. *Am.J Clin.Nutr* 60(3):430-436.

Atwater, W.O., Benedict, F.G. (1902). An experimental inquiry regarding the nutritive value of alcohol. *Mem Natl Acad Sci.* 8:235-295

Barnes, E.W., Cooke, N.J., King, A.J. & Passmore, R. (1965). Observations on the metabolism of alcohol in man. *Br.J.Nutr* 19(4):485-489.

Beier, J.I. & McClain, C.J. (2010). Mechanisms and cell signaling in alcoholic liver disease. *Biol.Chem.* 391(11):1249-1264.

Bellentani, S., Saccoccio, G., Costa, G., Tiribelli, C., Manenti, F., Sodde, M., Saveria, C.L., Sasso, F., Pozzato, G., Cristianini, G. & Brandi, G. (1997). Drinking habits as cofactors of risk for alcohol induced liver damage. The Dionysos Study Group. *Gut* 41(6):845-850.

Bergheim, I., Parlesak, A., Dierks, C., Bode, J.C. & Bode, C. (2003). Nutritional deficiencies in German middle-class male alcohol consumers: relation to dietary intake and severity of liver disease. *Eur.J.Clin Nutr* 57(3):431-438.

Bjorneboe, A., Bjorneboe, G.E., Bodd, E., Hagen, B.F., Kveseth, N. & Drevon, C.A. (1986). Transport and distribution of alpha-tocopherol in lymph, serum and liver cells in rats. *Biochim.Biophys.Acta* 889(3):310-315.

Bjorneboe, G.E., Bjorneboe, A., Hagen, B.F., Morland, J. & Drevon, C.A. (1987). Reduced hepatic alpha-tocopherol content after long-term administration of ethanol to rats. *Biochim.Biophys.Acta* 918(3):236-241.

Bjorneboe, G.E., Johnsen, J., Bjorneboe, A., Bache-Wiig, J.E., Morland, J. & Drevon, C.A. (1988a). Diminished serum concentration of vitamin E in alcoholics. *Ann.Nutr Metab* 32(2):56-61.

Bjorneboe, G.E., Johnsen, J., Bjorneboe, A., Marklund, S.L., Skylv, N., Hoiseth, A., Bache-Wiig, J.E., Morland, J. & Drevon, C.A. (1988b). Some aspects of antioxidant status in blood from alcoholics. *Alcohol Clin.Exp.Res.* 12(6):806-810.

Bode, J.C. (1980). Alcohol and the gastrointestinal tract. *Adv Intern Med Ped.* 45:1-75.

Bode, J.C., Bode, C. (1992). Alcohol malnutrition and the gastrointestinal tract. In: Watson, R.R., Watzl, B. (eds) *Nutrition and alcohol,* CRC Press Boca Raton, pp 403-428.

Burger, M., Bronstrup, A. & Pietrzik, K. (2004). Derivation of tolerable upper alcohol intake levels in Germany: a systematic review of risks and benefits of moderate alcohol consumption. *Prev.Med.* 39(1):111-127.

Clark, S.A., Stumpf, W.E. & Sar, M. (1981). Effect of 1, 25 dihydroxyvitamin D3 on insulin secretion. *Diabetes* 30(5):382-386.

Colditz, G.A., Giovannucci, E., Rimm, E.B., Stampfer, M.J., Rosner, B., Speizer, F.E., Gordis, E. & Willett, W.C. (1991). Alcohol intake in relation to diet and obesity in women and men. *Am.J.Clin Nutr* 54(1):49-55.

Cousins, R.J. (1994). Metal elements and gene expression. *Annu.Rev.Nutr* 14:449-469.

Cravo, M.L. & Camilo, M.E. (2000). Hyperhomocysteinemia in chronic alcoholism: relations to folic acid and vitamins B(6) and B(12) status. *Nutrition* 16(4):296-302.

Dalton, T.P., Bittel, D. & Andrews, G.K. (1997). Reversible activation of mouse metal response element-binding transcription factor 1 DNA binding involves zinc interaction with the zinc finger domain. *Mol.Cell Biol.* 17(5):2781-2789.

Dantzer, C., Wardle, J., Fuller, R., Pampalone, S.Z. & Steptoe, A. (2006). International study of heavy drinking: attitudes and sociodemographic factors in university students. *J.Am.Coll.Health* 55(2):83-89.

Day, C.P. (1997). Alcoholic liver disease: dose and threshold--new thoughts on an old topic. *Gut* 41(6):857-858.

Deutsche Hauptstelle für Suchtfragen (DHS). Available on: http://www.dhs.de/datenfakten/alkohol.html.

DiCecco, S.R. & Francisco-Ziller, N. (2006). Nutrition in alcoholic liver disease. *Nutr Clin Pract.* 21(3):245-254.

Dinda, P.K. & Beck, I.T. (1981). Ethanol-induced inhibition of glucose transport across the isolated brush-border membrane of hamster jejunum. *Dig.Dis.Sci.* 26(1):23-32.

Dinsmore, W., Callender, M.E., McMaster, D., Todd, S.J. & Love, A.H. (1985). Zinc absorption in alcoholics using zinc-65. *Digestion* 32(4):238-242.

Drevon, C.A. (1991). Absorption, transport and metabolism of vitamin E. *Free Radic.Res.Commun.* 14(4):229-246.

Dworkin, B., Rosenthal, W.S., Jankowski, R.H., Gordon, G.G. & Haldea, D. (1985). Low blood selenium levels in alcoholics with and without advanced liver disease. Correlations with clinical and nutritional status. *Dig.Dis.Sci.* 30(9):838-844.

Dworkin, B.M., Rosenthal, W.S., Stahl, R.E. & Panesar, N.K. (1988). Decreased hepatic selenium content in alcoholic cirrhosis. *Dig.Dis.Sci.* 33(10):1213-1217.

Farinati, F., Cardin, R., de, M.N., Della, L.G., Marafin, C., Lecis, E., Burra, P., Floreani, A., Cecchetto, A. & Naccarato, R. (1995). Iron storage, lipid peroxidation and glutathione turnover in chronic anti-HCV positive hepatitis. *J.Hepatol.* 22(4):449-456.

Figueiredo, F.A., Dickson, E.R., Pasha, T.M., Porayko, M.K., Therneau, T.M., Malinchoc, M., DiCecco, S.R., Francisco-Ziller, N.M., Kasparova, P. & Charlton, M.R. (2000). Utility of standard nutritional parameters in detecting body cell mass depletion in patients with end-stage liver disease. *Liver Transpl.* 6(5):575-581.

Flink, E.B. (1986). Magnesium deficiency in alcoholism. *Alcohol Clin Exp.Res.* 10(6):590-594.

Fonda, M.L., Brown, S.G. & Pendleton, M.W. (1989). Concentration of vitamin B6 and activities of enzymes of B6 metabolism in the blood of alcoholic and nonalcoholic men. *Alcohol Clin.Exp.Res.* 13(6):804-809.

Foster, L.H. & Sumar, S. (1997). Selenium in health and disease: a review. *Crit Rev.Food Sci.Nutr* 37(3):211-228.

Frayn, K.N., Coppack, S.W., Walsh, P.E., Butterworth, H.C., Humphreys, S.M. & Pedrosa, H.C. (1990). Metabolic responses of forearm and adipose tissues to acute ethanol ingestion. *Metabolism* 39(9):958-966.

French, S.W. (1992). Nutritional factors in the pathogenesis of alcoholic liver disease. In: Watson, R.R., Watzl, B. (eds) *Nutrition and alcohol*, CRC Press Boca Raton, pp 403-428.

French, S.W. & Castagna, J. (1967). Some effects of chronic ethanol feeding on vitamin B 6 deficiency in the rat. *Lab Invest* 16(4):526-531.

Fuhrman, M.P., Charney, P., Mueller, C.M. (2004). Hepatic proteins and nutrition assessment. *J Am Diet Assoc.* 104(8):1258-64.

Fujino, T., Kondo, J., Ishikawa, M., Morikawa, K. & Yamamoto, T.T. (2001). Acetyl-CoA synthetase 2, a mitochondrial matrix enzyme involved in the oxidation of acetate. *J.Biol.Chem.* 276(14):11420-11426.

Garfinkel, L. & Garfinkel, D. (1985). Magnesium regulation of the glycolytic pathway and the enzymes involved. *Magnesium* 4(2-3):60-72.

Gedik, O. & Akalin, S. (1986). Effects of vitamin D deficiency and repletion on insulin and glucagon secretion in man. *Diabetologia* 29(3):142-145.

Gruchow, H.W., Sobocinski, K.A., Barboriak, J.J. & Scheller, J.G. (1985). Alcohol consumption, nutrient intake and relative body weight among US adults. *Am.J Clin.Nutr* 42(2):289-295.

Halsted, C.H. (2004). Nutrition and alcoholic liver disease. *Semin.Liver Dis.* 24(3):289-304.

Halsted, C.H., Robles, E.A. & Mezey, E. (1971). Decreased jejunal uptake of labeled folic acid (3 H-PGA) in alcoholic patients: roles of alcohol and nutrition. *N.Engl.J Med.* 285(13):701-706.

Halsted, C.H., Robles, E.A. & Mezey, E. (1973). Intestinal malabsorption in folate-deficient alcoholics. *Gastroenterology* 64(4):526-532.

Haseba, T. & Ohno, Y. (2010). A new view of alcohol metabolism and alcoholism--role of the high-Km Class III alcohol dehydrogenase (ADH3). *Int.J.Environ.Res.Public Health* 7(3):1076-1092.

Hasse, J., Strong, S., Gorman, M.A. & Liepa, G. (1993). Subjective global assessment: alternative nutrition-assessment technique for liver-transplant candidates. *Nutrition* 9(4):339-343.

Hirsch, S., de Obaldia, N., Petermann, M., Rojo, P., Barrientos, C., Iturriaga, H., Bunout, D. (1991). Subjective global assessment of nutritional status: further validation. *Nutrition.* 7(1):35-7.

Howe, P., Meyer, B., Record, S. & Baghurst, K. (2006). Dietary intake of long-chain omega-3 polyunsaturated fatty acids: contribution of meat sources. *Nutrition* 22(1):47-53.

Institute of Alcohol Studies. (2010). *Binge Drinking – Nature, prevalence and causes.* London, UK; Available from: www.ias.org.uk/resources/factsheets/binge_drinking.pdf

Ioannou, G.N., Dominitz, J.A., Weiss, N.S., Heagerty, P.J. & Kowdley, K.V. (2004). The effect of alcohol consumption on the prevalence of iron overload, iron deficiency, and iron deficiency anemia. *Gastroenterology* 126(5):1293-1301.

Kamper-Jorgensen, M., Gronbaek, M., Tolstrup, J. & Becker, U. (2004). Alcohol and cirrhosis: dose--response or threshold effect? *J.Hepatol.* 41(1):25-30.

Kanazawa, S. & Herbert, V. (1985). Total corrinoid, cobalamin (vitamin B12), and cobalamin analogue levels may be normal in serum despite cobalamin in liver depletion in patients with alcoholism. *Lab Invest* 53(1):108-110.

Kang, Y.J. & Zhou, Z. (2005). Zinc prevention and treatment of alcoholic liver disease. *Mol.Aspects Med.* 26(4-5):391-404.

Kanny, D., Liu, Y. & Brewer, R.D. (2011). Binge drinking - United States, 2009. *MMWR Surveill Summ.* 60 Suppl:101-104.

Kawase, T., Kato, S. & Lieber, C.S. (1989). Lipid peroxidation and antioxidant defense systems in rat liver after chronic ethanol feeding. *Hepatology* 10(5):815-821.

Keiver, K. & Weinberg, J. (2003). Effect of duration of alcohol consumption on calcium and bone metabolism during pregnancy in the rat. *Alcohol Clin.Exp.Res.* 27(9):1507-1519.

Kesse, E., Clavel-Chapelon, F., Slimani, N. & van, L.M. (2001). Do eating habits differ according to alcohol consumption? Results of a study of the French cohort of the European Prospective Investigation into Cancer and Nutrition (E3N-EPIC). *Am.J Clin.Nutr* 74(3):322-327.

Kim, S.Y., Breslow, R.A., Ahn, J. & Salem, N., Jr. (2007). Alcohol consumption and fatty acid intakes in the 2001-2002 National Health and Nutrition Examination Survey. *Alcohol Clin.Exp.Res.* 31(8):1407-1414.

King J, Cousins RJ. (2005). In: Shils ME, Shike M, Ross AC, CaballeroB, Cousins RJ, editors. *Modern nutrition in health and disease,* 10th ed. Baltimore, MD: Lippincott Williams & Wilkins: 271-285.

Klipstein, F.A. & Lindenbaum, J. (1965). FOLATE DEFICIENCY IN CHRONIC LIVER DISEASE. *Blood* 25:443-456.

Klug, A. & Schwabe, J.W. (1995). Protein motifs 5. Zinc fingers. *FASEB J.* 9(8):597-604.

Kohgo, Y., Ohtake, T., Ikuta, K., Suzuki, Y., Torimoto, Y. & Kato, J. (2008). Dysregulation of systemic iron metabolism in alcoholic liver diseases. *J.Gastroenterol.Hepatol.* 23 Suppl 1:S78-S81.

Krebs, H.A., Freedland, R.A., Hems, R. & Stubbs, M. (1969). Inhibition of hepatic gluconeogenesis by ethanol. *Biochem.J.* 112(1):117-124.

Laitinen, K., Tahtela, R. & Valimaki, M. (1992). The dose-dependency of alcohol-induced hypoparathyroidism, hypercalciuria, and hypermagnesuria. *Bone Miner.* 19(1):75-83.

Laitinen, K. & Valimaki, M. (1991). Alcohol and bone. *Calcif.Tissue Int.* 49 Suppl:S70-S73.

Laitinen, K., Valimaki, M., Lamberg-Allardt, C., Kivisaari, L., Lalla, M., Karkkainen, M. & Ylikahri, R. (1990). Deranged vitamin D metabolism but normal bone mineral density in Finnish noncirrhotic male alcoholics. *Alcohol Clin.Exp.Res.* 14(4):551-556.

Lands WEM, Pawlosky RJ & Salem N Jr (1998). Alcoholism, antioxidant status and essential fatty acids. In *Antioxidants in Nutrition and Health,* pp. 299-344. (Anonymous). Boca Raton, FL: CRC Press].

Lands, W.E. & Zakhari, S. (1991). The case of the missing calories. *Am.J.Clin Nutr* 54(1):47-48.

Lelbach, W.K. (1975). Cirrhosis in the alcoholic and its relation to the volume of alcohol abuse. *Ann.N.Y.Acad.Sci.* 252:85-105.

Leo M A & Lieber C S (1982). Hepatic vitamin A depletion in alcoholic liver injury. *N.Engl.J Med.* 307:597-601.

Leo, M.A., Kim, C. & Lieber, C.S. (1986). Increased vitamin A in esophagus and other extrahepatic tissues after chronic ethanol consumption in the rat. *Alcohol Clin.Exp.Res.* 10(5):487-492.

Leo, M.A. & Lieber, C.S. (1988). Hypervitaminosis A: a liver lover's lament. *Hepatology* 8(2):412-417.

Leo, M.A. & Lieber, C.S. (1999). Alcohol, vitamin A, and beta-carotene: adverse interactions, including hepatotoxicity and carcinogenicity. *Am.J.Clin Nutr* 69(6):1071-1085.

Leo, M.A., Rosman, A.S. & Lieber, C.S. (1993). Differential depletion of carotenoids and tocopherol in liver disease. *Hepatology* 17(6):977-986.

Liangpunsakul, S. (2010). Relationship between alcohol intake and dietary pattern: findings from NHANES III. *World J Gastroenterol.* 16(32):4055-4060.

Lieber, C.S. (1984). Alcohol and the liver: 1984 update. *Hepatology* 4(6):1243-1260.

Lieber, C.S. (1991). Perspectives: do alcohol calories count? *Am.J.Clin Nutr* 54(6):976-982.

Lieber, C.S. (1994). Alcohol and the liver: 1994 update. *Gastroenterology* 106(4):1085-1105.

Lieber, C.S. (1997). Ethanol metabolism, cirrhosis and alcoholism. *Clin Chim.Acta* 257(1):59-84.

Lieber, C.S. (2003). Relationships between nutrition, alcohol use, and liver disease. *Alcohol Res.Health* 27(3):220-231.

Lieber, C.S. & DeCarli, L.M. (1970). Hepatic microsomal ethanol-oxidizing system. In vitro characteristics and adaptive properties in vivo. *J.Biol.Chem.* 245(10):2505-2512.

Lipscomb, W.N. & Strater, N. (1996). Recent Advances in Zinc Enzymology. *Chem.Rev.* 96(7):2375-2434.

Lumeng, L. (1978). The role of acetaldehyde in mediating the deleterious effect of ethanol on pyridoxal 5'-phosphate metabolism. *J Clin.Invest* 62(2):286-293.

Lumeng, L. & Li, T.K. (1974). Vitamin B6 metabolism in chronic alcohol abuse. Pyridoxal phosphate levels in plasma and the effects of acetaldehyde on pyridoxal phosphate synthesis and degradation in human erythrocytes. *J Clin.Invest* 53(3):693-704.

Lund, B., Sorensen, O.H., Hilden, M. & Lund, B. (1977). The hepatic conversion of vitamin D in alcoholics with varying degrees of liver affection. *Acta Med.Scand.* 202(3):221-224.

Manari, A.P., Preedy, V.R. & Peters, T.J. (2003). Nutritional intake of hazardous drinkers and dependent alcoholics in the UK. *Addict.Biol.* 8(2):201-210.

Mancinelli, R. & Ceccanti, M. (2009). Biomarkers in alcohol misuse: their role in the prevention and detection of thiamine deficiency. *Alcohol Alcohol* 44(2):177-182.

McClain, C.J., Marsano, L., Burk, R.F. & Bacon, B. (1991). Trace metals in liver disease. *Semin.Liver Dis.* 11(4):321-339.

McMartin, K.E., Collins, T.D., Eisenga, B.H., Fortney, T., Bates, W.R. & Bairnsfather, L. (1989). Effects of chronic ethanol and diet treatment on urinary folate excretion and development of folate deficiency in the rat. *J Nutr* 119(10):1490-1497.

Mezey, E. (1991). Interaction between alcohol and nutrition in the pathogenesis of alcoholic liver disease. *Semin.Liver Dis.* 11(4):340-348.

Morgan, M.Y. & Levine, J.A. (1988). Alcohol and nutrition. *Proc.Nutr Soc.* 47(2):85-98.

Müller, M.J. (1995). Hepatic fuel selection. *Proc Nutr Soc.* 54:139.

Müller, M.J. (1998). Hepatic energy and substrate metabolism: A possible metabolic basis for early nutritional support in cirrhotic patients. *Nutrition.* 14:30-38.

Müller, M.J. (1999). Alkohol: Kalorie oder leere Kalorie?. In: *Alkohol und Alkoholfolgekrankheiten Grundlagen – Diagnostik – Therapie,* Singer, M.V., Teyssen, S., pp. 85-94, Springer Berlin Heidelberg, ISBN 3-540-65094-6.

Nanji, A.A. & French, S.W. (1985). Relationship between pork consumption and cirrhosis. *Lancet* 1(8430):681-683.

National Institute on Alcohol Abuse and Alcoholism. (2007). *What colleges need to know now: An update on college drinking research.* (NIH Pub. No. 07-5010). Washington, DC: National

Nielsen, K., Kondrup, J., Martinsen, L., Stilling, B. & Wikman, B. (1993). Nutritional assessment and adequacy of dietary intake in hospitalized patients with alcoholic liver cirrhosis. *Br.J.Nutr* 69(3):665-679.

Pekkanen, L. & Rusi, M. (1979). The effects of dietary niacin and riboflavin on voluntary intake and metabolism of ethanol in rats. *Pharmacol.Biochem Behav.* 11(5):575-579.

Pirola, R.C. & Lieber, C.S. (1972). The energy cost of the metabolism of drugs, including ethanol. *Pharmacology* 7(3):185-196.

Plauth, M., Cabre, E., Riggio, O., ssis-Camilo, M., Pirlich, M., Kondrup, J., Ferenci, P., Holm, E., Vom, D.S., Muller, M.J. & Nolte, W. (2006). ESPEN Guidelines on Enteral Nutrition: Liver disease. *Clin Nutr* 25(2):285-294.

Prasad, A.S. (1995). Zinc: an overview. *Nutrition* 11(1 Suppl):93-99.

Reinus, J.F., Heymsfield, S.B., Wiskind, R., Casper, K. & Galambos, J.T. (1989). Ethanol: relative fuel value and metabolic effects in vivo. *Metabolism* 38(2):125-135.

Rissanen, A., Sarlio-Lahteenkorva, S., Alfthan, G., Gref, C.G., Keso, L. & Salaspuro, M. (1987). Employed problem drinkers: a nutritional risk group? *Am.J.Clin Nutr* 45(2):456-461.

Rodríguez-Moreno, F., González-Reimers, E., Santolaria-Fernández, F., Galindo-Martín, L., Hernandez-Torres, O., Batista-López, N., Molina-Perez, M. (1997). Zinc, copper, manganese, and iron in chronic alcoholic liver disease. *Alcohol.* 14(1):39-44.

Rylander, R., Megevand, Y., Lasserre, B., Amstutz, W. & Granbom, S. (2001). Moderate alcohol consumption and urinary excretion of magnesium and calcium. *Scand.J.Clin Lab Invest* 61(5):401-405.

Salen, N. Jr., Olsson, N.U. (1997). Abnormalities in essential fatty acid status in alcoholism. In *Handbook of Essential Fatty Acid Biology : Biochemistry, Physiology and Behavioral Neurobiology*, pp. 67-87. (Anonymous). Totowa, NJ: Humana Press].

Sampson, H.W. (1997). Alcohol, osteoporosis, and bone regulating hormones. *Alcohol Clin.Exp.Res.* 21(3):400-403.

Schuhmacher, M., Domingo, J.L. & Corbella, J. (1994). Zinc and copper levels in serum and urine: relationship to biological, habitual and environmental factors. *Sci.Total Environ.* 148(1):67-72.

Shaw, S., Jayatilleke, E., Herbert, V. & Colman, N. (1989). Cleavage of folates during ethanol metabolism. Role of acetaldehyde/xanthine oxidase-generated superoxide. *Biochem J* 257(1):277-280.

Soberon, S., Pauley, M.P., Duplantier, R., Fan, A. & Halsted, C.H. (1987). Metabolic effects of enteral formula feeding in alcoholic hepatitis. *Hepatology* 7(6):1204-1209.

Sonko, B.J., Prentice, A.M., Murgatroyd, P.R., Goldberg, G.R., van de Ven, M.L., Coward, W.A. (1994). Effect of alcohol on postmeal fat storage. *Am J Clin Nutr.* 59(3):619-625.

Stal, P. & Hultcrantz, R. (1993). Iron increases ethanol toxicity in rat liver. *J.Hepatol.* 17(1):108-115.

Stickel, F., Hoehn, B., Schuppan, D. & Seitz, H.K. (2003). Review article: Nutritional therapy in alcoholic liver disease. *Aliment.Pharmacol.Ther.* 18(4):357-373.

Sullivan, J.F. (1962). Effect of alcohol on urinary zinc excretion. *Q.J.Stud.Alcohol* 23:216-220.

Suter, P.M. (2005). Alkohol und Ernährung. In: *Alkohol und Alkoholfolgekrankheiten Grundlagen - Diagnostik - Therapie,* Singer, M.V., Teyssen, S., pp. 326-348, Springer Berlin Heidelberg, ISBN 978-3-540-22552-2.

Suter, P.M., Hasler, E. & Vetter, W. (1997). Effects of alcohol on energy metabolism and body weight regulation: is alcohol a risk factor for obesity? *Nutr Rev.* 55(5):157-171.

Suter, P.M., Schutz, Y. & Jequier, E. (1992). The effect of ethanol on fat storage in healthy subjects. *N.Engl.J.Med.* 326(15):983-987.

Suzuki, Y., Saito, H., Suzuki, M., Hosoki, Y., Sakurai, S., Fujimoto, Y. & Kohgo, Y. (2002). Up-regulation of transferrin receptor expression in hepatocytes by habitual alcohol drinking is implicated in hepatic iron overload in alcoholic liver disease. *Alcohol Clin Exp.Res.* 26(8 Suppl):26S-31S.

Tamura, T. & Halsted, C.H. (1983). Folate turnover in chronically alcoholic monkeys. *J Lab Clin.Med.* 101(4):623-628.

Tanner, A.R., Bantock, I., Hinks, L., Lloyd, B., Turner, N.R. & Wright, R. (1986). Depressed selenium and vitamin E levels in an alcoholic population. Possible relationship to hepatic injury through increased lipid peroxidation. *Dig.Dis.Sci.* 31(12):1307-1312.

Thomson, M., Fulton, M., Elton, R.A., Brown, S., Wood, D.A. & Oliver, M.F. (1988). Alcohol consumption and nutrient intake in middle-aged Scottish men. *Am.J Clin.Nutr* 47(1):139-145.

Toniolo, P., Riboli, E. & Cappa, A.P. (1991). A community study of alcohol consumption and dietary habits in middle-aged Italian women. *Int.J Epidemiol.* 20(3):663-670.

Tsukamoto, H., Horne, W., Kamimura, S., Niemela, O., Parkkila, S., Yla-Herttuala, S. & Brittenham, G.M. (1995). Experimental liver cirrhosis induced by alcohol and iron. *J.Clin Invest* 96(1):620-630.

Turner, R.T., Aloia, R.C., Segel, L.D., Hannon, K.S. & Bell, N.H. (1988). Chronic alcohol treatment results in disturbed vitamin D metabolism and skeletal abnormalities in rats. *Alcohol Clin.Exp.Res.* 12(1):159-162.

Valberg, L.S., Flanagan, P.R., Ghent, C.N. & Chamberlain, M.J. (1985). Zinc absorption and leukocyte zinc in alcoholic and nonalcoholic cirrhosis. *Dig.Dis.Sci.* 30(4):329-333.

Van Haaren, M.R.T., Hendriks, H.F.J. (1999). Alkoholstoffwechsel. In: *Alkohol und Alkoholfolgekrankheiten Grundlagen - Diagnostik - Therapie,* Singer, M.V., Teyssen, S., pp. 95-107, Springer Berlin Heidelberg, ISBN 3-540-65094-6.

Wacker, W.E. & Parisi, A.F. (1968b). Magnesium metabolism. *N.Engl.J.Med.* 278(12):658-663, 278(13):712-717, 278(14):772-776.

Watson, W.H., Song, Z., Kirpich, I.A., Deaciuc, I.V., Chen, T. & McClain, C.J. (2011). Ethanol exposure modulates hepatic S-adenosylmethionine and S-adenosylhomocysteine levels in the isolated perfused rat liver through changes in the redox state of the NADH/NAD(+) system. *Biochim.Biophys.Acta* 1812(5):613-618.

World Health Organitation (WHO). (1994). *Lexicon of alcohol and drug terms.* [online]. Geneva, Switzerland: WHO Office of Publications; Available from: www.who.int/substance_abuse/terminology/who_lexicon/en/

Wood, B. , Breen, K.J. (1979). Vitamin deficiency in alcoholism with particular reference to thiamine deficiency. *Clinical and Experimental pharmacology and Physiology* 6:457.

Wu, A., Chanarin, I., Slavin, G. & Levi, A.J. (1975). Folate deficiency in the alcoholic--its relationship to clinical and haematological abnormalities, liver disease and folate stores. *Br.J Haematol.* 29(3):469-478.

Zakhari, S. (2006). Overview: how is alcohol metabolized by the body? *Alcohol Res.Health* 29(4):245-254.

Zakhari, S. & Li, T.K. (2007). Determinants of alcohol use and abuse: Impact of quantity and frequency patterns on liver disease. *Hepatology* 46(6):2032-2039.

Zhao, M., Matter, K., Laissue, J.A., ZimmermannA. (1996). Copper/zinc and manganese superoxide dismutases in alcoholic liver disease: immunohistochemical quantitation. *Histol Histopathol.* 11(4):899-907.

2

Gender Difference in Alcoholic Liver Disease

Ichiro Shimizu, Mari Kamochi,
Hideshi Yoshikawa and Yoshiyuki Nakayama
Showa Clinic, Kohoku-ku, Yokohama, Kanagawa, Japan

1. Introduction

Alcoholic liver disease occurs after prolonged heavy drinking, particularly among persons who are physically dependent on alcohol. Alcoholic liver disease is pathologically classified into three forms: fatty liver (hepatic steatosis), alcoholic hepatitis, and cirrhosis. There is considerable overlap among these conditions. The incidence of alcoholic liver disease increases in a dose-dependent manner proportionally to the cumulative alcoholic intake. Alcoholism is increasing among females, owing to a decline in the social stigma attached to drinking and to the ready availability of alcohol in supermarkets. In general, however, males have a greater opportunity for drinking. In the United States, the National Comorbidity Survey estimated that, at some time in their lives, 6.4% of females and 12.5% of males will meet the criteria for alcoholic abuse (Kessler et al., 1994). The Italian longitudinal study on aging showed that 42% of elderly females and 12% of elderly males were lifelong abstainers (Buja et al., 2010). In Japan, based on data from the National Nutrition Survey, heavy drinkers with a daily consumption exceeded 40 g of ethanol per day for females and 60 g of ethanol per day for males were more frequently observed in males (Figure 1). Despite the male predominance for alcoholism, chronic alcohol consumption induces more rapid and more severe liver injury in females than males.

In contrast, the progression of hepatic fibrosis in chronic hepatitis B and C appears to be slower in females than in males (Poynard et al., 1997; Poynard et al., 2003; Rodriguez-Torres et al., 2006; Wright et al., 2003). Hepatic fibrosis is fibrous scarring of the liver in which excessive collagens build up along with the duration and extent of persistence of liver injury. In other words, overproduced collagens are deposited in injured areas instead of destroyed hepatocytes. Moreover, females, especially before menopause, produce antibodies against hepatitis B virus (HBV) surface antigen (HBsAg) and HBV e antigen (HBeAg) at higher frequency than males (Furusyo et al., 1999; Zacharakis et al., 2005). In chronic infection with hepatitis C virus (HCV), the clearance rate of blood HCV RNA appears to be higher in females (Bakr et al., 2006). Most asymptomatic carriers of HCV with persistent normal alanine aminotransferase (ALT) are females and have a good prognosis with a low risk of progression of hepatic fibrosis to the end-stage cirrhosis and its complications such as hepatocellular carcinoma (HCC) (Gholson et al., 1997; Puoti et al., 2002). The menopause is associated with accelerated progression of hepatic fibrosis, and the HCC risk is inversely related to the age at natural menopause (Shimizu, 2003; Shimizu et al., 2007a).

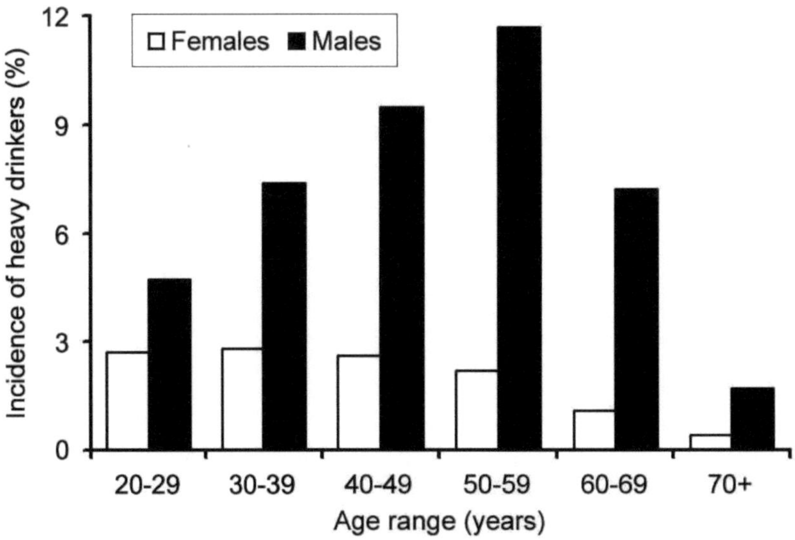

Fig. 1. Incidence of heavy drinkers with a daily consumption exceeded 40 g of ethanol per day for females and 60 g of ethanol per day for males based on data in 2002 from the National Nutrition Survey in Japan.

The "female paradox" observed in patients with alcoholic liver disease in comparison with chronic viral hepatitis is based on susceptibility by females to liver damage from smaller quantities of ethanol.

2. Alcoholic liver disease in females

The amount of alcohol required producing hepatitis or cirrhosis varies among individuals, but as little as 40 g/day (Table 1) for 10 years is associated with an increased incidence of cirrhosis. There is considerable evidence to suggest that females require less total alcohol consumption (20 g ethanol/day) to produce clinically significant liver disease. Indeed, it is reported that the lowest point of weekly alcohol intake that helps to develop liver disease was higher in males (168-324 g) than in females (84-156 g), and that, in the case of heavy drinkers with a weekly consumption of 336-492 g, the relative risk for alcoholic liver disease was 3.7 in males and 7.3 in females, while it was 1.0 in the group with a weekly consumption of 12-72 g (Becker et al., 1996). Thus, safe drinking guidelines recommend that females do not drink more than 20 g ethanol per day, and males not more than 40 g ethanol. A common, reasonable recommendation is not to exceed 70 g of ethanol a week.

Whisky	60 ml	20 g
Wine	200 ml	20 g
Beer	500 ml	20 g

Table 1. Alcohol (ethanol) equivalents.

The incidence of alcoholic liver disease correlates with the national per capita consumption of ethanol derived from sales of beer, wine and spirits (Figure 2). For instance, in France, the

United Kingdom and Germany, the annual per capita (average consumed by each person) ethanol consumption is over 9 litres per person per year, but in Asia such as China and Japan, it is 4 to 6.5 litres per person per year. Ethanol is metabolized by hepatic alcohol dehydrogenase (ADH) and the hepatic microsomal ethanol oxidizing system (MEOS) to acetaldehyde, which is subsequently converted by aldehyde dehydrogenase (ALDH) to acetate. The accumulation of acetaldehyde leads to the clinical syndrome of flushing, nausea and vomiting. Isoenzymes of ALDH with low activities are common among Asian populations and are associated with lower rates of alcoholism. These persons experience a similar flushing syndrome after consuming ethanol. This inhibits Asian populations from taking alcohol and is a negative risk for the development of alcoholic liver disease (Tanaka et al., 1996).

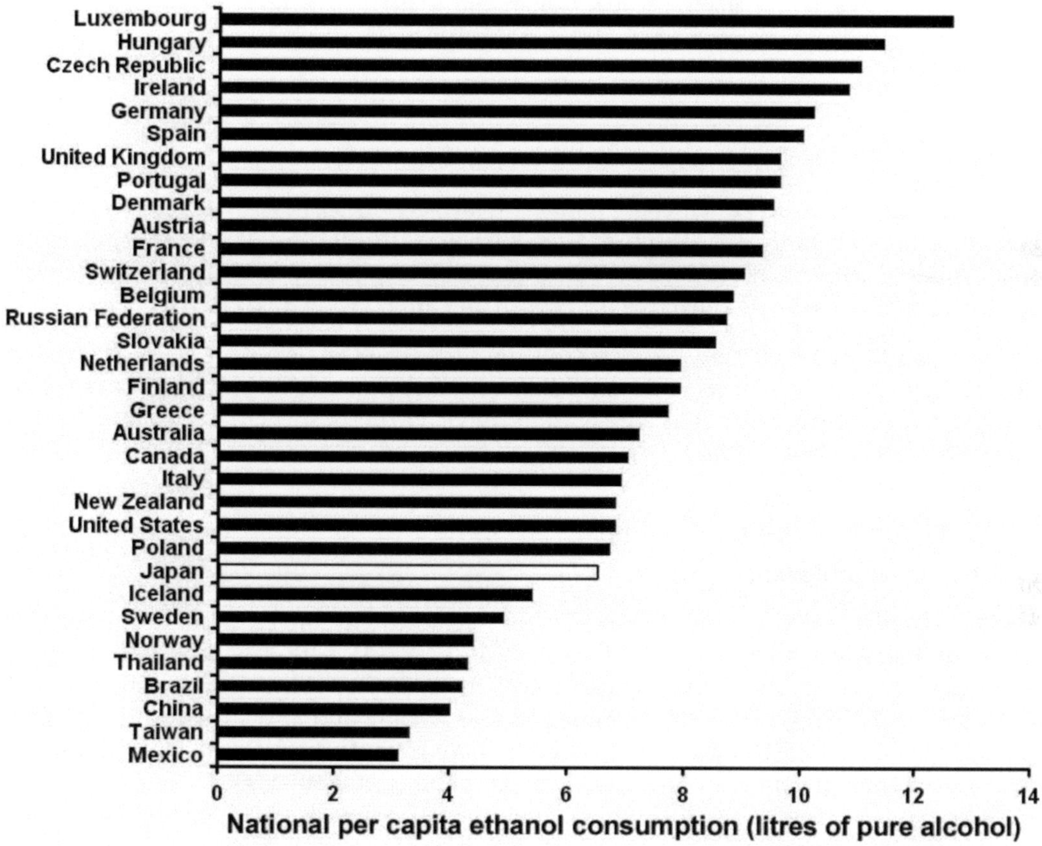

Fig. 2. The annual per capita (average consumed by each person) consumption of ethanol derived from sales of beer, wine and spirits (whisky, brandy, vodka, rum, gin and all other spirits) in the world (National Tax Agency, 2008).

In a study on the sex difference in Japanese patients hospitalized in Tokushima, western Japan, the incidence of alcoholic cirrhosis was 9-fold higher in males than females (Figure 3). However, females develop higher blood ethanol levels following a standard dose, at least in part, because of a smaller mean apparent volume of ethanol distribution. Moreover, sex differences in hepatic metabolism with increased production of acetaldehyde may contribute

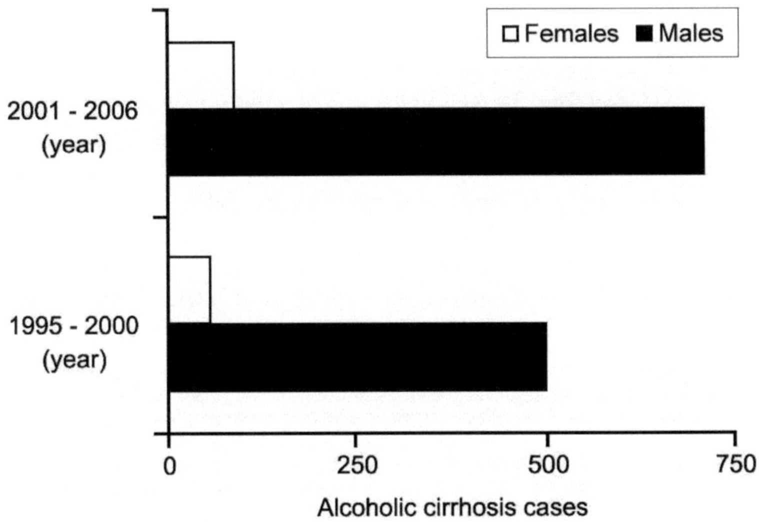

Fig. 3. Male-to-female ratio in Japanese patients with alcoholic cirrhosis. Male-to-female ratio in alcoholic cirrhosis was examined from 1995 to 2000 and from 2001 to 2006 in 1,005 Japanese patients (mean age 59.5 years, 10.4% females) hospitalized in Tokushima, western Japan. The subjects were seronegative for HBsAg and antibody against HCV.

to vulnerability of females to alcohol consumption (Eriksson et al., 1996) (see below), suggesting that chronic alcohol consumption may induce more rapid and more severe liver injury in females than males. Females with alcoholic cirrhosis survive a shorter time than males (Sherlock & Dooley, 2002).

3. Alcoholic liver injury and oxidative stress

3.1 Ethanol hepatotoxicity

Alcoholic liver injury is mainly due to ethanol hepatotoxicity linked to its metabolism by means of the ADH and cytochrome P450 2E1 (CYP2E1) pathways and the resulting production of toxic acetaldehyde (Figure 4). CYP2E1 is the key enzyme of the MEOS, and it is involved in the oxygenation of substrates such as ethanol and fatty acids. Although most ethanol is oxidized by ADH, CYP2E1 assumes a more important role in ethanol oxidation at elevated levels of ethanol or after chronic consumption of ethanol. CYP2E1 has a very high NADPH oxidase activity. NADPH/NADH oxidase is a primary source of reactive oxygen species (ROS) production in non-phagocytic cells such as hepatic stellate cells (HSCs) in the space of Disse (Figure 5). Therefore, excess of ethanol and fatty acids and their metabolism by means of CYP2E1 pathway produce extensively ROS, which cause oxidative stress with lipid peroxidation and membrane damage, leading to cell death. ROS and products of lipid peroxidation activate not only inflammatory cells including neutrophils, macrophages and Kupffer cells (hepatic resident macrophages), but HSCs as well. In the injured liver, HSCs are regarded as the primary target cells for inflammatory and oxidative stimuli, and undergo proliferation and transformation into myofibroblast-like cells. These HSCs are activated cells and are responsible for much of the collagen synthesis observed during hepatic fibrosis to cirrhosis.

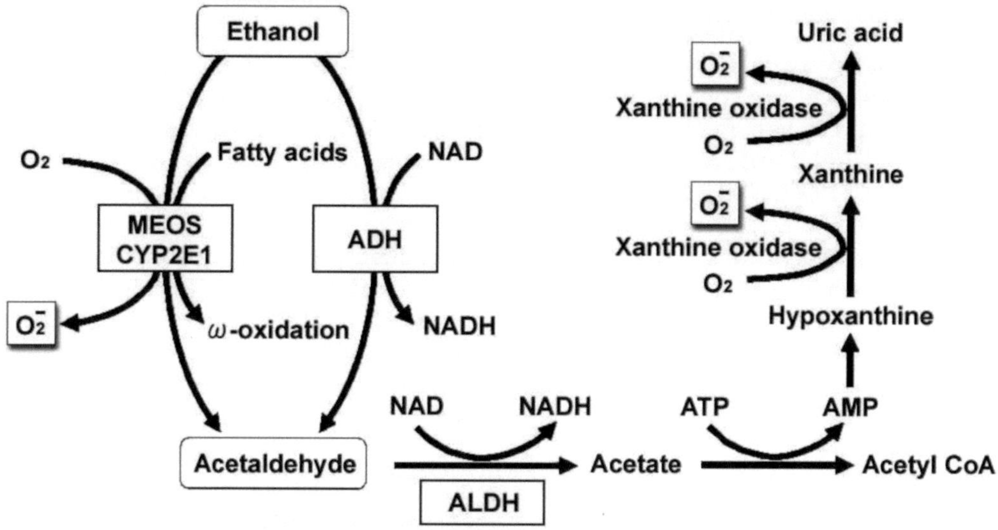

Fig. 4. Ethanol oxidation by alcohol dehydrogenase (ADH) and the hepatic microsomal ethanol oxidizing system (MEOS), which involves cytochrome P450 2E1 (CYP2E1), produces acetaldehyde (Shimizu, 2009). CYP2E1 produces ROS (superoxide, O_2^-). Acetaldehyde is converted by aldehyde dehydrogenase (ALDH) to acetate. Both reactions of ethanol to acetaldehyde and then acetate reduce nicotinamide adenine dinucleotide (NAD) to its reduced form (NADH). Excess NADH causes inhibition of fatty acid oxidation, leading to fat accumulation (hepatic steatosis).

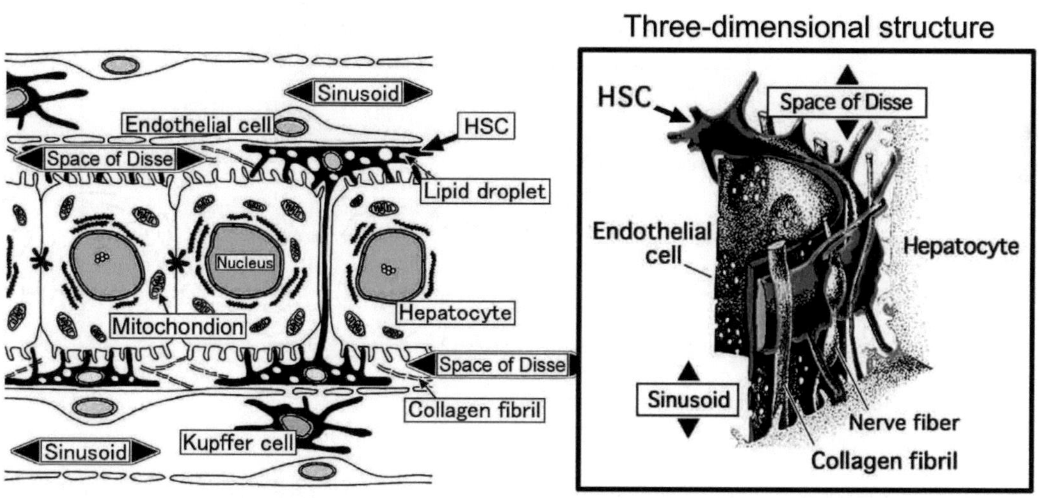

Fig. 5. Schema of the sinusoidal wall of the liver. Schematic representation of hepatic stellate cells (HSCs) was based on the studies by Wake (Wake, 1999). Kupffer cells (hepatic resident macrophages) rest on fenestrated endothelial cells. HSCs are located in the space of Disse in close contact with endothelial cells and hepatocytes, functioning as the primary retinoid storage area. Collagen fibrils course through the space of Disse between endothelial cells and the cords of hepatocytes.

3.2 Excess fatty acids lead to hepatic steatosis

Increased lipid peroxidation and accumulation of end products of lipid peroxidation are commonly observed in alcoholic liver disease and non-alcoholic fatty liver disease (NAFLD) based on studies of human alcohol-related liver injury and animal models of diet-induced hepatic steatosis and drug-induced steatohepatitis (Berson et al., 1998; Letteron et al., 1993; Letteron et al., 1996). Fatty liver is the result of the deposition of triglycerides via the accumulation of fatty acids in hepatocytes. In the progression of fatty liver disease, lipid peroxidation products are generated because of impaired β-oxidation of the accumulated fatty acids. The major site for fatty acid β-oxidation (degradation of fatty acids) in the liver is hepatocyte mitochondria (Figure 6). Key mediators of impaired fatty acid β-oxidation include a reduced mitochondrial electron transport (respiratory chain dysfunction). In addition to impaired mitochondrial β-oxidation of fatty acids, an activity of CYP2E1 in the

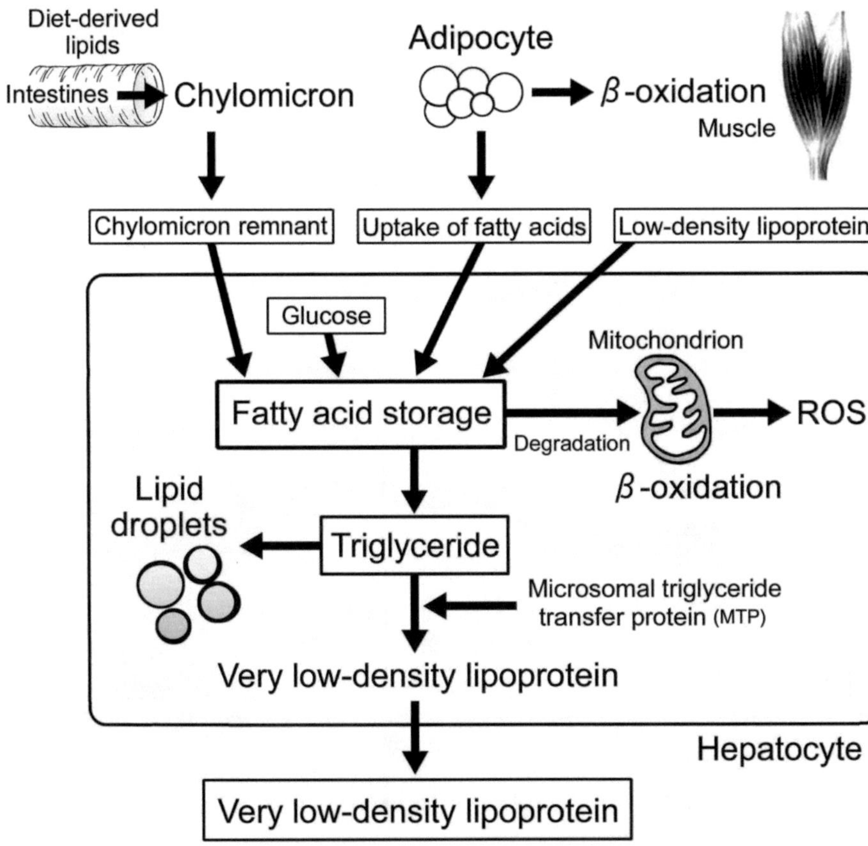

Fig. 6. Increased hepatic uptake of free fatty acids, increased triglyceride synthesis, and impaired transport of very low-density lipoprotein (triglyceride-rich lipoprotein) into the blood mainly contribute to the accumulation of hepatocellular triglycerides. Microsomal trigyceride transfer protein (MTP) is essential for the secretion of very low-density lipoprotein. Excess triglycerides are stored as lipid droplets in hepatocytes, which in turn results in a preferential shift to fatty acid degradation (β-oxidation), leading to the formation of ROS and lipid peroxidation products.

microsomes is increased. Elevated CYP2E1 and mitochondrial defects result in an increase in the ROS formation and lipid peroxidation products. ROS and lipid peroxidation in turn cause further mitochondrial dysfunction and oxidative stress, thus contributing to cell death via ROS-induced DNA injury and membrane lipid peroxidation and discharge of products of lipid peroxidation, malondialdehyde (MDA) and 4-hydroxynonecal (HNE), into the space of Disse. MDA and HNE besides ROS are able to activate inflammatory cells (neutrophils, macrophages and Kupffer cells) and HSCs. Activated inflammatory cells in turn produce chemokines as well as tumor necrosis factor-α (TNF-α) and ROS. Chemokines such as monocytes chemoattractant protein-1 (MCP-1) and interleukin-8 (IL-8) attract neutrophils, lymphocytes, monocytes, macrophages, and Kupffer cells to inflammatory sites, leading to the persistent liver injury.

3.3 CYP2E1

Oxidation of ethanol through the ADH and CYP2E1 pathways produces acetaldehyde which is also toxic to the hepatocyte mitochondria. Acetaldehyde aggravates oxidative stress by binding to reduced glutathione, an antioxidant, and promoting its leakage, which triggers an inflammatory response of the host. This involves the activation of Kupffer cells and the attraction of inflammatory cells to injured sites. The inflammatory cells in the liver produce transforming growth factor-β (TGF-β) and proinflammatory mediators including TNF-α and ROS, leading to oxidative tress and hepatic fibrosis. Thus, TNF-α mediates not only the early stages of alcoholic liver disease but also the transition to more advanced stages of liver damage.

Reactions of ethanol converted to acetaldehyde and subsequently acetate reduce nicotinamide adenine dinucleotide (NAD) to its reduced form (NADH). Excess NADH causes a number of metabolic disorders, including stimulation of the fatty acid synthesis and inhibition of the Krebs cycle and of its fatty acid oxidation (Lieber, 2004). The stimulation of the fatty acid synthesis and inhibition of fatty acid oxidation favor fat accumulation (hepatic steatosis) and hyperlipidemia.

CYP2E1 activity is elevated in the livers of obese animals (Raucy et al., 1991) and non-alcoholic steatohepatitis (NASH) patients (Weltman et al., 1998) as well as patients with alcoholic liver disease. The role of CYP2E1 in fatty acid metabolism supports the concept of a nutritional role for CYP2E1. Indeed, besides its ethanol-oxidizing activity, CYP2E1 catalyzes fatty acid ω-hydroxylations (microsomal ω-oxidation of fatty acids) and metabolizes ketones. Fatty acids and ketones increase especially in obesity and diabetes, and their excess up-regulates CYP2E1. CYP2E1 leaks ROS as part of its operation, and when increased ROS production exceed the cellular antioxidant defense systems, excess ROS result in oxidative stress with its pathologic consequences. This is true when excess alcohol has to be metabolized, as in alcoholic steatohepatitis, or when CYP2E1 is confronted by an excess of fatty acids and ketones associated with obesity, diabetes, or both, resulting in NASH (Lieber, 2004).

4. Endotoxin in alcoholic liver injury

Alcohol ingestion disrupts gastrointestinal barrier function and subsequently induces the diffusion of luminal bacterial products including bacterial lipopolysaccharides (endotoxins) into the portal vein. Experiments using animals show direct evidence of increased translocation of endotoxin from the gut lumen into the portal bloodstream caused by ethanol (Mathurin et al., 2000). Acute ethanol ingestion, especially at high concentrations, facilitates the absorption of endotoxin from rat small intestine via an increase in intestinal permeability, which may play an important role in endotoxemia observed in alcoholic liver injury (Tamai et al., 2000). Increased endotoxin levels in the portal blood are essential for initiation and progression of alcoholic liver disease (Bode & Bode, 2005).

Bacterial translocation from the gastrointestinal tract, namely spillover endotoxemia, is important in the relationship between endotoxin and hepatotoxicity in the reticuloendothelial system such as monocytes-macrophages and Kupffer cells. Gut-derived endotoxin activates Kupffer cells, which produce proinflammatory mediators such as TNF-α and ROS. The ability of Kupffer cells to eliminate and detoxify various exogenous and endogenous substances including endotoxin is an important physiological regulatory function (Figure 7).

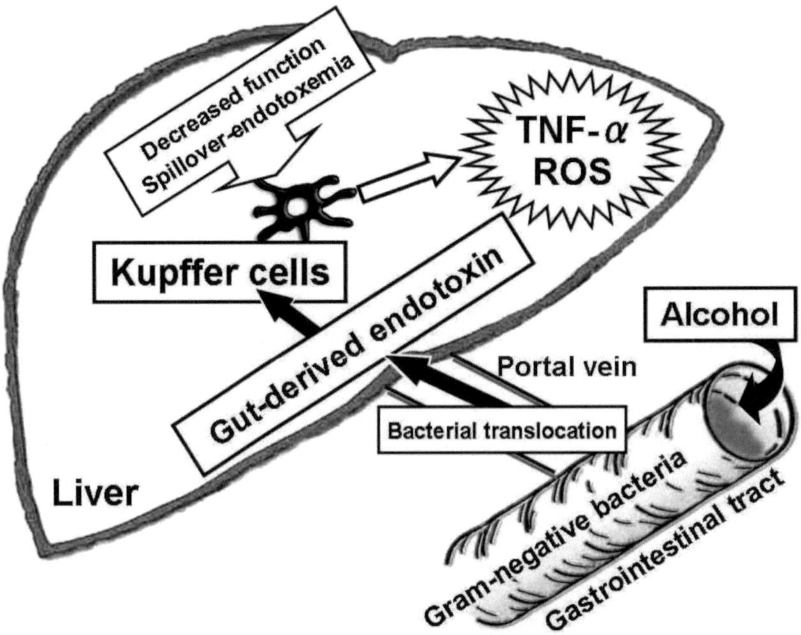

Fig. 7. Activation of Kupffer cells by gut-derived endotoxin plays a pivotal role in alcoholic liver injury (Shimizu, 2009). Following chronic alcohol ingestion, endotoxin, also called lipopolysaccharide, released from intestinal gram-negative bacteria moves from gastrointestinal tract (gut) into the liver via the portal bloodstream.

Like chronic ethanol feeding, TNF-α cytotoxicity is also with alteration of mitochondrial function. The mitochondria of TNF-α-exposed cells overproduce ROS derived from the respiratory chain. The mitochondria themselves then become the targets of ROS, thus setting up a cycle of injury (Nagata et al., 2007). In addition to ROS production, TNF-α prompts the opening of the mitochondrial permeability transition (MPT). The MPT is the regulatable opening of a large and non-specific pore across the outer and inner mitochondrial membrane. Ethanol may also increase the susceptibility of MPT induction by TNF-α at the mitochondrial level, possibly through an increase in ROS production caused by respiratory chain dysfunction and/or CYP2E1 (Pastorino & Hoek, 2000).

Ethanol-induced oxidative stress is the result of the combined impairment of antioxidant defense and the ROS production by the mitochondrial electron transport chain, the ethanol-induced CYP2E1 and activated phagocyte such as macrophages and Kupffer cells (Albano, 2006). Indirectly, chronic ethanol ingestion may augment oxidative stress by decreasing antioxidant defenses such as reducing glutathione peroxidase and glutathione homeostasis (Figure 8).

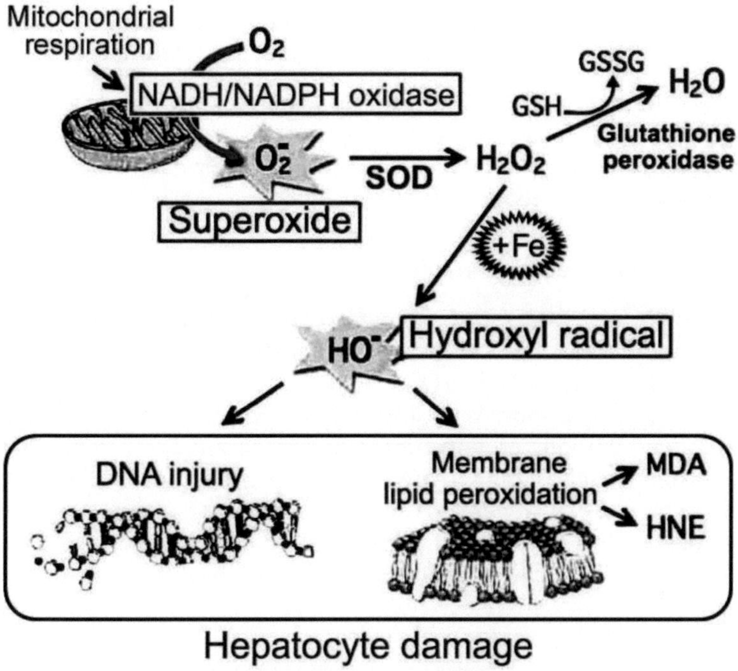

Fig. 8. Oxidative stress and hepatocyte damage (Shimizu and Ito, 2007). A primary source of reactive oxygen species (ROS) production is mitochondrial NADPH/NADH oxidase. Hydrogen peroxide (H_2O_2) is converted to a highly reactive ROS, the hydroxyl radical, in the presence of transition metals such as iron (+Fe) and copper. The hydroxyl radical induces DNA cleavage and lipid peroxidation in the structure of membrane phospholipids, leading to cell death and discharge of products of lipid peroxidation, malondialdehyde (MDA) and 4-hydroxynonenal (HNE) into the space of Disse. Cells have comprehensive antioxidant protective systems, including SOD, glutathione peroxidase and glutathione (GSH). Upon oxidation, GSH forms glutathione disulfide (GSSG).

5. Sex difference of ADH and CYP2E1 via growth hormone and estrogens

5.1 Gastric ADH in females

After an equivalent dose of alcohol, females have higher blood ethanol levels than males (Nolen-Hoeksema, 2004). There are multiple explanations for this. First, females are generally smaller than males so the same dose of alcohol leads to higher blood alcohol levels for females than males. Second, female body water content is smaller than male per kilogram of body weight. Thus, a dose of ethanol is distributed in a smaller volume of water in females than in males, leading to somewhat higher concentrations of ethanol in female blood (Frezza et al., 1990).

Third, the first pass metabolism of alcohol in the stomach may lead to higher blood alcohol levels in females than males. In the stomach, alcohol is metabolized with the enzyme gastric ADH. The stomach thus acts as a barrier against the penetration of alcohol into the body, by retaining and breaking down part of the alcohol (Nolen-Hoeksema, 2004). Gastric ADH activity is lower in females than in males; one study found that for a given alcohol dose, male ADH levels were two times higher than female levels, and in turn, female blood alcohol levels were higher than those of males (Frezza et al., 1990).

This sex difference in metabolism of alcohol appears to hold for younger adults but not older adults. ADH activity decreases with age, particularly for males, leading to similar blood alcohol concentrations in older males and females, or even higher concentrations in older males than older females (Nolen-Hoeksema, 2004).

5.2 Growth hormone secretion in females

The profile of growth hormone secretion pattern shows clear sex dimorphism (Ameen & Oscarsson, 2003). In female rats, the growth hormone is continuously secreted, and the hormone levels are always detectable in the circulation, while, in male rats, it is secreted by episodic bursts every 3.5 to 4 hours with low or undetectable levels between peaks (Shapiro et al., 1995). Integrated 24-hour growth hormone secretion (Clasey et al., 2001) and fasting blood growth hormone levels (Figure 9) are higher in women than in men. Growth hormone secretion is stimulated by estrogens (Ameen & Oscarsson, 2003). Oral and high-dose transdermal estrogen administration in menopausal women increases integrated 24-hour growth hormone secretion (Friend et al., 1996).

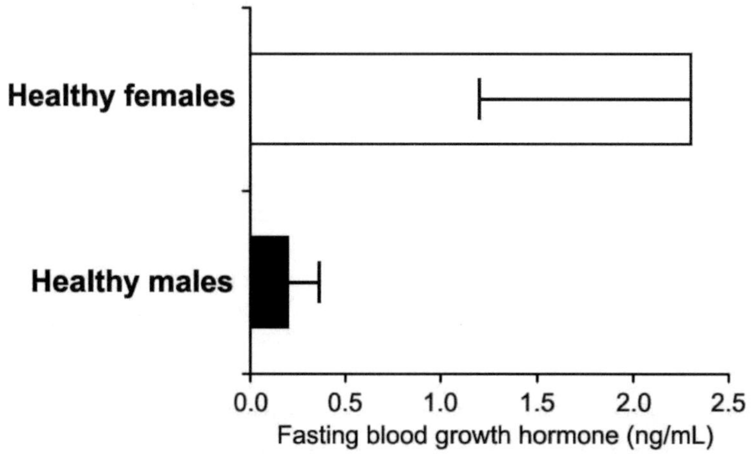

Fig. 9. Fasting mean blood levels of growth hormone in 15 premenopausal women (mean age 41.3 years) and 15 age-matched men (mean age 41.1 years) of healthy non-obese (body mass index ≥ 18.5 to 24.9 kg/m²) individuals. The subjects had no history of alcohol abuse (defined as an alcohol intake >20 g/day).

Interestingly, growth hormone increases ADH activity in the liver. The steady exposure of hepatocytes in cultures to growth hormone resulting in increased ADH activity resembles the female pattern of growth hormone secretion (Potter et al., 1993). ADH activity is higher in female rats and mice than in their male counterparts (Mezey, 2000). Thus, increased rates of the resulting production of toxic acetaldehyde in females compared with males may be responsible for the known increased susceptibility to alcohol-induced liver injury by females. Females are more likely to progress from alcoholic hepatitis to cirrhosis even if they abstain.

5.3 Endotoxin after ethanol in females

Endotoxin-stimulated monocytes in males produce more TNF-α as compared to females (Bouman et al., 2004). Like Kupffer cells, monocytes stimulated by endotoxin induce proinflammatory cytokines and ROS. In studies using animals, however, the stimulation of Kupffer cells by estrogen increased sensitivity to endotoxin after ethanol (Ikejima et al., 1998). It appears that monocytes-macrophages respond differently to endotoxins compared to Kupffer cells as far as the signaling pathways are concerned (Schultze et al., 1999). The estrogen addition to ethanol ingestion enhanced TNF-α production in Kupffer cells via elevation of the blood endotoxin level and hepatic endotoxin receptor (CD14) expression, resulting in increased inflammatory activity in the liver (Yin et al., 2000). The administration of ethanol in female rats induced the hepatic activity of CYP2E1, and the ethanol-induced CYP2E1 activity was reduced by the treatment with antiestrogen (Jarvelainen et al., 2001). Because activity of cytochrome P-450 (CYP) isoenzymes is regulated by circulating growth hormone, sex differences in growth hormone secretion profiles account for a different expression pattern of hepatic CYP isoenzymes between females and males (Agrawal & Shapiro, 2001).

6. Favorable role of female factors in chronic viral hepatitis

Clinical observations and death statistics support the view that chronic hepatitis C and B appears to progress more rapidly in males than in females (Poynard et al., 1997; Poynard et al., 2003; Rodriguez-Torres et al., 2006; Wright et al., 2003), and that cirrhosis is largely a disease of men and postmenopausal women with the exception of classically autoimmune liver diseases, such as primary biliary cirrhosis and chronic autoimmune hepatitis (Shimizu, 2003). HCV infections are more common than HBV infections in Japan and Western countries, and are recognized as a major causative factor of chronic hepatitis, cirrhosis, and HCC. According to a report of the International Agency for Research on Cancer (Brannstrom et al., 1999), the male:female ratio of the age-standardized incidence per 100,000 of liver cancer worldwide is 2.9 : 1, and in Asia (particularly in China, Japan, and Taiwan), the incidence of liver cancer is high and it accounts for half of all liver cancer cases in the world.

The prevalence of HBsAg is reported to be higher in males than in females throughout the world (Blumberg et al., 1972). In a prospective follow-up study of up to 19 years on HBsAg carriers in Okinawa in Japan, clearance of HBsAg was found more frequently in females (7.8%) than in males (5.8%) (Furusyo et al., 1999). Seroconversion from HBeAg to its antibody (anti-HBe) occurs more frequently in females than in males (Zacharakis et al.,

2005). In chronic HCV infection, the clearance rate of blood HCV RNA appears to be higher in females (Bakr et al., 2006). Demographic data from the United States (Gholson et al., 1997), Europe (France and Italy) (Puoti et al., 2002; Renou et al., 2002), and Japan (Okanoue et al., 2005) show that most HCV carriers with persistently normal ALT (asymptomatic carriers) are females, and have a good prognosis with a low risk of progression to cirrhosis and HCC. The menopause is associated with accelerated progression of hepatic fibrosis, and the HCC risk is inversely related to the age at natural menopause (Shimizu, 2003; Shimizu et al., 2007a). Chronic HCV- and HBV-infected patients of female sex and under 50 years old, namely premenopausal women are least vulnerable to HCC (Shimizu, 2009).

Premenopausal women have lower hepatic iron stores and a decreased production of proinflammatory cytokines such as TNF-α (Clerici et al., 1991; Pfeilschifter et al., 2002; Shimizu et al., 2007b). Iron is essential for life, but is toxic in excess, because it produces ROS that react readily with lipids and DNA, leading to cell death and DNA mutagenesis. An experimental animal study showed that hepatic steatosis spontaneously becomes evident in an aromatase-deficient mouse, which lacks the intrinsic ability to produce estrogen and is impaired with respect to hepatocellular fatty acid β-oxidation. Estrogen replacement reduces hepatic steatosis and restores the impairment in mitochondrial and peroxisomal fatty acid β-oxidation to a wild-type level (Nemoto et al., 2000). In addition, tamoxifen is a well known antiestrogen used in the hormone treatment of estrogen receptor-positive breast cancer, and it has been shown to be associated with an increased risk of developing fatty liver and NASH in such patients (Oien et al., 1999; Van et al., 1996). Estrogens are potent endogenous antioxidant (Lacort et al., 1995; Yoshino et al., 1987), suppresses hepatic fibrosis in animal models, and attenuates induction of redox sensitive transcription factors, hepatocyte apoptosis and HSC activation by inhibiting the generation of ROS and TGF-β in primary cultures (Itagaki et al., 2005; Lu et al., 2004; Shimizu et al., 1999; Yasuda et al., 1999; Zhou et al., 2001). Variant estrogen receptors are expressed in HCC patients and, to a greater extent, in male patients with chronic liver disease than in female patients, even at an early stage of chronic liver disease (Villa et al., 1995; Villa et al., 1998). The occurrence of variant estrogen receptors leads to the loss of estrogen responsiveness. These lines of evidence suggest that the greater progression of hepatic fibrosis and HCC in men and postmenopausal women may be due, at least in part, to both a lower production of estrogen and a lower response to the action of estrogen.

7. Heavy alcohol intake and HCC

Chronic alcohol intake (mostly heavy alcohol use of more than 50 g/day) and alcoholic cirrhosis have long been recognized as a cause of HCC. In alcoholic cirrhosis, the risk of HCC is about 1% per a year. Most HCC cases are in males. There are no clinical or pathological differences compared with HCC complicating chronic HBV and HCV infection. However, it is not certain whether alcohol is a true carcinogen. Several epidemiologic studies among alcoholics show a high prevalence of HBV markers (16%-70%) and HCV markers (10%-20%) as compared with a background prevalence of close to 5% and less than 1%, respectively (Bosch et al., 2004). These prevalences are even higher in HCC cases who are also alcoholics (27% to 81% of HBV markers and 50% to 77% of HCV markers), suggesting a complex interaction between alcohol and viral infections in the etiology of HCC (Di Bisceglie et al., 1998).

Case-control studies have shown that, as a result of the synergy between alcohol intake and HCV infection, the risk of liver cancer is increased approximately 2- to 4-fold among cases drinking more 60-80 g/day of alcohol (Fattovich et al., 2004). The presumed basis for this is that both alcohol and HCV infection independently promote the development of cirrhosis. In a longitudinal cohort study of cirrhotic patients with HCV infection, heavy alcohol intake (>65 g/day) was an independent factor for the development of HCC, increasing the risk approximately 3-fold (Aizawa et al., 2000).

A case-control study also shows a synergism between alcohol drinking and HBV infection on the risk of HCC, increasing the risk approximately 2-fold for HBsAg-positive subject of both sexes who drink more than 60 g/day of ethanol compared with HBsAg-positive non-drinkers (Donato et al., 2006). In a longitudinal cohort study of patients with HBV-related cirrhosis, heavy alcohol intake was associated with a 3-fold increased risk for HCC (Ikeda et al., 1998).

Studies in northern Italy and Greece estimated that the attributable fraction of high levels of alcohol consumption, once adjusted for HBV and HCV status, were 45% in Italy (Donato et al., 1997) and 15% in Greece (Kuper et al., 2000). In low-risk populations, heavy alcohol intake may account for the majority of the HCC cases who are seronegative for HBV and HCV markers.

8. Conclusion

A large body of evidence has been accumulated suggesting that increased oxidative stress is an essential step in the development of hepatic fibrogenesis and carcinogenesis. Environmental and lifestyle risk factors such as HCV and HBV infection and heavy alcohol intake lead to increased oxidative stress, which in general occurs more frequently in males. Moreover, biological female sex factors such as estrogens, hepatic iron storage status, and growth hormone play antioxidative and cytoprotective roles in the functional and morphological modulation of the liver physiopathology. However, it should be noted that females consistently drink less than males and appear to suffer serious negative consequences of alcohol consumption earlier and to a greater degree than males. Specifically, chronic alcohol consumption induces more rapid and more severe liver injury in females than males. The "female paradox" observed in patients with alcoholic liver disease in comparison with chronic viral hepatitis is based on susceptibility by females to liver damage from smaller quantities of ethanol. Being female or male is an important basic human variable that affects health and liver disease throughout the life span. Sex is defined as female or male according to their biological functions, while gender is shaped by environment and experience. Better knowledge of the basic mechanisms underlying the sex-associated differences during hepatic fibrogenesis and carciogenesis may open up new avenues for the prevention and treatment of chronic liver disease.

9. References

Agrawal AK & Shapiro BH . (2001). Intrinsic signals in the sexually dimorphic circulating growth hormone profiles of the rat. Mol Cell Endocrinol 173:167-181.

Aizawa Y, Shibamoto Y, Takagi I, Zeniya M & Toda G . (2000). Analysis of factors affecting the appearance of hepatocellular carcinoma in patients with chronic hepatitis C. A long term follow-up study after histologic diagnosis. Cancer 89:53-59.

Albano E . (2006). Alcohol, oxidative stress and free radical damage. Proc Nutr Soc 65:278-290.

Ameen C & Oscarsson J . (2003). Sex difference in hepatic microsomal triglyceride transfer protein expression is determined by the growth hormone secretory pattern in the rat. Endocrinology 144:3914-3921.

Bakr I, Rekacewicz C, El HM, Ismail S, El DM, El-Kafrawy S, Esmat G, Hamid MA, Mohamed MK & Fontanet A . (2006). Higher clearance of hepatitis C virus infection in females compared with males. Gut 55:1183-1187.

Becker U, Deis A, Sorensen TI, Gronbaek M, Borch-Johnsen K, Muller CF, Schnohr P & Jensen G . (1996). Prediction of risk of liver disease by alcohol intake, sex, and age: a prospective population study. Hepatology 23:1025-1029.

Berson A, De B, V, Letteron P, Robin MA, Moreau C, El Kahwaji J, Verthier N, Feldmann G, Fromenty B & Pessayre D . (1998). Steatohepatitis-inducing drugs cause mitochondrial dysfunction and lipid peroxidation in rat hepatocytes. Gastroenterology 114:764-774.

Blumberg BS, Sutnick AI, London WT & Melartin L . (1972). Sex distribution of Australia antigen. Arch Intern Med 130:227-231.

Bode C & Bode JC . (2005). Activation of the innate immune system and alcoholic liver disease: effects of ethanol per se or enhanced intestinal translocation of bacterial toxins induced by ethanol? Alcohol Clin Exp Res 29:166S-171S.

Bosch FX, Ribes J, Diaz M & Cleries R . (2004). Primary liver cancer: worldwide incidence and trends. Gastroenterology 127:S5-S16.

Bouman A, Schipper M, Heineman MJ & Faas M . (2004). 17beta-estradiol and progesterone do not influence the production of cytokines from lipopolysaccharide-stimulated monocytes in humans. Fertil Steril 82 Suppl 3:1212-1219.

Brannstrom M, Friden BE, Jasper M & Norman RJ . (1999). Variations in peripheral blood levels of immunoreactive tumor necrosis factor alpha (TNFalpha) throughout the menstrual cycle and secretion of TNFalpha from the human corpus luteum. Eur J Obstet Gynecol Reprod Biol 83:213-217.

Buja A, Scafato E, Sergi G, Maggi S, Suhad MA, Rausa G, Coin A, Baldi I, Manzato E, Galluzzo L, Enzi G & Perissinotto E . (2010). Alcohol consumption and metabolic syndrome in the elderly: results from the Italian longitudinal study on aging. Eur J Clin Nutr 64:297-307.

Clasey JL, Weltman A, Patrie J, Weltman JY, Pezzoli S, Bouchard C, Thorner MO & Hartman ML . (2001). Abdominal visceral fat and fasting insulin are important predictors of 24-hour GH release independent of age, gender, and other physiological factors. J Clin Endocrinol Metab 86:3845-3852.

Clerici E, Bergamasco E, Ferrario E & Villa ML . (1991). Influence of sex steroids on the antigen-specific primary antibody response in vitro. J Clin Lab Immunol 34:71-78.

Di Bisceglie AM, Carithers RL, Jr. & Gores GJ . (1998). Hepatocellular carcinoma. Hepatology 28:1161-1165.

Donato F, Gelatti U, Limina RM & Fattovich G . (2006). Southern Europe as an example of interaction between various environmental factors: a systematic review of the epidemiologic evidence. Oncogene 25:3756-3770.

Donato F, Tagger A, Chiesa R, Ribero ML, Tomasoni V, Fasola M, Gelatti U, Portera G, Boffetta P & Nardi G . (1997). Hepatitis B and C virus infection, alcohol drinking, and hepatocellular carcinoma: a case-control study in Italy. Brescia HCC Study. Hepatology 26:579-584.

Eriksson CJ, Fukunaga T, Sarkola T, Lindholm H & Ahola L . (1996). Estrogen-related acetaldehyde elevation in women during alcohol intoxication. Alcohol Clin Exp Res 20:1192-1195.

Fattovich G, Stroffolini T, Zagni I & Donato F . (2004). Hepatocellular carcinoma in cirrhosis: incidence and risk factors. Gastroenterology 127:S35-S50.

Frezza M, di PC, Pozzato G, Terpin M, Baraona E & Lieber CS . (1990). High blood alcohol levels in women. The role of decreased gastric alcohol dehydrogenase activity and first-pass metabolism. N Engl J Med 322:95-99.

Friend KE, Hartman ML, Pezzoli SS, Clasey JL & Thorner MO . (1996). Both oral and transdermal estrogen increase growth hormone release in postmenopausal women--a clinical research center study. J Clin Endocrinol Metab 81:2250-2256.

Furusyo N, Hayashi J, Sawayama Y, Kishihara Y & Kashiwagi S . (1999). Hepatitis B surface antigen disappearance and hepatitis B surface antigen subtype: a prospective, long-term, follow-up study of Japanese residents of Okinawa, Japan with chronic hepatitis B virus infection. Am J Trop Med Hyg 60:616-622.

Gholson CF, Morgan K, Catinis G, Favrot D, Taylor B, Gonzalez E & Balart L . (1997). Chronic hepatitis C with normal aminotransferase levels: a clinical histologic study. Am J Gastroenterol 92:1788-1792.

Ikeda K, Saitoh S, Suzuki Y, Kobayashi M, Tsubota A, Fukuda M, Koida I, Arase Y, Chayama K, Murashima N & Kumada H . (1998). Interferon decreases hepatocellular carcinogenesis in patients with cirrhosis caused by the hepatitis B virus: a pilot study. Cancer 82:827-835.

Ikejima K, Enomoto N, Iimuro Y, Ikejima A, Fang D, Xu J, Forman DT, Brenner DA & Thurman RG . (1998). Estrogen increases sensitivity of hepatic Kupffer cells to endotoxin. Am J Physiol 274:G669-G676.

Itagaki T, Shimizu I, Cheng X, Yuan Y, Oshio A, Tamaki K, Fukuno H, Honda H, Okamura Y & Ito S . (2005). Opposing effects of oestradiol and progesterone on intracellular pathways and activation processes in the oxidative stress induced activation of cultured rat hepatic stellate cells. Gut 54:1782-1789.

Jarvelainen HA, Lukkari TA, Heinaro S, Sippel H & Lindros KO . (2001). The antiestrogen toremifene protects against alcoholic liver injury in female rats. J Hepatol 35:46-52.

Kessler RC, McGonagle KA, Zhao S, Nelson CB, Hughes M, Eshleman S, Wittchen HU & Kendler KS . (1994). Lifetime and 12-month prevalence of DSM-III-R psychiatric disorders in the United States. Results from the National Comorbidity Survey. Arch Gen Psychiatry 51:8-19.

Kuper H, Tzonou A, Kaklamani E, Hsieh CC, Lagiou P, Adami HO, Trichopoulos D & Stuver SO . (2000). Tobacco smoking, alcohol consumption and their interaction in the causation of hepatocellular carcinoma. Int J Cancer 85:498-502.

Lacort M, Leal AM, Liza M, Martin C, Martinez R & Ruiz-Larrea MB . (1995). Protective effect of estrogens and catecholestrogens against peroxidative membrane damage in vitro. Lipids 30:141-146.

Letteron P, Duchatelle V, Berson A, Fromenty B, Fisch C, Degott C, Benhamou JP & Pessayre D . (1993). Increased ethane exhalation, an in vivo index of lipid peroxidation, in alcohol-abusers. Gut 34:409-414.

Letteron P, Fromenty B, Terris B, Degott C & Pessayre D . (1996). Acute and chronic hepatic steatosis lead to in vivo lipid peroxidation in mice. J Hepatol 24:200-208.

Lieber CS . (2004). Alcoholic fatty liver: its pathogenesis and mechanism of progression to inflammation and fibrosis. Alcohol 34:9-19.

Lu G, Shimizu I, Cui X, Itonaga M, Tamaki K, Fukuno H, Inoue H, Honda H & Ito S . (2004). Antioxidant and antiapoptotic activities of idoxifene and estradiol in hepatic fibrosis in rats. Life Sci 74:897-907.

Mathurin P, Deng QG, Keshavarzian A, Choudhary S, Holmes EW & Tsukamoto H . (2000). Exacerbation of alcoholic liver injury by enteral endotoxin in rats. Hepatology 32:1008-1017.

Mezey E . (2000). Influence of sex hormones on alcohol metabolism. Alcohol Clin Exp Res 24:421.

Nagata K, Suzuki H & Sakaguchi S . (2007). Common pathogenic mechanism in development progression of liver injury caused by non-alcoholic or alcoholic steatohepatitis. J Toxicol Sci 32:453-468.

National Tax Agency . 2008. National Tax Agency Report 2008. Tokyo, Japan.

Nemoto Y, Toda K, Ono M, Fujikawa-Adachi K, Saibara T, Onishi S, Enzan H, Okada T & Shizuta Y . (2000). Altered expression of fatty acid-metabolizing enzymes in aromatase- deficient mice. J Clin Invest 105:1819-1825.

Nolen-Hoeksema S . (2004). Gender differences in risk factors and consequences for alcohol use and problems. Clin Psychol Rev 24:981-1010.

Oien KA, Moffat D, Curry GW, Dickson J, Habeshaw T, Mills PR & MacSween RN . (1999). Cirrhosis with steatohepatitis after adjuvant tamoxifen. Lancet 353:36-37.

Okanoue T, Makiyama A, Nakayama M, Sumida Y, Mitsuyoshi H, Nakajima T, Yasui K, Minami M & Itoh Y . (2005). A follow-up study to determine the value of liver biopsy and need for antiviral therapy for hepatitis C virus carriers with persistently normal serum aminotransferase. J Hepatol 43:599-605.

Pastorino JG & Hoek JB . (2000). Ethanol potentiates tumor necrosis factor-alpha cytotoxicity in hepatoma cells and primary rat hepatocytes by promoting induction of the mitochondrial permeability transition. Hepatology 31:1141-1152.

Pfeilschifter J, Koditz R, Pfohl M & Schatz H . (2002). Changes in Proinflammatory Cytokine Activity after Menopause. Endocr Rev 23:90-119.

Potter JJ, Yang VW & Mezey E . (1993). Regulation of the rat class I alcohol dehydrogenase gene by growth hormone. Biochem Biophys Res Commun 191:1040-1045.

Poynard T, Bedossa P & Opolon P . (1997). Natural history of liver fibrosis progression in patients with chronic hepatitis C. Lancet 349:825-832.

Poynard T, Mathurin P, Lai CL, Guyader D, Poupon R, Tainturier MH, Myers RP, Muntenau M, Ratziu V, Manns M, Vogel A, Capron F, Chedid A & Bedossa P . (2003). A comparison of fibrosis progression in chronic liver diseases. J Hepatol 38:257-265.

Puoti C, Castellacci R, Montagnese F, Zaltron S, Stornaiuolo G, Bergami N, Bellis L, Precone DF, Corvisieri P, Puoti M, Minola E & Gaeta GB . (2002). Histological and virological features and follow-up of hepatitis C virus carriers with normal aminotransferase levels: the Italian prospective study of the asymptomatic C carriers (ISACC). J Hepatol 37:117-123.

Raucy JL, Lasker JM, Kraner JC, Salazar DE, Lieber CS & Corcoran GB . (1991). Induction of cytochrome P450IIE1 in the obese overfed rat. Mol Pharmacol 39:275-280.

Renou C, Halfon P, Pol S, Cacoub P, Jouve E, Bronowicki JP, Arpurt JP, Rifflet H, Picon M, Causse X, Canva V, Denis J, Tran A, Bourliere M, Ouzan D, Pariente A, Dantin S, Alric L, Cartier V, Reville M & Caillat-Zucman S . (2002). Histological features and HLA class II alleles in hepatitis C virus chronically infected patients with persistently normal alanine aminotransferase levels. Gut 51:585-590.

Rodriguez-Torres M, Rios-Bedoya CF, Rodriguez-Orengo J, Fernandez-Carbia A, Marxuach-Cuetara AM, Lopez-Torres A, Salgado-Mercado R & Brau N . (2006). Progression to cirrhosis in Latinos with chronic hepatitis C: differences in Puerto Ricans with and without human immunodeficiency virus coinfection and along gender. J Clin Gastroenterol 40:358-366.

Schultze RL, Gangopadhyay A, Cay O, Lazure D & Thomas P . (1999). Tyrosine kinase activation in LPS stimulated rat Kupffer cells. Cell Biochem Biophys 30:287-301.

Shapiro BH, Agrawal AK & Pampori NA . (1995). Gender differences in drug metabolism regulated by growth hormone. Int J Biochem Cell Biol 27:9-20.

Sherlock S & Dooley J . 2002. Diseases of the liver and biliary system. Blackwell Science, Oxford.

Shimizu I . (2003). Impact of estrogens on the progression of liver disease. Liver Int 23:63-69.

Shimizu I & Ito S . (2007). Protection of estrogens against the progression of chronic liver disease. Hepatol Res 37:239-247.

Shimizu I . 2009. Female Hepatology: favorable role of female factors in chronic liver disease. Nova Science, Hauppauge, New York.

Shimizu I, Kohno N, Tamaki K, Shono M, Huang HW, He JH & Yao DF . (2007a). Female hepatology: favorable role of estrogen in chronic liver disease with hepatitis B virus infection. World J Gastroenterol 13:4295-4305.

Shimizu I, Kohno N, Tamaki K, Shono M, Huang HW, He JH & Yao DF . (2007b). Female hepatology: favorable role of estrogen in chronic liver disease with hepatitis B virus infection. World J Gastroenterol 13:4295-4305.

Shimizu I, Mizobuchi Y, Shiba M, Ma Y-R, Horie T, Liu F & Ito S . (1999). Inhibitory effect of estradiol on activation of rat hepatic stellate cells in vivo and in vitro. Gut 44:127-136.

Tamai H, Kato S, Horie Y, Ohki E, Yokoyama H & Ishii H . (2000). Effect of acute ethanol administration on the intestinal absorption of endotoxin in rats. Alcohol Clin Exp Res 24:390-394.

Tanaka F, Shiratori Y, Yokosuka O, Imazeki F, Tsukada Y & Omata M . (1996). High incidence of ADH2*1/ALDH2*1 genes among Japanese alcohol dependents and patients with alcoholic liver disease. Hepatology 23:234-239.

Van HM, Rahier J & Horsmans Y . (1996). Tamoxifen-induced steatohepatitis. Ann Intern Med 124:855-856.

Villa E, Camellini L, Dugani A, Zucchi F, Grottola A, Merighi A, Buttafoco P, Losi L & Manenti F . (1995). Variant estrogen receptor messenger RNA species detected in human primary hepatocellular carcinoma. Cancer Res 55:498-500.

Villa E, Dugani A, Moles A, Camellini L, Grottola A, Buttafoco P, Merighi A, Ferretti I, Esposito P, Miglioli L, Bagni A, Troisi R, De Hemptinne B, Praet M, Callea F &

Manenti F . (1998). Variant liver estrogen receptor transcripts already occur at an early stage of chronic liver disease. Hepatology 27:983-988.

Wake K . (1999). Cell-cell organization and functions of 'sinusoids' in liver microcirculation system. J Electron Microsc 48:89-98.

Weltman MD, Farrell GC, Hall P, Ingelman-Sundberg M & Liddle C . (1998). Hepatic cytochrome P450 2E1 is increased in patients with nonalcoholic steatohepatitis. Hepatology 27:128-133.

Wright M, Goldin R, Fabre A, Lloyd J, Thomas H, Trepo C, Pradat P & Thursz M . (2003). Measurement and determinants of the natural history of liver fibrosis in hepatitis C virus infection: a cross sectional and longitudinal study. Gut 52:574-579.

Yasuda M, Shimizu I, Shiba M & Ito S . (1999). Suppressive effects of estradiol on dimethylnitrosamine-induced fibrosis of the liver in rats [see comments]. Hepatology 29:719-727.

Yin M, Ikejima K, Wheeler MD, Bradford BU, Seabra V, Forman DT, Sato N & Thurman RG . (2000). Estrogen is involved in early alcohol-induced liver injury in a rat enteral feeding model. Hepatology 31:117-123.

Yoshino K, Komura S, Watanabe I, Nakagawa Y & Yagi K . (1987). Effect of estrogens on serum and liver lipid peroxide levels in mice. J Clin Biochem Nutr 3:233-239.

Zacharakis GH, Koskinas J, Kotsiou S, Papoutselis M, Tzara F, Vafeiadis N, Archimandritis AJ & Papoutselis K . (2005). Natural history of chronic HBV infection: a cohort study with up to 12 years follow-up in North Greece (part of the Interreg I-II/EC-project). J Med Virol 77:173-179.

Zhou Y, Shimizu I, Lu G, Itonaga M, Okamura Y, Shono M, Honda H, Inoue S, Muramatsu M & Ito S . (2001). Hepatic stellate cells contain the functional estrogen receptor beta but not the estrogen receptor alpha in male and female rats. Biochem Biophys Res Commun 286:1059-1065.

3

Innate Immunity in Alcohol Liver Disease

João-Bruno Soares and Pedro Pimentel-Nunes
Department of Physiology, Faculty of Medicine, University of Oporto
Portugal

1. Introduction

Excessive ingestion of alcohol is one of the major causes of chronic liver disease worldwide. Alcoholic liver disease (ALD) encompasses a broad spectrum of diseases ranging from steatosis (fatty liver), steatohepatitis, fibrosis, cirrhosis to hepatocarcinoma. Almost all heavy drinkers develop fatty liver; however, only up to 30% of heavy drinkers may develop more several forms of chronic liver injury such as alcoholic hepatitis, fibrosis, cirrhosis, and hepatocellular carcinoma (O'Shea et al., 2010). Despite extensive research, cellular and molecular mechanisms contributing to the pathogenesis of ALD remain to be fully elucidated. Classically, direct hepatotoxicity and production of reactive oxygen species (ROS) induced by alcohol and its metabolites (e.g. acetaldehyde, acetate) are considered the major causative factors. Nevertheless, growing evidence suggests innate immunity also plays an important role in the pathogenesis of ALD (Byun & Jeong, 2010; Gao et al., 2011; Miller et al., 2011).

In this chapter we discuss the association between innate immunity and ALD. Specifically, we discuss the following topics: i) role of liver in innate immunity; ii) mechanisms of alcohol-induced dysregulation of innate immunity; iii) role of dysregulation of innate immunity in the pathogenesis of ALD; iv) modulation of innate immunity in the treatment of ALD. Additionally, we also discuss the role of innate immunity impairment in ALD-associated infection risk. In this topic, we detail the data of our recent study on Toll-like receptor (TLR)2- and 4-mediated immune response in patients with alcoholic cirrhosis.

2. Role of liver in innate immunity

Innate immunity is an important first line of defense against infection, quickly responding to potential attacks by pathogens. It consists of anatomic barriers (e.g., skin, epidermis, dermis, and mucous membranes), physiologic barriers (e.g., temperature, low pH, oxygen), humoral factors (e.g., pepsin, lysozyme, anti-microbial substances, interferons, complement), phagocytic cells (e.g., neutrophils and macrophages), and lymphocyte cells (e.g., natural killer [NK] and NKT cells). Many of these barriers and factors can prevent or destroy the invading pathogens nonspecifically. However, recent evidence suggests that innate immunity can also specifically detect infection through pattern-recognition receptors (PRRs) that recognize specific structures, called pathogen-associated molecular patterns (PAMPs), that are expressed by invading pathogens. Many PAMPs have been identified, including bacterial carbohydrates (e.g., lipopolysaccharide or LPS, mannose), bacterial peptides (flagellin), peptidoglycans and lipoteichoic acids (from Gram-positive bacteria), *N*-formylmethionine, lipoproteins and fungal glucans, and nucleic acids (e.g., bacterial or viral DNA or RNA). The PRRs can be divided into 3 categories: secreted PRRs, membrane-bound PRRs, and phagocytic PRRs. Secreted PRRs are a group of proteins that kill pathogens through complement activation and opsonization of microbial cells for phagocytosis. Secreted PRRs include complements, pentraxins, and peptidoglycan-recognition proteins, which are mainly produced by hepatocytes and secreted into the blood stream. Membrane-bound or intracellular PRRs include TLRs, nucleotide-binding oligomerization domain (NOD)-like receptors, and retinoic acid-induced gene I-like helicases. Phagocytic (or endocytic) PRRs which are expressed on the surface of macrophages, neutrophils, and dendritic cells can bind directly to pathogens, and this is followed by phagocytosis into lysosomal compartments and elimination. These phagocytic PRRs include scavenger receptors, macrophage mannose receptors, and β-glucan receptors (Janeway & Medzhitov, 2002).

Blood circulating from the intestines to the liver is rich in bacterial products, environmental toxins, and food antigens. To effectively and quickly defend against potentially toxic agents without launching harmful immune responses, the liver relies on its strong immune system. Interestingly, increasing evidence has suggested that the immune system in the liver consists of predominantly innate immunity (Gao et al., 2008). First, the liver is responsible for the biosynthesis of 80–90% innate proteins including complements, secreted PRRs and acute phase proteins. Second, the liver contains a large number of Kupffer cells (KCs), which account for 80-90% of the total population of fixed tissue macrophages in the body. KCs, in combination with liver sinusoidal cells, are responsible for clearance of soluble macromolecules and insoluble waste in the body. Third, liver lymphocytes are enriched in innate immune cells including NK and NKT cells. Human intrahepatic lymphocyte population contain about 30% to 50% NK cells and up to 10% NKT cells. Fourth, liver non-parenchymal cells also express high levels of membrane-bound PRRs, such as TLRs. Finally and interestingly, the adaptive immunity in the liver seems less active because the liver is a major site to induce T cell apoptosis.

3. Dysregulation of innate immunity in ALD

Growing evidence suggests alcohol induces dysregulation of innate immunity through three main mechanisms: i) activation of LPS/TLR4 signalling pathway; ii) activation of complement system; iii) inhibition of innate immunity cells, namely NK cells.

3.1 Activation of LPS/TLR4 signalling pathway

LPS is a component of Gram-negative bacteria cell wall. It consists of hydrophilic polysaccharides of the core and O-antigen and a hydrophobic lipid A component. This hydrophobic component corresponds to the conserved molecular pattern of LPS and is the main inducer of biological responses to LPS. TLR4, a member of human TLR family, is the receptor of LPS. Stimulation of TLR4 by LPS involves the participation of several molecules [LPS binding protein (LBP), cluster of differentiation-14 (CD14) and myeloid differentiation-2 (MD-2)] (figure 1). LBP (a soluble protein) extracts LPS from the bacterial membrane and shuttles it to CD14 (a glycosylphosphatidylinositol-anchored protein, which also exists in a soluble form). CD14 then transfers the LPS to MD-2 (a soluble protein that non-covalently associates with the extracellular domain of TLR4). Binding of LPS to MD-2 induces a conformational change in MD-2 which then allows the complex MD-2-TLR4 to bind to a second TLR4 receptor thus achieving TLR4 homo-dimerisation and signalling.

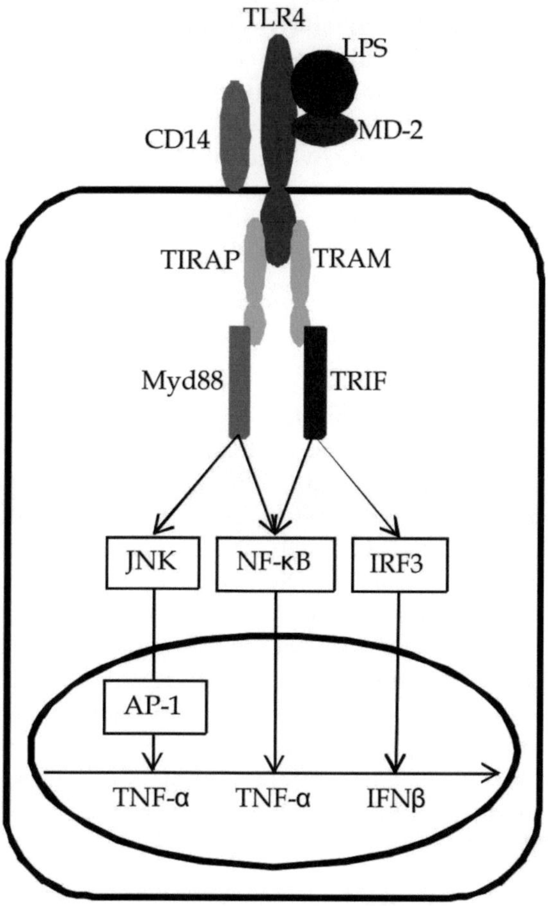

Fig. 1. Overview of LPS/TLR4 signalling pathway. Stimulation of TLR4 by LPS involves the participation of several molecules (LBP, CD14 and MD-2). Activation of TLR4 induces two downstream signalling pathways. First, the MyD88-dependent pathway is initiated by recruitment of TIRAP and MyD88 to the TLR4 complex which leads to early-phase activation of NF-κB and subsequent induction of the expression of NF-κB-controlled genes including pro-inflammatory cytokines (TNF-α). The MyD88-dependent pathway can also activate JNK, leading to transcription of several genes including TNF-α, via activation of AP-1. Second, the MyD88-independent pathway is initiated by recruitment of TRAM and TRIF to the TLR4 complex, followed by late activation of NF-κB complex and activation of IRF3 which leads to the transcription of IFN-β as well as other interferon-induced genes. See text for abbreviations.

Activation of TLR4 induces two downstream signalling pathways (figure 1). First, the MyD88-dependent pathway is initiated by recruitment of TIR domain-containing adaptor protein (TIRAP) and myeloid differentiation factor 88 (MyD88) to the TLR4 complex which leads to early-phase activation of nuclear factor-κB (NF-κB) and subsequent induction of the expression of NF-κB-controlled genes including pro-inflammatory cytokines [tumor necrosis factor-α (TNF-α), interleukin-6 (IL-6)] and chemokines [monocyte chemotactic protein-1 (MCP-1)] genes. The MyD88-dependent pathway can also activate c-Jun N-terminal kinase (JNK), leading to activator protein-1 (AP-1) activation that initiates the transcription of genes involved in regulation of cell proliferation, morphogenesis, apoptosis, and differentiation. Second, the MyD88-independent pathway is initiated by recruitment of TIR-domain containing adaptor inducing interferon-β (TRIF) and TRIF-related adaptor molecule (TRAM) to the TLR4 complex, followed by late activation of NF-κB complex and activation of interferon regulatory factor 3 (IRF3) which leads to the transcription of interferon-β (IFN-β) as well as other interferon-induced genes (Lu et al., 2008).

Most parenchymal and non-parenchymal liver cells express TLR4. Nonetheless, with the exception of KCs, the amount of TLR4 expression and the level of responsiveness to LPS in most liver cells appear to be low in non-inflamed liver (Su et al., 2000; Zarember & Godowski, 2002).

Several studies suggest that chronic alcohol ingestion can enhance hepatic LPS/TLR4 signalling through increase of portal and systemic levels of LPS and upregulation and sensitization of hepatic TLR4 (Soares et al., 2010). Chronic ingestion of alcohol leads to a strong elevation of portal and systemic levels of LPS in animal models and humans (Mathurin et al., 2000; Parlesak et al., 2000). The elevation of LPS levels appears to be predominantly caused by two mechanisms. First, alcohol exposure can promote the growth of Gram-negative bacteria in the intestine, which leads to enhanced production of LPS (Hauge et al., 1997). Second, alcohol metabolism by Gram-negative bacteria and intestinal epithelial cells can result in accumulation of acetaldehyde, which in turn can increase intestinal permeability by opening intestinal tight junctions. Increased intestinal permeability can lead to increased transfer of LPS from the intestine to portal and systemic circulation (Purohit et al., 2008). Furthermore, chronic alcohol consumption upregulates hepatic TLR4 and sensitizes it to LPS to enhance TNF-α production, a process known as *priming* (Gustot et al., 2006).

Besides LPS, TLR4 also senses endogenous ligands initiating danger signals, such as high mobility group box 1 (HMGB1), hyaluronan, heat shock protein 60 and free fatty acids (C12:0, C14:0, C16:0, and C18:0) (Erridge, 2010). In particular, HMGB1 has been shown to be released from damaged hepatocytes and contribute to liver injury (Tsung et al., 2005). Due to the association of many endogenous ligands with tissue injury, they are termed damage-associated molecular patterns (DAMPs). Interestingly, recent studies show that many of the proposed endogenous TLR4 ligands may also have the capacity to bind and transport LPS and/or enhance the sensitivity of cells to LPS, suggesting that many of these molecules may be more accurately described as PAMP-binding molecules or PAMP-sensitizing molecules, rather than genuine ligands of TLR4 (Erridge, 2010). Therefore, these endogenous ligands, namely HMGB1, may enhance TLR4 signalling in ALD.

3.2 Activation of complement system

The complement system is a component of innate immunity that consists of multiple plasma proteins which act to fight infection by opsonizing pathogens, inducing inflammatory responses, enhancing antibody responses, and attacking some pathogens directly. Activation of the complement cascade relies on cleavage of a zymogen to yield an active enzyme that in turns cleaves and activates the next zymogen in the cascade. Through this series of cleavage and enzyme activation, the immune system is able to produce a wide-reaching response to few stimulation events (Gasque, 2004). The complement system is activated by three different pathways: classical, lectin and alternative pathways (figure 2). The classical pathway is activated by IgM- or IgG-containing immune complexes. The lectin pathway is activated when mannose-binding lectin binds its receptor, mannose, which is expressed by microbial pathogens. The alternative pathway is activated by C3b-coated pathogens. The three pathways converge at the generation of a C3 convertase that cleaves C3 to C3a and C3b. C3b is an opsonizing protein that coats pathogen surfaces to facilitate their uptake and destruction by phagocytes. C3b can also activate alternative pathway or associate to C3 convertase forming C5 convertase that cleaves C5 to C5a and C5b. C3a and C5a lead to increased migration of phagocytes to the site of infection and induce mast cells to release histamine and TNF-α, which contribute to the enhancement of inflammatory response. C5b forms with C6, C7, C7, C8 and C9 the membrane-attack complex that destroys certain pathogens by disrupting their membrane integrity (Gasque, 2004).

The liver (primarily hepatocytes) is a major site that biosynthesizes complement components found in plasma. Hepatocytes are also primarily responsible for the biosynthesis of several complement regulator proteins found in plasma, such as factor I, factor H, and the C1 inhibitor. Additionally, cells in the liver also express complement factor receptors, as well as intrinsic regulatory proteins (Qin & Gao, 2006).

A growing body of evidence in mouse models suggests that alcohol exposure results in activation of the complement system and inhibition of regulatory proteins. Chronic alcohol feeding to mice for 4-6 weeks increases activation of C3, as evidenced by increased C3a in the circulation (Pritchard et al., 2007), as well as increased accumulation of C3 or its proteolytic end product C3b/iC3b/C3c in liver (Jarvelainen et al., 2002; Roychowdhury et al., 2009). In rats, chronic alcohol exposure increases C3 activity and decreases expression of Crry, the rat homologue of the complement inhibitory protein CD55/DAF (decay-accelerating factor), and CD59 in the liver (Jarvelainen et al., 2002).

Complement is activated early in the progression of alcohol-induced liver injury, prior to detectable increases in ALT/AST or accumulation of hepatic triglycerides (Roychowdhury et al., 2009). Early activation of complement contributes to increased inflammatory cytokine expression, mediated via the activation of the anaphylatoxin receptors, C3aR (C3a receptor) and C5aR (C5a receptor), on KCs (Roychowdhury et al., 2009). The contribution of each pathway of complement activation in response to alcohol exposure is still unclear. It has been suggested that alcohol-induced increase in LPS levels may contribute to activation of complement via the alternative pathway (Jarvelainen et al., 2002). Recent evidence shows that alcohol feeding activates the classical complement pathway via C1q binding to apoptotic cells in the liver, suggesting that the classical complement pathway also contributes to complement activation in the pathogenesis of ALD (Cohen et al., 2010). It is also likely that activation of complement by any mechanism will initiate the alternative pathway-mediated feedback loop (Gasque, 2004). Further studies are still needed to elucidate the specific role of each pathway of complement activation in response to alcohol exposure.

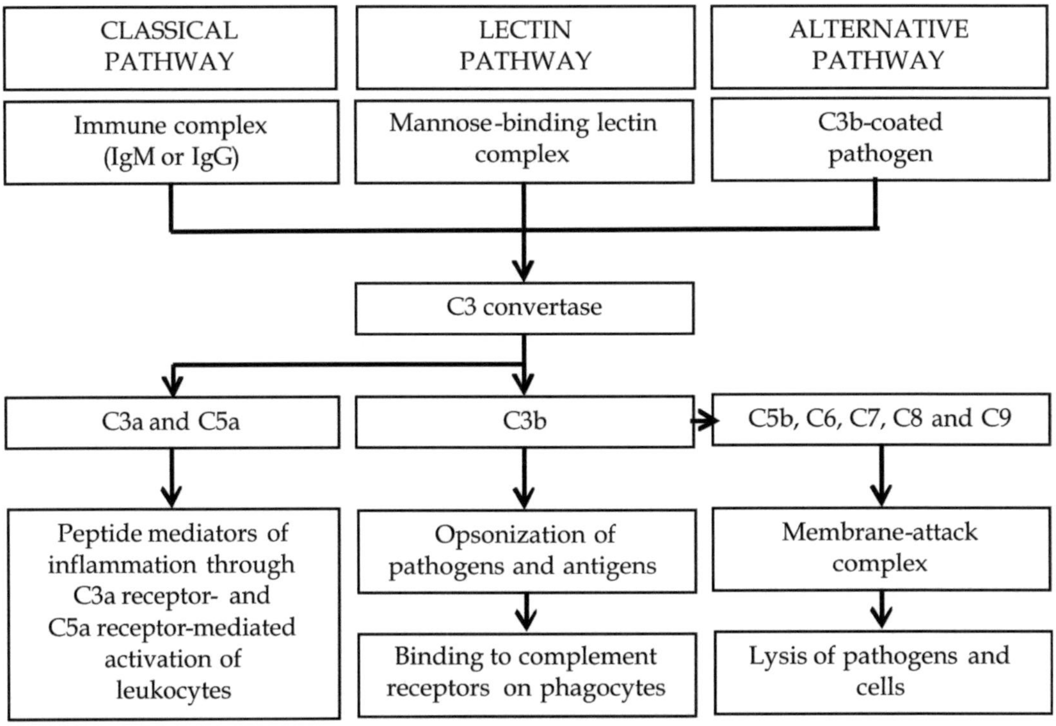

Fig. 2. Overview of complement system. The complement system is activated by three different pathways: the classical, lectin and alternative pathways. The classical pathway is activated by IgM- or IgG-containing immune complexes. The lectin pathway is activated when mannose-binding lectin bind its receptor, mannose, which is expressed by microbial pathogens. The alternative pathway is activated by C3b-coated pathogens. The three pathways converge at the generation of a C3 convertase that cleaves C3 to C3a and C3b. C3b is an opsonizing protein that coats pathogen surfaces to facilitate their uptake and destruction by phagocytes. C3b can also activate alternative pathway or associate to C3 convertase forming C5 convertase that cleaves C5 to C5a and C5b. C3a and C5a lead to increased migration of phagocytes to the site of infection and induce mast cells to release histamine and TNF-α, which contribute to the enhancement of inflammatory response. C5b forms with C6, C7, C7, C8 and C9 the membrane-attack complex that destroys certain pathogens by disrupting their membrane integrity.

3.3 Inhibition of NK cells

Over last several decades, many studies have shown that liver lymphocytes are rich in NK cells and that these cells play an important role in innate immune response against tumors and microbial pathogens including viruses, bacteria and parasites (Gao et al., 2009). NK cells can kill virus-infected cells and tumor cells via releasing granules containing granzyme and perforin, death ligand as TNF-related apoptosis-inducing ligand (TRAIL) and a variety of proinflammatory cytokines such as IFN-γ and TNF-α (Gao et al., 2009). Increasing evidence suggests that NK cells may also be involved in the pathogenesis of liver injury, fibrosis, and regeneration. For example, it has been shown that activation of NK cells inhibits liver fibrosis *in vivo* (Melhem et al., 2006).

Chronic alcohol consumption inhibits NK cells and such inhibition likely contributes to the pathogenesis of ALD. The inhibitory effect of chronic alcohol consumption on NK cells function has been observed for many years in alcoholic patients and rodents fed alcohol diets (Cook et al., 1997). This inhibitory effect is mediated by multiple mechanisms. First, chronic alcohol consumption directly attenuates NK cell cytotoxicity against activated hepatic stellate cells (HSCs) via down regulation of NK cell-associated molecules such as TRAIL, Natural killer group 2, member D (NKG2D) and interferon-γ (IFN-γ) (Jeong et al., 2008). Second, chronic alcohol consumption indirectly attenuates NK cell killing activity by stimulating HSCs to produce transforming growth factor-β (TGF-β), an inhibitor of NK cells (Jeong et al., 2008), by elevating serum levels of corticosterone, which inhibits NK cells functions (Arjona et al., 2004), and by reducing central and peripheral levels of opioid peptide β-endorphin that can induce NK cells activation (Boyadjieva et al., 2004). Third, chronic alcohol exposure renders activated HSCs resistant to NK cell killing, because it induces higher expression of suppressor of cytokine signaling 1 (SOCS1) and ROS that inhibit IFN-γ activation of signal transducer and activator of transcription 1 (STAT1) (Jeong et al., 2008). Lastly, alcohol consumption blocks NK cells release from the bone marrow and enhances splenic NK cell apoptosis (Zhang & Meadows, 2009).

4. Role of dysregulation of innate immunity in ALD

Recent studies have revealed how alcohol-induced dysregulation of innate immunity may contribute to the pathogenesis of ALD (figure 3).

4.1 Alcoholic liver steatosis

Alcoholic liver steatosis corresponds to fat accumulation in hepatocytes, which is the result of unbalanced fat metabolism characterized by decreased mitochondrial lipid oxidation and enhanced synthesis of triglycerides. This unbalancing may be related with increased nicotinamide adenine dinucleotide (NADH)/NAD^+ ratio (Fromenty et al., 1997), increased sterol regulatory element-binding protein-1 (SREBP-1) activity (You et al., 2004), decreased peroxisome proliferator-activated receptor-α (PPAR-α) activity (Ip et al., 2003) and decreased AMP-activated protein kinase (AMPK) activity (You et al., 2004).

In addition to these mechanisms, growing evidence suggests alcohol-induced dysregulation of innate immunity may also contribute to alcohol-induced liver steatosis, mainly through increased TNF-α production by KCs in response to LPS. Increased expression of TNF-α has been observed in alcoholic liver steatosis of mice (Pritchard et al., 2007) and absence of its receptor (TNF-α R1) activity inhibits the development of alcoholic liver steatosis (Yin et al., 1999). In addition, it has been reported that TNF-α has a potential to increase mRNA expression of SREBP-1, a potent transcription factor of fat synthesis, in the liver of mice and to stimulate the maturation of SREBP-1 in human hepatocytes, respectively (Endo et al., 2007). In contrast, IL-6 produced by KCs in response to LPS has been shown to protect against alcoholic liver steatosis via activation of signal transducer and activator of transcription 3 (STAT3), consequently inhibiting of SREBP-1 gene expression in hepatocytes (El-Assal et al., 2004). Interestingly, chronic alcohol exposure inhibits IL-6 activation of STAT3 in hepatocytes and thus can counterbalance the protective effective of IL-6 (Weng et al., 2008).

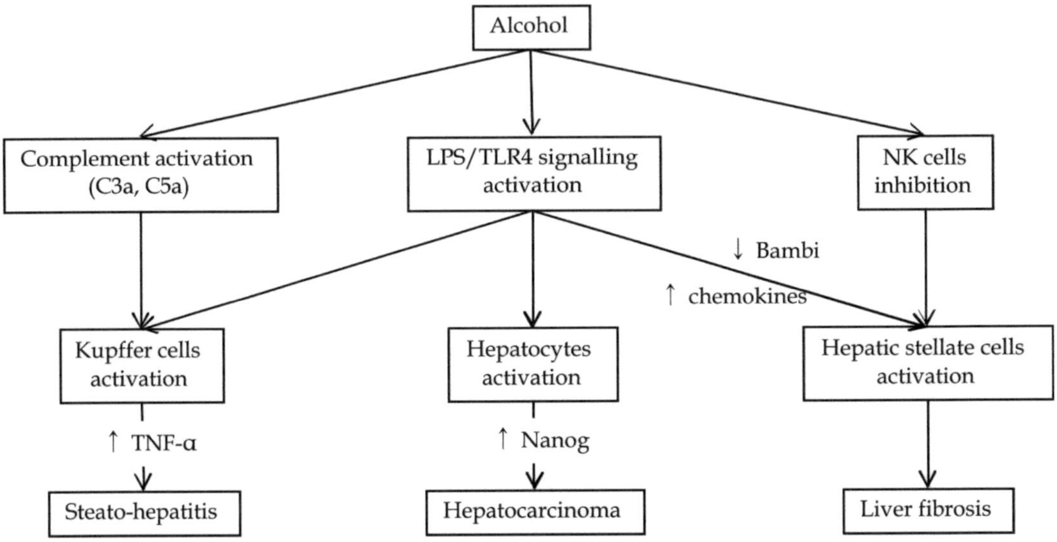

Fig. 3. Overview of the role of alcohol-induced innate immunity dysregulation in the pathogenesis of ALD. Chronic alcohol consumption activates complement system (C3a, C5a) and LPS/TLR4 signalling pathway on KCs, which produce large amounts of pro-inflammatory cytokines, including TNF-α, leading to liver steatosis and inflammation. LPS/TLR4 signalling pathway activation on hepatocytes may lead to hepatocarcinoma through expression of Nanog gene. LPS/TLR4 signalling pathway activation on HSCs contributes to liver fibrosis via two independent mechanisms: it induces the secretion of chemokines from HSCs leading to chemotaxis of KCs which secrete the profibrogenic cytokine TGF-β; additionally, it augments TGF-β signalling on HSCs via down-regulation of the TGF-β pseudoreceptor Bambi. Inhibition of NK cells during chronic alcohol consumption also contributes to alcoholic liver fibrosis, since NK cells have anti-fibrotic effects through suppression of HSCs. See text for abbreviations.

In addition to alcohol-induced activation of LPS/TLR4 signalling pathway, alcohol-induced inhibition of NK cell cytotoxicity against HSCs can also contribute liver steatosis as HSCs have been shown to stimulate accumulation of fat in hepatocyte (Jeong et al., 2008). It has been shown that chronic alcohol drinking activates HSCs to produce 2-arachidonoylglycerol (2-AG), one of endocannabinoids, which, activating its receptor, cannabinoid receptor 1 (CB1R) on hepatocytes increases the expression of SREPB-1 and fatty acid synthase (FAS) but decreased AMPK activation, consequently leading to accumulation of fat in hepatocytes. These data, however, are provided by a single study and require further studies.

4.2 Alcoholic liver steatohepatitis

Alcoholic steatohepatitis (ASH) refers to infiltration of liver by inflammatory cells, mainly granulocytes, in addition to fat accumulation. The recruitment of inflammatory cells seems to be related with the production of cytokines, chemokines and ROS. Although this production was historically linked to direct hepatotoxicity of alcohol and its metabolites, recent evidence suggest that alcohol-induced LPS/TLR4 signalling can also contribute to this production and be a key player in the pathogenesis of ASH. Exposure to LPS during chronic alcohol consumption results in increased production of inflammatory mediators (TNF-α, IL-1, IL-6 and IL-8) as well as in induction of ROS, which subsequently aggravate steatohepatitis (Arteel, 2003). The role of LPS/TLR4 signalling pathway in the pathogenesis of ASH is further supported by studies showing that inhibition of LPS/TLR4 signalling, by altering intestinal microbiota and LPS production (through the use of antibiotics or probiotics) or suppressing TLR4, LBP or CD14 genes expression, protects against ASH. Indeed treatment with antibiotics or probiotics suppresses alcohol-induced liver injury by reducing LPS circulating levels (Adachi et al., 1995; Nanji et al., 1994). Studies in knockout mouse models have shown that chronic alcohol feeding in mice deficient of TLR4, LBP or CD14 results in attenuation of alcohol-induced liver injury despite elevated LPS circulating levels (Uesugi et al., 2001; Uesugi et al., 2002; Yin et al., 2001).

Recent studies have clarified the cellular and molecular pathways by which LPS/TLR4 signalling promotes ASH. KCs have been established as a crucial cellular target of LPS in ASH as demonstrated by a strong reduction of alcoholic liver injury following depletion of KCs with gadolium chloride (Adachi et al., 1994). Moreover, it was shown that disruption of the TLR4 downstream signaling molecule MyD88 in mice failed to prevent ASH (Hritz et al., 2008), while disruption of the MyD88-indepdenent signaling molecule TRIF in mice abolished ASH (Zhao et al., 2008), suggesting that the MyD88-independent pathway contributes to TLR4-mediated alcoholic liver injury. Further studies suggest that TRIF/IRF-3 plays a critical role in alcohol-induced transactivation of the TNF-α gene in KCs/macrophages *in vitro* and *in vivo*, thereby initiating alcoholic liver injury (Zhao et al., 2008). Furthermore, it was also shown that TLR4 deficiency prevented hepatic alcohol-induced production of inflammatory mediators (TNF-α and IL-6), TLR4 coreceptors (CD14 and MD2) and ROS by cytochrome P450 and the nicotinamide adenine dinucleotide phosphate (NADPH) complexes (Hritz et al., 2008). These data suggest that TLR4-mediated alcoholic liver injury is carried out by increased inflammatory mediators (TNF-α and IL-6) and ROS production and that there is a crosstalk between oxidative stress and TLR4 pathways in ALD. This is further supported by studies showing that mice deficient in p47phox, the main cytosolic component of NADPH complex, show an absence of free-radical production, NF-kB activation, TNF-α mRNA induction and liver pathology after alcohol treatment (Kono et al., 2000) and that inhibition of NADPH complex prevents upregulation of TLR4 and sensitization to LPS-induced liver injury (Gustot et al., 2006). Taken together these data suggest that activation of TLR4 in KCs by LPS is a key pathogenetic mediator of ASH, through production of inflammatory cytokines and ROS.

In addition to alcohol-induced activation of LPS/TLR4 signalling pathway, alcohol-induced activation of complement can also contribute to ASH. This is mainly supported by studies showing that mice deficient in C3 and C5 are protected against alcohol-induced increases in hepatic triglycerides and circulating ALT, respectively (Pritchard et al., 2007) and that chronic alcohol-induced liver injury is exacerbated in mice lacking CD55/DAF, a complement regulatory protein, compared to wild-type controls (Pritchard et al., 2007). At present, the molecular mechanisms by which C3 and C5 contribute to ASH are not fully understood and require further studies.

4.3 Alcoholic liver fibrosis

Alcoholic liver fibrosis is characterized by excessive deposition of extracelular matrix components due to increased matrix production and decreased matrix degradation (Henderson & Iredale, 2007). Several studies have highlighted the central role of HSCs in the production of extracellular matrix and the promotion of liver fibrosis.

Alcohol contributes to activation of HSCs by several mechanisms, including upregulation of collagen transcription in HSCs by acetaldehyde or ROS from alcohol-exposed hepatocytes. Recently, alcohol-induced innate immunity dysregulation has also been shown to contribute to liver fibrosis, mainly through activation of LPS/TLR4 signalling in HSCs and inhibition of NK cells, as discussed below (figure 4).

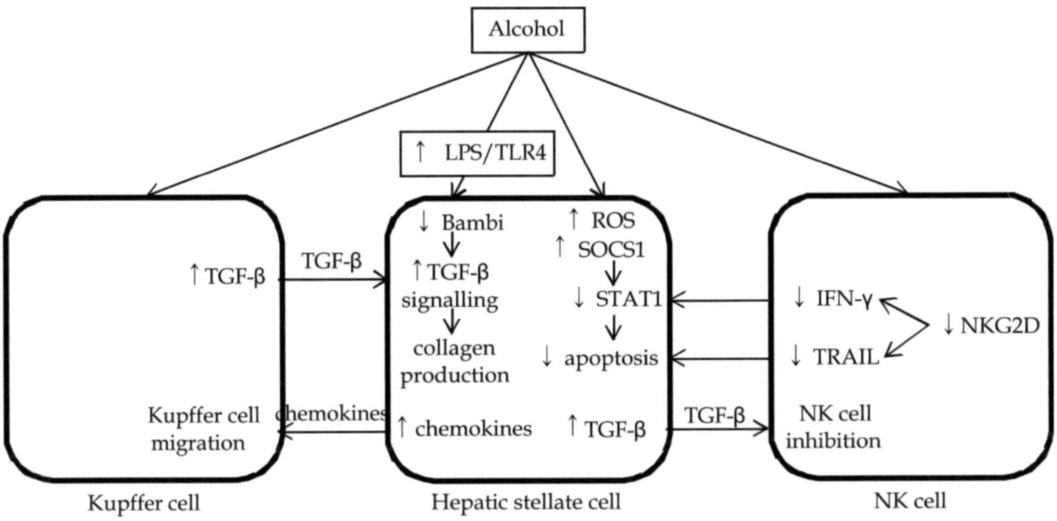

Fig. 4. Overview of the role of alcohol-induced innate immunity dysregulation in liver fibrosis. LPS/TLR4 signalling pathway activation on HSCs induces the secretion of chemokines that lead to chemotaxis of KCs which secrete the profibrogenic cytokine TGF-β (in a TLR4-independent manner); additionally, it augments TGF-β signalling on HSCs via down-regulation of the TGF-β pseudoreceptor Bambi. Chronic alcohol consumption directly attenuates NK cell cytotoxicity against activated HSCs via down regulation of NK cell-associated molecules such as NKG2D, TRAIL and IFN-γ. Alcohol also renders HSCs resistant to NK cell killing, because it induces higher expression of ROS and SOCS1 that inhibit IFN-γ activation of STAT1 and apoptosis. Finally, alcohol stimulates HSCs to produce TGF-β, an inhibitor of NK cells. ↓, decrease; ↑, increase. See text for abbreviations.

The crucial role of LPS/TLR4 signalling in liver fibrosis is supported by studies showing that inhibition of LPS/TLR4 signalling by altering intestinal microbiota and LPS production (through use of antibiotics or probiotics) or suppressing TLR4, LBP or CD14 genes expression protects against liver fibrosis. It has been shown that antibiotics prevent fibrosis induced by CCl4 treatment or a choline-deficient diet (MCDD), and that LPS enhances hepatic fibrosis induced by a MCDD (Luckey et al., 1954; Rutenburg et al., 1957). Treatment of mice with nonabsorbable broad-spectrum antibiotics also resulted in a clear reduction in the fibrotic response of mice, upon bile duct ligation (Seki et al., 2007). Recently, Velayudham et al showed that VSL#3 (a probiotic) protects against MCDD–induced liver fibrosis, through modulation of collagen expression and inhibition of TGF-β expression and signalling (Velayudham et al., 2009). TLR4-, LBP- and CD14-deficient mice also have demonstrated the crucial role for the LPS–TLR4 pathway in hepatic fibrogenesis (Isayama et al., 2006; Seki et al., 2007). TLR4-mutant mice display a profound reduction in hepatic fibrogenesis in three different experimental models of biliary and toxic fibrosis (Seki et al., 2007). LBP- and CD14-deficient mice also have a marked reduction of hepatic fibrosis upon bile duct ligation (Isayama et al., 2006).

In a recent study, Seki et al analyzed the cell-specific molecular mechanism underlying the role of LPS/TLR4 on liver fibrosis (Seki et al., 2007). They showed that chimeric mice that contain TLR4-mutant KCs and TLR4-intact HSCs developed significant fibrosis and the mice that contain TLR4-intact KCs and TLR4-mutant HSCs developed minimal fibrosis after bile duct ligation, indicating that TLR4 on HSCs, but not on KCs, is crucial for hepatic fibrosis. Notably, KCs are essential for fibrosis by producing TGF-β independent of TLR4. TLR4-activated HSCs produce CC-chemokines [chemokine ligand (CCL)2, CCL3, and CCL4] and express adhesion molecules [inter-cellular adhesion molecule-1 (ICAM-1) and vascular cell adhesion molecule-1 (VCAM-1)] that recruit KCs to the site of injury. Simultaneously, TLR4 signalling downregulates the TGF-β decoy receptor (Bambi) to boost TGF-β signalling and allow for unrestricted activation of HSCs by KCs, leading to hepatic fibrosis. Finally, by using adenoviral vectors expressing an inhibitor of NF-κB kinase (IκB)-superrepressor and knockout mice for MyD88 and the adapter molecule TRIF, the authors demonstrated that TLR4-dependent down-regulation of Bambi is mediated via a pathway involving MyD88 and NF-κB, but not TRIF. In summary, they demonstrated that LPS/TLR4 signalling acts in a profibrogenic manner via two independent mechanisms: it induces the secretion of chemokines from HSCs and chemotaxis of KCs which secrete the profibrogenic cytokine TGF-β (in a TLR4-independent manner); additionally, TLR4-dependent signals augment TGF-β signalling on HSCs via down-regulation of the TGF-β pseudoreceptor Bambi.

The strong association of the LPS/TLR4 signalling pathway and liver fibrosis has been recently confirmed in patients with chronic hepatitis C virus (HCV) infection by studying TLR4 single nucleotide polymorphisms (SNPs). Huang et al conducted a gene centric functional genome scan in patients with chronic HCV infection, which yielded a Cirrhosis Risk Score signature consisting of seven SNPs that may predict the risk of developing cirrhosis (Huang et al., 2007). Among these, a major CC allele of TLR4 encoding a threonine at amino acid 399 (p.T399I) was the second most predictive SNP among the seven, indicating a protective role in fibrosis progression of its c.1196C>T (rs4986791) variant at this location (p.T399I), along with another highly cosegregated c.896A>G (rs4986790) SNP located at coding position 299 (p.D299G). In a subsequent study the same group examined the functional linkage of these SNPs to HSCs responses (Guo et al., 2009). They showed that both HSCs from TLR4-deficient mice and a human HSC line (LX-2) reconstituted with either TLR4 D299G and/or T399I complementary DNAs were hyporesponsive to LPS stimulation compared to those expressing wild-type TLR4, as assessed by the expression and secretion of LPS-induced inflammatory and chemotactic cytokines (i.e., MCP-1, IL-6), downregulation of Bambi expression and activation of NF-κB–responsive luciferase reporter. In addition, spontaneous apoptosis, as well as apoptosis induced by pathway inhibitors of NF-κB, extracellular signal-regulated kinase (ERK), and phosphatidylinositol 3-kinase were greatly increased in HSCs from either TLR4-deficient or Myd88-deficient mice, as well as in murine HSCs expressing D299G and/or T399I SNPs (Guo et al., 2009). Thus, the protective effect of the TLR4 SNP (c.1196C>T [rs4986791, p.T399I]) is explained at least in part by its ability to increase apoptosis and decrease fibrogenic signalling in HSCs. Recently, Li et al expanded the list of TLR4 SNPs that are independently associated with the risk of liver fibrosis progression and the development of cirrhosis (Li et al., 2009). Taken together these data suggest LPS/TLR4 signalling in HSCs is essential for liver fibrosis development, by stimulating production chemokines that recruit KCs and at the same time allowing for unrestricted activation of HSCs by KCs-derived TGF-β.

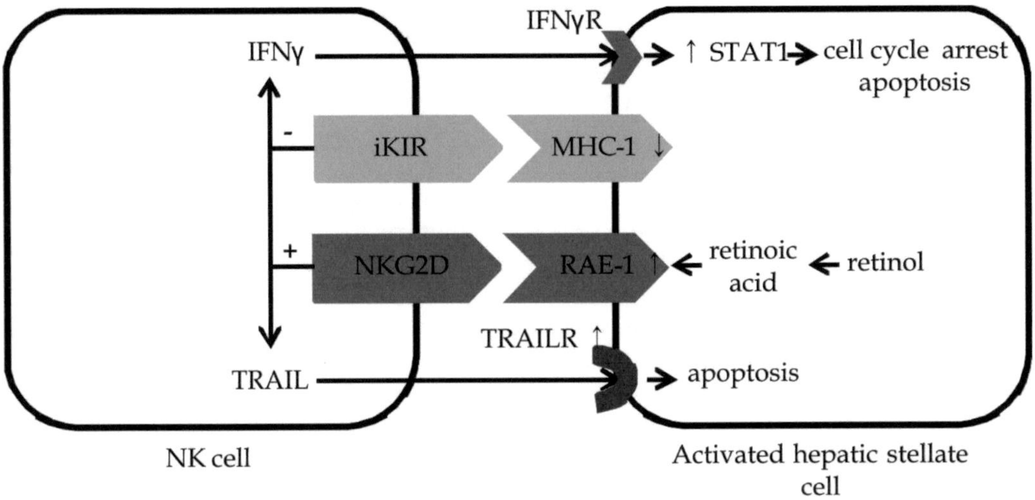

Fig. 5. Mechanisms of killing of activated stellate cells by NK cells. NK cells kill early activated HSCs but not quiescent HSCs. This is because early activated HSCs express increased RAE-1 via retinol metabolism, a NK cell-activating ligand of NKG2D, but express MHC-I, a NK cell-inhibitory ligand of iKIR, thus activating NK cells. After activation, NK cells initiate killing of activated HSCs through releasing of TRAIL, which targets TRAILR that is upregulated on activated HSCs, and IFN-γ, which targets IFN-γR on HSCs to induce cell cycle arrest and apoptosis in a STAT1-dependent manner. ↓, decrease; ↑, increase. See text for abbreviations.

In addition to alcohol-induced activation of LPS/TLR4 signalling pathway, alcohol-induced NK cells inhibition, can also lead liver fibrosis as these cells have been shown to have anti-fibrotic effects via multiple mechanisms (figure 5). Interestingly, NK cells directly kill early activated HSCs but not quiescent HSCs (Melhem et al., 2006; Radaeva et al., 2006; Radaeva et al., 2007). This is because early activated HSCs express increased retinoic acid early inducible gene 1 (RAE-1) via retinol metabolism, a NK cell-activating ligand of NKG2D but express decreased class I major histocompatibilty complex (MHC-I), a NK cell-inhibitory ligand of inhibitory killer immunoglobulin-related receptor (iKIR), thus activating NK cells (Radaeva et al., 2007; Taimr et al., 2003). After activation, NK cells initiate killing of activated HSCs through releasing of TRAIL, which targets TRAIL receptor (TRAILR) that is upregulated on activated HSCs, and IFN-γ, which targets IFN-γ receptor (IFN-γR) on HSCs to induce cell cycle arrest and apoptosis in a STAT1-dependetent manner (Baroni et al., 1996; Jeong et al., 2006). The crucial role of alcohol-induced NK cells inhibition on alcoholic liver fibrosis has been suggested by the finding that attenuated NK cell cytotoxicity against HSCs in alcohol-fed mice contributed to acceleration of liver fibrosis associated with CCl(4) treatment (Jeong et al., 2008).

Few studies have evaluated the role of complement in alcoholic liver fibrosis. By using intercross studies in animal models of liver fibrosis, Hillebrandt et al (Hillebrandt et al., 2005) demonstrated that C5 plays an important role in promoting liver fibrogenesis via targeting C5aR on activated HSCs and KC in mice, because C5 deficiency resulted in lowered liver fibrosis, whereas overexpression of the C5 gene resulted in increased liver fibrosis. Thus, C5 activation during alcohol consumption, as discussed above, likely also contributes to the development of alcoholic liver fibrosis. In addition, Hillebrandt et al (Hillebrandt et al., 2005) also reported that two C5 htSNPs (rs 2300929 and rs17611) are associated with the high risk for developing advanced fibrosis in patients with chronic HCV infection. At present, the molecular mechanisms by which the C5 contributes to liver fibrosis are not fully understood and require further studies.

4.4 Hepatocarcinoma

Hepatocarcinoma is a complication of ALD, which always develops in a cirrhotic liver. Thus, alcoholic liver cirrhosis is a premalignant condition with approximately fourfold increase in the risk of hepatocarcinoma. The five-year cumulative incidence of hepatocarcinoma reaches 8%. In addition, clinical and epidemiological evidence implicates long-term alcohol consumption in accelerating HCV-mediated tumorigenesis (Hassan et al., 2002). A recent study provided evidence that TLR4 mediates the synergism between alcohol and HCV in hepatic oncogenesis (Machida et al., 2009). Machida et al studied the molecular mechanism of synergism between alcohol and HCV, using mice with hepatocyte-specific transgenic expression of the HCV nonstructural protein NS5A, which is known to have a cryptic *trans*-acting activity for cellular gene promoters. They demonstrated that NS5A and alcohol synergistically induce hepatocellular damage and transformation via accentuated and/or sustained activation of TLR4 signalling, which results from HCV NS5A-induced hepatic TLR4 expression and alcohol-induced endotoxaemia. Additionally, Nanog, a stem cell marker, was identified as a novel downstream gene transcriptionally induced by activated TLR4 signalling, that is largely responsible for TLR4-mediated liver tumor development.

Taken together these data suggest TLR4 signalling in hepatocytes may constitute the link between alcoholic liver cirrhosis and hepatocarcinoma.

5. Role of innate immunity impairment in ALD infection risk

Patients with ALD are particularly susceptible to infections, with increased morbidity and mortality from sepsis, mainly in the presence of cirrhosis (Linderoth et al., 2006; Navasa et al., 1999). We and others have shown that in advanced stages of alcoholic liver disease the alcohol-induced pro-inflammatory state is replaced by a state of *immune paralysis* that can greatly decrease the innate immune response of immunological cells (Lin et al., 2007; Pimentel-Nunes et al., 2010; Wasmuth et al., 2005). These data support the hypothesis that patients with alcoholic cirrhosis are likely to have underlying immune dysfunction, particularly innate immunity dysfunction that makes them susceptible to increased risk of infections.

Homman et al have shown that acquired C3 deficiency and decreased haemolytic complement function predisposes to infection and increased mortality in patients with alcoholic cirrhosis (Homann et al., 1997).

Recently we evaluated *ex vivo* TLR2- and TLR4-mediated innate immune response in patients with stable well-compensated alcoholic cirrhosis (Pimentel-Nunes et al., 2010). Namely, we evaluated TNF-α production by peripheral blood monocytes (PM) primary cultures after stimulation with the TLR2/TLR6 ligand zymosan and the TLR2/TLR1 ligand lipopeptide, as well as with the TLR4 ligand LPS. We found an attenuated TLR2 response to zymosan and lipopetide whereas the TLR4-mediated response to LPS was not significantly different to controls. We also studied a subset of patients with decompensated liver disease, where in addition to the blunted TLR2 response, the TLR4 response to LPS was also defective. Interestingly, we could not find any changes in protein or mRNA expression of TLRs between PM of patients and controls, which suggest that this blunted TLR2- and TLR4-response probably implies dysfunction in intracellular signalling pathways. To further clarify the molecular mechanisms underlying the selective attenuation of TLR2-mediated innate immune response in patients with stable compensated alcoholic cirrhosis, the differential effect of zymosan and LPS in PM stimulation on TLR2 and TLR4 gene expression was analyzed. In fact, zymosan and LPS stimulation has distinct effects on TLR2 and TLR4 expression levels. Whereas zymosan-mediated TLR2 stimulation induced a downregulation of both TLR2 and TLR4, LPS-mediated TLR4 stimulation was accompanied by a selective upregulation of TLR2 and a downregulation of TLR4. These differences could be related to distinct intracellular pathway activation. In fact, although TLR2 and TLR4 share most of its intracellular pathways, TLR4 also activates MyD88-independent pathways.

Other authors also found a decrease TLR2- and TLR4- response in immune cells, particularly in advanced stages of disease, that was associated with decreased, normal or increased levels of TLRs, depending on the study (Riordan et al., 2003; Stadlbauer et al., 2008; Stadlbauer et al., 2009; Tazi et al., 2006; Testro et al., 2009; Wasmuth et al., 2005). The data of these studies are compared in table 1. Analyzing all these studies, we conclude that decreased TLRs levels are insufficient to alter TLR function. Instead blunted TLRs response probably implies dysfunction in intracellular signalling pathways. Actually, in our study, we found blunted TLR2 activation that was independent of TLR2 levels (Pimentel-Nunes et al., 2010). Furthermore, we have shown *in vitro* that TLR2 and/or TLR4 agonists change the expression levels of these receptors (Pimentel-Nunes et al., 2010). Hence, we believe that the frequent episodes of bacteraemia that occur in cirrhosis, by changing TLR expression on immune cells, can help explain these discrepancies concerning TLR expression. This also might be the reason why Stadlbauer et al (Stadlbauer et al., 2008), using probiotics, promoted the decrease, and Testro et al (Testro et al., 2009), using antibiotics, the increase in TLR4 levels, both trending towards normal levels of expression. Possibly, these two different therapeutic agents decrease episodes of bacteraemia, consequently with less fluctuation of TLR levels. Why they restored TLR4 function remains unclear because expression levels cannot explain the results from these two studies.

Taking in consideration data from all these studies several conclusions can be made. Firstly, the data point to important role of bacterial translocation, endotoxaemia and alteration of TLR2 and TLR4 signalling providing potential biomarkers to identify patients at risk of infection and potential targets for intervention. Secondly, our study (Pimentel-Nunes et al., 2010) and others (Riordan et al., 2003) clearly suggest a blunted TLR2 function even in the early stages of cirrhosis, which may help explain the growing risk of Gram-positive bacteria infection in these patients. Thirdly, at least in advanced cirrhosis, TLR4 impairment is also present (Pimentel-Nunes et al., 2011). Fourthly, taking together the discrepancies in the expression levels of TLRs, it appears that other factors, probably intracellular, are fundamental to this immunodeficiency. Finally, this process may be reversible with antibiotics and/or probiotics (Stadlbauer et al., 2008; Testro et al., 2009). However, further studies are needed before generalization since Riordan et al. (Riordan et al., 2003) showed that the use of a symbiotic (mixture of probiotic and probiotic) further compromised TLR2 function, in contrast to the positive immunological effects obtained by Stadlbauer et al. (Stadlbauer et al., 2008) and Testro et al. (Testro et al., 2009).

Study	Cirrhotic population	Cell	TLR2 expression	TLR4 expression	TLR function	Therapeutic intervention
Riordan et al., 2003†	Stable (n=36) several etiologies	PBMC	↑	=	TLR4 = TLR2 ↓	Symbiotic ↑ TLR2 levels and ↓ function
Wasmuth et al., 2005	Advanced (n=27) alcohol	PM	NE	NE	TLR4 ↓	NE
Tazi et al., 2006‡	Advanced (n=48) alcohol	PM	NE	↓	TLR4 ↑	NE
Lin et al., 2007	Stable (n=64) several etiologies	PM	NE	NE	TLR4 ↓ only in Child C	NE
Stadlbauer et al., 2008†	Stable (n=12) alcohol	PN	↑	↑	TLR4 =§	Probiotic decreased TLR4 levels to normal§
Pimentel-Nunes et al., 2010*,†	Stable (n=26) and advanced (n=5) alcohol	PM	=	=	TLR4 =;↓ only in unstable; TLR2 ↓	NE
Testro et al., 2009†	Advanced (n=41) alcohol	PBMC	=	TLR4 ↓ in patients without ATB	TLR4 apparently ↓ in patients without ATB; TLR2 =	ATB increased TLR4 levels to normal with increase of function

*TLRs quantified by RNA.
†TLRs quantified by flow cytometry.
‡TLR4 quantified by Western blotting.
§Despite presenting decrease phagocytic capacity, stimulated TNF-α in culture was not different to controls and probiotic restored phagocytic capacity.
ATB, antibiotics; PBMC, peripheral blood mononuclear cell; PM, peripheral monocytes; PN, peripheral neutrophils; NE, not evaluated; = , equal to controls; ↓, decrease when compared with controls; ↑, increase when compared with controls. Adapted with permission from Liver Int 2011;31:140-1.

Table 1. Review of the studies about the role of TLR2 and TLR4 in cirrhotic patients according to TLR expression and function (considered as TNF-α production in culture).

6. Modulation of innate immunity in the treatment of ALD

Recently, a number of different approaches that modulate innate immunity, mainly LPS/TLR4 signalling pathway, have been developed and studied in the treatment of ALD (Petrasek et al., 2010). Among these approaches, two of them, modulation of LPS release by probiotics or antibiotics and interference with cytokines induced by TLR4 signalling, have progressed into clinical trials in patients with ALD.

Modulation of intestinal microbiota using probiotics has been shown to reduce bacterial translocation, circulating LPS levels in animal models, and bacterial infection, a marker for bacterial translocation, in patients with liver cirrhosis (Petrasek et al., 2010). In liver cirrhosis, probiotics have shown positive effects on several parameters including the improvement of liver function, prevention of infection, improvement of the hyperdynamic circulation and prevention of hepatic encephalopathy (Liu et al., 2004). Beneficial effects of probiotics have been reported in an animal model of alcohol-induced liver injury (Nanji et al., 1994) and of LPS-induced liver injury (Ewaschuk et al., 2007; Osman et al., 2007). Patients with alcoholic liver cirrhosis treated with *Lactobacillus casei Shirota* three times daily for 4 weeks showed restoration of deranged neutrophil phagocytic capacity, compared to controls (Stadlbauer et al., 2008). A recent open-label pilot trial showed that a 5-day administration of *Bifidobacterium bifidum* and *Lactobacillus plantarum* in alcohol-addicted psychiatric patients with mild alcoholic hepatitis ameliorated serum markers of liver injury to a significantly higher extent compared to control group treated with abstinence only (Kirpich et al., 2008). However, not all studies associate probiotics with improvement, since in the study from Riordan et al, the use of symbiotic (mixture of probiotic and prebiotic) further compromised TLR2 function (Riordan et al., 2003). Other problem with probiotics is that the number of studies is relatively small and many of these are uncontrolled studies. The large number of probiotic strains and combinations of strains represents other important problem, and it will require additional studies to confirm and ideally compare the efficacy of these probiotic strains.

A second approach to reduce TLR4 ligand is the treatment with antibiotics to achieve selective intestinal decontamination of Gram-negative bacteria, the predominant source of LPS. Selective intestinal decontamination has been shown to reduce bacterial translocation in many studies performed in rats (Runyon et al., 1995). Importantly, norfloxacin administration reduced the 1 year probability of developing spontaneous bacterial peritonitis (SBP), hepatorenal syndrome, and improved the 3 month and 1 year probability of survival compared with placebo (Fernandez et al., 2007). While the reduction of SBP in norfloxacin treated patients is a direct consequence of reducing bacterial strains in the microbiota responsible for spontaneous peritonitis, some of the positive effect on mortality are likely SBP-independent and related to reducing bacterial translocation and circulating levels of LPS (Fernandez et al., 2007). One problem with antibiotics is the severe consequences of long-term antibiotics treatment. Rifaximin may help to solve this problem (Butterworth, 2011). Rifaximin is a minimally absorbed oral antimicrobial agent that is concentrated in the gastrointestinal tract, has broad-spectrum in vitro activity against gram-positive and gram-negative aerobic and anaerobic enteric bacteria, and has a low risk of inducing bacterial resistance. In randomized studies, rifaximin was more effective than nonabsorbable disaccharides and had efficacy that was equivalent to or greater than that of other antibiotics used in the treatment of acute hepatic encephalopathy. Furthermore, with minimal systemic bioavailability, rifaximin may be more conducive to long-term use than other, more bioavailable antibiotics with detrimental side effects.

These data suggest that modulation of the bowel flora may play a role in the pathogenesis and treatment of ALD and indicate a need for larger and rigorously designed clinical trials to support the use of probiotics or antibiotics in treatment of ALD.

While the role of TNF-α in the development of ALD has been well characterized, clinical investigations of the therapeutic efficacy of antibodies to TNF-α (e.g., infliximab) to treat patients with acute alcoholic hepatitis have generated variable results (Naveau et al., 2004; Tilg et al., 2003). There is particular concern about off-target effects of completely inhibiting TNF-α function. For example, since TNF-α is a critical component of immunity, infectious disease is a primary concern during TNF-α therapy (Naveau et al., 2004). Moreover, TNF-α is required for normal liver regeneration as hepatocyte proliferation in response to injury is impaired in mice lacking TNF-α receptors (Yamada et al., 1997). Etanercept, a TNF-α neutralizing antibody, appeared to increase short-term survival of patients with alcoholic hepatitis in a small pilot study (Menon et al., 2004), although a subsequent randomized, placebo-controlled trial conducted by the same investigators showed a worse 6-month survival rate in the group treated with etanercept than in the placebo group (Boetticher et al., 2008). Thus, it seems very unlikely that inhibition of TNF-α may become a therapeutic target in ALD, especially at the long-term.

7. Conclusion

In summary, the liver is an organ with predominant innate immunity function. Dysregulation of many components of innate immunity in the liver due to chronic alcohol consumption likely contributes additively or synergistically to alcohol-induced liver disease. Chronic alcohol consumption activates LPS/TLR4 signalling pathway on KCs, which produce large amounts of pro-inflammatory cytokines, including TNF-α, leading to liver steatosis and inflammation. Alcohol-induced LPS/TLR4 signalling pathway activation also contributes to alcoholic liver fibrosis via two independent mechanisms: it induces the secretion of chemokines from HSCs and chemotaxis of KCs which secrete the profibrogenic cytokine TGF-β; additionally, TLR4-dependent signals augment TGF-β signalling on HSCs via down-regulation of the TGF-β pseudoreceptor Bambi. Inhibition of NK cells during chronic alcohol consumption also seem to contribute to alcoholic liver fibrosis, since NK cells have anti-fibrotic effects through suppression of HSCs. Activation of LPS/TLR4 signalling pathway on hepatocytes may also contribute to hepatocarcinoma development, through activation of Nanog gene. In contrast to activation LPS/TLR4 signalling pathway and inhibition of NK cells, the role of complement activation in the pathogenesis of ALD remains largely obscure. Few studies suggest that alcohol-induced complement activation may contribute to liver steatosis, inflammation and fibrosis, but more studies are needed to clarify the underlying mechanisms.

Alcohol-induced dysregulation of innate immunity also seem to contribute to the increased risk of infections of patients with alcoholic cirrhosis, as we and others have demonstrated a blunted response of immune cells to TLR2/4 ligands, probably associated with compromised intracellular signalling, in these patients.

Modulation of innate immunity, mainly of LPS/TLR4 signalling through the use of probiotics or antibiotics, may play a role in the treatment of ALD, but we need for larger and rigorously designed clinical trials to support the use of probiotics or antibiotics in treatment of ALD. Inhibition of TNF-α has produced variable results in the treatment of ALD and may be associated with serious off-target effects.

Although, in the last decade, we have gain significant insight over the role of alcohol-induced innate immunity dysregulation in ALD, further research is still needed to further clarify and identify the interrelationships between innate immunity components involved in ALD. Examples of questions for future studies are:

1. Which is the role of other TLRs than TLR2 and TLR4 in the development of ALD?
2. Which is the role of DAMPs (HMGB1, heat shock proteins) and Myd88-independent pathway in ALD progression?
3. Which are the molecular mechanisms by which complement system contribute to alcohol-induced liver steatosis, inflammation and fibrosis?
4. Which are the molecular mechanisms underlying blunted response of immune cells to TLR2/4 ligands in patients with alcoholic cirrhosis?
5. Is there any correlation between TLR4 SNPs and the progression of ALD?
6. Which is the effect in ALD of neutralization of LPS or LPS-signalling through the use of TLR4 anatgonists (e.g., CyP, CRX-526, Eritoran), or LPS signalling interfering molecules (e.g., TAK-242, besifloxacin, compound K)?

The answers to these questions may help us identify novel therapeutic targets to treat ALD.

8. Acknowledgment

The authors greatly appreciate Dr. Raquel Gonçalves and Prof. Mário-Dinis Ribeiro for critical reading of the chapter.

9. References

Adachi, Y.; Bradford, B.U.; Gao, W.; Bojes, H.K. & Thurman, R.G. (1994). Inactivation of Kupffer cells prevents early alcohol-induced liver injury. *Hepatology*. Vol.20, No.2, pp. 453-460, ISSN 0270-9139

Adachi, Y.; Moore, L.E.; Bradford, B.U.; Gao, W. & Thurman, R.G. (1995). Antibiotics prevent liver injury in rats following long-term exposure to ethanol. *Gastroenterology*. Vol.108, No.1, pp. 218-224, ISSN 0016-5085

Arjona, A.; Boyadjieva, N. & Sarkar, D.K. (2004). Circadian rhythms of granzyme B, perforin, IFN-gamma, and NK cell cytolytic activity in the spleen: effects of chronic ethanol. *J Immunol*. Vol.172, No.5, pp. 2811-2817, ISSN 0022-1767

Arteel, G.E. (2003). Oxidants and antioxidants in alcohol-induced liver disease. *Gastroenterology*. Vol.124, No.3, pp. 778-790, ISSN 0016-5085

Baroni, G.S.; D'Ambrosio, L.; Curto, P.; Casini, A.; Mancini, R.; Jezequel, A.M. & Benedetti, A. (1996). Interferon gamma decreases hepatic stellate cell activation and extracellular matrix deposition in rat liver fibrosis. *Hepatology*. Vol.23, No.5, pp. 1189-1199, ISSN 0270-9139

Boetticher, N.C.; Peine, C.J.; Kwo, P.; Abrams, G.A.; Patel, T.; Aqel, B.; Boardman, L.; Gores, G.J.; Harmsen, W.S.; McClain, C.J.; Kamath, P.S. & Shah, V.H. (2008). A randomized, double-blinded, placebo-controlled multicenter trial of etanercept in the treatment of alcoholic hepatitis. *Gastroenterology*. Vol.135, No.6, pp. 1953-1960, ISSN 1528-0012

Boyadjieva, N.I.; Chaturvedi, K.; Poplawski, M.M. & Sarkar, D.K. (2004). Opioid antagonist naltrexone disrupts feedback interaction between mu and delta opioid receptors in splenocytes to prevent alcohol inhibition of NK cell function. *J Immunol.* Vol.173, No.1, pp. 42-49, ISSN 0022-1767

Butterworth, R.F. (2011). Editorial: rifaximin and minimal hepatic encephalopathy. *Am J Gastroenterol.* Vol.106, No.2, pp. 317-318, ISSN 1572-0241

Byun, J.S. & Jeong, W.I. (2010). Involvement of hepatic innate immunity in alcoholic liver disease. *Immune Netw.* Vol.10, No.6, pp. 181-187, ISSN 2092-6685

Cohen, J.I.; Roychowdhury, S.; McMullen, M.R.; Stavitsky, A.B. & Nagy, L.E. (2010). Complement and alcoholic liver disease: role of C1q in the pathogenesis of ethanol-induced liver injury in mice. *Gastroenterology.* Vol.139, No.2, pp. 664-674, 674 e661, ISSN 1528-0012

El-Assal, O.; Hong, F.; Kim, W.H.; Radaeva, S. & Gao, B. (2004). IL-6-deficient mice are susceptible to ethanol-induced hepatic steatosis: IL-6 protects against ethanol-induced oxidative stress and mitochondrial permeability transition in the liver. *Cell Mol Immunol.* Vol.1, No.3, pp. 205-211, ISSN 1672-7681

Endo, M.; Masaki, T.; Seike, M. & Yoshimatsu, H. (2007). TNF-alpha induces hepatic steatosis in mice by enhancing gene expression of sterol regulatory element binding protein-1c (SREBP-1c). *Exp Biol Med (Maywood).* Vol.232, No.5, pp. 614-621, ISSN 1535-3702

Erridge, C. (2010). Endogenous ligands of TLR2 and TLR4: agonists or assistants? *J Leukoc Biol.* Vol.87, No.6, pp. 989-999, ISSN 1938-3673

Ewaschuk, J.; Endersby, R.; Thiel, D.; Diaz, H.; Backer, J.; Ma, M.; Churchill, T. & Madsen, K. (2007). Probiotic bacteria prevent hepatic damage and maintain colonic barrier function in a mouse model of sepsis. *Hepatology.* Vol.46, No.3, pp. 841-850, ISSN 0270-9139

Fernandez, J.; Navasa, M.; Planas, R.; Montoliu, S.; Monfort, D.; Soriano, G.; Vila, C.; Pardo, A.; Quintero, E.; Vargas, V.; Such, J.; Gines, P. & Arroyo, V. (2007). Primary prophylaxis of spontaneous bacterial peritonitis delays hepatorenal syndrome and improves survival in cirrhosis. *Gastroenterology.* Vol.133, No.3, pp. 818-824, ISSN 0016-5085

Fromenty, B.; Berson, A. & Pessayre, D. (1997). Microvesicular steatosis and steatohepatitis: role of mitochondrial dysfunction and lipid peroxidation. *J Hepatol.* Vol.26 Suppl 1, pp. 13-22, ISSN 0168-8278

Gao, B.; Jeong, W.I. & Tian, Z. (2008). Liver: An organ with predominant innate immunity. *Hepatology.* Vol.47, No.2, pp. 729-736, ISSN 1527-3350

Gao, B.; Radaeva, S. & Park, O. (2009). Liver natural killer and natural killer T cells: immunobiology and emerging roles in liver diseases. *J Leukoc Biol.* Vol.86, No.3, pp. 513-528, ISSN 1938-3673

Gao, B.; Seki, E.; Brenner, D.A.; Friedman, S.; Cohen, J.I.; Nagy, L.; Szabo, G. & Zakhari, S. (2011). Innate immunity in alcoholic liver disease. *Am J Physiol Gastrointest Liver Physiol.* Vol.300, No.4, pp. G516-525, ISSN 1522-1547

Gasque, P. (2004). Complement: a unique innate immune sensor for danger signals. *Mol Immunol.* Vol.41, No.11, pp. 1089-1098, ISSN 0161-5890

Guo, J.; Loke, J.; Zheng, F.; Hong, F.; Yea, S.; Fukata, M.; Tarocchi, M.; Abar, O.T.; Huang, H.; Sninsky, J.J. & Friedman, S.L. (2009). Functional linkage of cirrhosis-predictive single nucleotide polymorphisms of Toll-like receptor 4 to hepatic stellate cell responses. *Hepatology.* Vol.49, No.3, pp. 960-968, ISSN 1527-3350

Gustot, T.; Lemmers, A.; Moreno, C.; Nagy, N.; Quertinmont, E.; Nicaise, C.; Franchimont, D.; Louis, H.; Deviere, J. & Le Moine, O. (2006). Differential liver sensitization to toll-like receptor pathways in mice with alcoholic fatty liver. *Hepatology*. Vol.43, No.5, pp. 989-1000, ISSN 0270-9139

Hassan, M.M.; Hwang, L.Y.; Hatten, C.J.; Swaim, M.; Li, D.; Abbruzzese, J.L.; Beasley, P. & Patt, Y.Z. (2002). Risk factors for hepatocellular carcinoma: synergism of alcohol with viral hepatitis and diabetes mellitus. *Hepatology*. Vol.36, No.5, pp. 1206-1213, ISSN 0270-9139

Hauge, T.; Persson, J. & Danielsson, D. (1997). Mucosal bacterial growth in the upper gastrointestinal tract in alcoholics (heavy drinkers). *Digestion*. Vol.58, No.6, pp. 591-595, ISSN 0012-2823

Henderson, N.C. & Iredale, J.P. (2007). Liver fibrosis: cellular mechanisms of progression and resolution. *Clin Sci (Lond)*. Vol.112, No.5, pp. 265-280, ISSN 1470-8736

Hillebrandt, S.; Wasmuth, H.E.; Weiskirchen, R.; Hellerbrand, C.; Keppeler, H.; Werth, A.; Schirin-Sokhan, R.; Wilkens, G.; Geier, A.; Lorenzen, J.; Kohl, J.; Gressner, A.M.; Matern, S. & Lammert, F. (2005). Complement factor 5 is a quantitative trait gene that modifies liver fibrogenesis in mice and humans. *Nat Genet*. Vol.37, No.8, pp. 835-843, ISSN 1061-4036

Homann, C.; Varming, K.; Hogasen, K.; Mollnes, T.E.; Graudal, N.; Thomsen, A.C. & Garred, P. (1997). Acquired C3 deficiency in patients with alcoholic cirrhosis predisposes to infection and increased mortality. *Gut*. Vol.40, No.4, pp. 544-549, ISSN 0017-5749

Hritz, I.; Mandrekar, P.; Velayudham, A.; Catalano, D.; Dolganiuc, A.; Kodys, K.; Kurt-Jones, E. & Szabo, G. (2008). The critical role of toll-like receptor (TLR) 4 in alcoholic liver disease is independent of the common TLR adapter MyD88. *Hepatology*. Vol.48, No.4, pp. 1224-1231, ISSN 1527-3350

Huang, H.; Shiffman, M.L.; Friedman, S.; Venkatesh, R.; Bzowej, N.; Abar, O.T.; Rowland, C.M.; Catanese, J.J.; Leong, D.U.; Sninsky, J.J.; Layden, T.J.; Wright, T.L.; White, T. & Cheung, R.C. (2007). A 7 gene signature identifies the risk of developing cirrhosis in patients with chronic hepatitis C. *Hepatology*. Vol.46, No.2, pp. 297-306, ISSN 0270-9139

Ip, E.; Farrell, G.C.; Robertson, G.; Hall, P.; Kirsch, R. & Leclercq, I. (2003). Central role of PPARalpha-dependent hepatic lipid turnover in dietary steatohepatitis in mice. *Hepatology*. Vol.38, No.1, pp. 123-132, ISSN 0270-9139

Isayama, F.; Hines, I.N.; Kremer, M.; Milton, R.J.; Byrd, C.L.; Perry, A.W.; McKim, S.E.; Parsons, C.; Rippe, R.A. & Wheeler, M.D. (2006). LPS signaling enhances hepatic fibrogenesis caused by experimental cholestasis in mice. *Am J Physiol Gastrointest Liver Physiol*. Vol.290, No.6, pp. G1318-1328, ISSN 0193-1857

Janeway, C.A., Jr. & Medzhitov, R. (2002). Innate immune recognition. *Annu Rev Immunol*. Vol.20, pp. 197-216, ISSN 0732-0582

Jarvelainen, H.A.; Vakeva, A.; Lindros, K.O. & Meri, S. (2002). Activation of complement components and reduced regulator expression in alcohol-induced liver injury in the rat. *Clin Immunol*. Vol.105, No.1, pp. 57-63, ISSN 1521-6616

Jeong, W.I.; Osei-Hyiaman, D.; Park, O.; Liu, J.; Batkai, S.; Mukhopadhyay, P.; Horiguchi, N.; Harvey-White, J.; Marsicano, G.; Lutz, B.; Gao, B. & Kunos, G. (2008). Paracrine activation of hepatic CB1 receptors by stellate cell-derived endocannabinoids mediates alcoholic fatty liver. *Cell Metab*. Vol.7, No.3, pp. 227-235, ISSN 1550-4131

Jeong, W.I.; Park, O. & Gao, B. (2008). Abrogation of the antifibrotic effects of natural killer cells/interferon-gamma contributes to alcohol acceleration of liver fibrosis. *Gastroenterology*. Vol.134, No.1, pp. 248-258, ISSN 1528-0012

Jeong, W.I.; Park, O.; Radaeva, S. & Gao, B. (2006). STAT1 inhibits liver fibrosis in mice by inhibiting stellate cell proliferation and stimulating NK cell cytotoxicity. *Hepatology*. Vol.44, No.6, pp. 1441-1451, ISSN 0270-9139

Kirpich, I.A.; Solovieva, N.V.; Leikhter, S.N.; Shidakova, N.A.; Lebedeva, O.V.; Sidorov, P.I.; Bazhukova, T.A.; Soloviev, A.G.; Barve, S.S.; McClain, C.J. & Cave, M. (2008). Probiotics restore bowel flora and improve liver enzymes in human alcohol-induced liver injury: a pilot study. *Alcohol*. Vol.42, No.8, pp. 675-682, ISSN 1873-6823

Kono, H.; Rusyn, I.; Yin, M.; Gabele, E.; Yamashina, S.; Dikalova, A.; Kadiiska, M.B.; Connor, H.D.; Mason, R.P.; Segal, B.H.; Bradford, B.U.; Holland, S.M. & Thurman, R.G. (2000). NADPH oxidase-derived free radicals are key oxidants in alcohol-induced liver disease. *J Clin Invest*. Vol.106, No.7, pp. 867-872, ISSN 0021-9738

Li, Y.; Chang, M.; Abar, O.; Garcia, V.; Rowland, C.; Catanese, J.; Ross, D.; Broder, S.; Shiffman, M.; Cheung, R.; Wright, T.; Friedman, S.L. & Sninsky, J. (2009). Multiple variants in toll-like receptor 4 gene modulate risk of liver fibrosis in Caucasians with chronic hepatitis C infection. *J Hepatol*. Vol.51, No.4, pp. 750-757, ISSN 0168-8278

Lin, C.Y.; Tsai, I.F.; Ho, Y.P.; Huang, C.T.; Lin, Y.C.; Lin, C.J.; Tseng, S.C.; Lin, W.P.; Chen, W.T. & Sheen, I.S. (2007). Endotoxemia contributes to the immune paralysis in patients with cirrhosis. *J Hepatol*. Vol.46, No.5, pp. 816-826, ISSN 0168-8278

Linderoth, G.; Jepsen, P.; Schonheyder, H.C.; Johnsen, S.P. & Sorensen, H.T. (2006). Short-term prognosis of community-acquired bacteremia in patients with liver cirrhosis or alcoholism: A population-based cohort study. *Alcohol Clin Exp Res*. Vol.30, No.4, pp. 636-641, ISSN 0145-6008

Liu, Q.; Duan, Z.P.; Ha, D.K.; Bengmark, S.; Kurtovic, J. & Riordan, S.M. (2004). Synbiotic modulation of gut flora: effect on minimal hepatic encephalopathy in patients with cirrhosis. *Hepatology*. Vol.39, No.5, pp. 1441-1449, ISSN 0270-9139

Lu, Y.C.; Yeh, W.C. & Ohashi, P.S. (2008). LPS/TLR4 signal transduction pathway. *Cytokine*. Vol.42, No.2, pp. 145-151, ISSN 1096-0023

Luckey, T.D.; Reyniers, J.A.; Gyorgy, P. & Forbes, M. (1954). Germfree animals and liver necrosis. *Ann N Y Acad Sci*. Vol.57, No.6, pp. 932-935, ISSN 0077-8923

Machida, K.; Tsukamoto, H.; Mkrtchyan, H.; Duan, L.; Dynnyk, A.; Liu, H.M.; Asahina, K.; Govindarajan, S.; Ray, R.; Ou, J.H.; Seki, E.; Deshaies, R.; Miyake, K. & Lai, M.M. (2009). Toll-like receptor 4 mediates synergism between alcohol and HCV in hepatic oncogenesis involving stem cell marker Nanog. *Proc Natl Acad Sci U S A*. Vol.106, No.5, pp. 1548-1553, ISSN 1091-6490

Mathurin, P.; Deng, Q.G.; Keshavarzian, A.; Choudhary, S.; Holmes, E.W. & Tsukamoto, H. (2000). Exacerbation of alcoholic liver injury by enteral endotoxin in rats. *Hepatology*. Vol.32, No.5, pp. 1008-1017, ISSN 0270-9139

Melhem, A.; Muhanna, N.; Bishara, A.; Alvarez, C.E.; Ilan, Y.; Bishara, T.; Horani, A.; Nassar, M.; Friedman, S.L. & Safadi, R. (2006). Anti-fibrotic activity of NK cells in experimental liver injury through killing of activated HSC. *J Hepatol*. Vol.45, No.1, pp. 60-71, ISSN 0168-8278

Menon, K.V.; Stadheim, L.; Kamath, P.S.; Wiesner, R.H.; Gores, G.J.; Peine, C.J. & Shah, V. (2004). A pilot study of the safety and tolerability of etanercept in patients with alcoholic hepatitis. *Am J Gastroenterol*. Vol.99, No.2, pp. 255-260, ISSN 0002-9270

Miller, A.M.; Horiguchi, N.; Jeong, W.I.; Radaeva, S. & Gao, B. (2011). Molecular mechanisms of alcoholic liver disease: innate immunity and cytokines. *Alcohol Clin Exp Res*. Vol.35, No.5, pp. 787-793, ISSN 1530-0277

Nanji, A.A.; Khettry, U. & Sadrzadeh, S.M. (1994). Lactobacillus feeding reduces endotoxemia and severity of experimental alcoholic liver (disease). *Proc Soc Exp Biol Med*. Vol.205, No.3, pp. 243-247, ISSN 0037-9727

Navasa, M.; Fernandez, J. & Rodes, J. (1999). Bacterial infections in liver cirrhosis. *Ital J Gastroenterol Hepatol*. Vol.31, No.7, pp. 616-625, ISSN 1125-8055

Naveau, S.; Chollet-Martin, S.; Dharancy, S.; Mathurin, P.; Jouet, P.; Piquet, M.A.; Davion, T.; Oberti, F.; Broet, P. & Emilie, D. (2004). A double-blind randomized controlled trial of infliximab associated with prednisolone in acute alcoholic hepatitis. *Hepatology*. Vol.39, No.5, pp. 1390-1397, ISSN 0270-9139

O'Shea, R.S.; Dasarathy, S. & McCullough, A.J. (2010). Alcoholic liver disease. *Hepatology*. Vol.51, No.1, pp. 307-328, ISSN 1527-3350

Osman, N.; Adawi, D.; Ahrne, S.; Jeppsson, B. & Molin, G. (2007). Endotoxin- and D-galactosamine-induced liver injury improved by the administration of Lactobacillus, Bifidobacterium and blueberry. *Dig Liver Dis*. Vol.39, No.9, pp. 849-856, ISSN 1590-8658

Parlesak, A.; Schafer, C.; Schutz, T.; Bode, J.C. & Bode, C. (2000). Increased intestinal permeability to macromolecules and endotoxemia in patients with chronic alcohol abuse in different stages of alcohol-induced liver disease. *J Hepatol*. Vol.32, No.5, pp. 742-747, ISSN 0168-8278

Petrasek, J.; Mandrekar, P. & Szabo, G. (2010). Toll-like receptors in the pathogenesis of alcoholic liver disease. *Gastroenterol Res Pract*. Vol.2010, pp. ISSN 1687-630X

Pimentel-Nunes, P.; Roncon-Albuquerque, R., Jr.; Dinis-Ribeiro, M. & Leite-Moreira, A.F. (2011). Role of Toll-like receptor impairment in cirrhosis infection risk: are we making progress? *Liver Int*. Vol.31, No.1, pp. 140-141, ISSN 1478-3231

Pimentel-Nunes, P.; Roncon-Albuquerque, R., Jr.; Goncalves, N.; Fernandes-Cerqueira, C.; Cardoso, H.; Bastos, R.P.; Marques, M.; Marques, C.; Alexandre Sarmento, J.; Costa-Santos, C.; Macedo, G.; Pestana, M.; Dinis-Ribeiro, M. & Leite-Moreira, A.F. (2010). Attenuation of toll-like receptor 2-mediated innate immune response in patients with alcoholic chronic liver disease. *Liver Int*. Vol.30, No.7, pp. 1003-1011, ISSN 1478-3231

Pritchard, M.T.; McMullen, M.R.; Stavitsky, A.B.; Cohen, J.I.; Lin, F.; Medof, M.E. & Nagy, L.E. (2007). Differential contributions of C3, C5, and decay-accelerating factor to ethanol-induced fatty liver in mice. *Gastroenterology*. Vol.132, No.3, pp. 1117-1126, ISSN 0016-5085

Purohit, V.; Bode, J.C.; Bode, C.; Brenner, D.A.; Choudhry, M.A.; Hamilton, F.; Kang, Y.J.; Keshavarzian, A.; Rao, R.; Sartor, R.B.; Swanson, C. & Turner, J.R. (2008). Alcohol, intestinal bacterial growth, intestinal permeability to endotoxin, and medical consequences: summary of a symposium. *Alcohol*. Vol.42, No.5, pp. 349-361, ISSN 0741-8329

Qin, X. & Gao, B. (2006). The complement system in liver diseases. *Cell Mol Immunol*. Vol.3, No.5, pp. 333-340, ISSN 1672-7681

Radaeva, S.; Sun, R.; Jaruga, B.; Nguyen, V.T.; Tian, Z. & Gao, B. (2006). Natural killer cells ameliorate liver fibrosis by killing activated stellate cells in NKG2D-dependent and tumor necrosis factor-related apoptosis-inducing ligand-dependent manners. *Gastroenterology*. Vol.130, No.2, pp. 435-452, ISSN 0016-5085

Radaeva, S.; Wang, L.; Radaev, S.; Jeong, W.I.; Park, O. & Gao, B. (2007). Retinoic acid signaling sensitizes hepatic stellate cells to NK cell killing via upregulation of NK cell activating ligand RAE1. *Am J Physiol Gastrointest Liver Physiol*. Vol.293, No.4, pp. G809-816, ISSN 0193-1857

Riordan, S.M.; Skinner, N.; Nagree, A.; McCallum, H.; McIver, C.J.; Kurtovic, J.; Hamilton, J.A.; Bengmark, S.; Williams, R. & Visvanathan, K. (2003). Peripheral blood mononuclear cell expression of toll-like receptors and relation to cytokine levels in cirrhosis. *Hepatology*. Vol.37, No.5, pp. 1154-1164, ISSN 0270-9139

Roychowdhury, S.; McMullen, M.R.; Pritchard, M.T.; Hise, A.G.; van Rooijen, N.; Medof, M.E.; Stavitsky, A.B. & Nagy, L.E. (2009). An early complement-dependent and TLR-4-independent phase in the pathogenesis of ethanol-induced liver injury in mice. *Hepatology*. Vol.49, No.4, pp. 1326-1334, ISSN 1527-3350

Runyon, B.A.; Borzio, M.; Young, S.; Squier, S.U.; Guarner, C. & Runyon, M.A. (1995). Effect of selective bowel decontamination with norfloxacin on spontaneous bacterial peritonitis, translocation, and survival in an animal model of cirrhosis. *Hepatology*. Vol.21, No.6, pp. 1719-1724, ISSN 0270-9139

Rutenburg, A.M.; Sonnenblick, E.; Koven, I.; Aprahamian, H.A.; Reiner, L. & Fine, J. (1957). The role of intestinal bacteria in the development of dietary cirrhosis in rats. *J Exp Med*. Vol.106, No.1, pp. 1-14, ISSN 0022-1007

Seki, E.; De Minicis, S.; Osterreicher, C.H.; Kluwe, J.; Osawa, Y.; Brenner, D.A. & Schwabe, R.F. (2007). TLR4 enhances TGF-beta signaling and hepatic fibrosis. *Nat Med*. Vol.13, No.11, pp. 1324-1332, ISSN 1078-8956

Soares, J.-B.; Pimentel-Nunes, P.; Roncon-Albuquerque, R. & Leite-Moreira, A. (2010). The role of lipopolysaccharide/toll-like receptor 4 signaling in chronic liver diseases. *Hepatol Int*. Vol.4, No.4, pp. 659-672, ISSN 1936-0533

Stadlbauer, V.; Mookerjee, R.P.; Hodges, S.; Wright, G.A.; Davies, N.A. & Jalan, R. (2008). Effect of probiotic treatment on deranged neutrophil function and cytokine responses in patients with compensated alcoholic cirrhosis. *J Hepatol*. Vol.48, No.6, pp. 945-951, ISSN 0168-8278

Stadlbauer, V.; Mookerjee, R.P.; Wright, G.A.; Davies, N.A.; Jurgens, G.; Hallstrom, S. & Jalan, R. (2009). Role of Toll-like receptors 2, 4, and 9 in mediating neutrophil dysfunction in alcoholic hepatitis. *Am J Physiol Gastrointest Liver Physiol*. Vol.296, No.1, pp. G15-22, ISSN 0193-1857

Su, G.L.; Klein, R.D.; Aminlari, A.; Zhang, H.Y.; Steinstraesser, L.; Alarcon, W.H.; Remick, D.G. & Wang, S.C. (2000). Kupffer cell activation by lipopolysaccharide in rats: role for lipopolysaccharide binding protein and toll-like receptor 4. *Hepatology*. Vol.31, No.4, pp. 932-936, ISSN 0270-9139

Taimr, P.; Higuchi, H.; Kocova, E.; Rippe, R.A.; Friedman, S. & Gores, G.J. (2003). Activated stellate cells express the TRAIL receptor-2/death receptor-5 and undergo TRAIL-mediated apoptosis. *Hepatology*. Vol.37, No.1, pp. 87-95, ISSN 0270-9139

Tazi, K.A.; Quioc, J.J.; Saada, V.; Bezeaud, A.; Lebrec, D. & Moreau, R. (2006). Upregulation of TNF-alpha production signaling pathways in monocytes from patients with advanced cirrhosis: possible role of Akt and IRAK-M. *J Hepatol*. Vol.45, No.2, pp. 280-289, ISSN 0168-8278

Testro, A.G.; Gow, P.J.; Angus, P.W.; Wongseelashote, S.; Skinner, N.; Markovska, V. & Visvanathan, K. (2009). Effects of antibiotics on expression and function of Toll-like receptors 2 and 4 on mononuclear cells in patients with advanced cirrhosis. *J Hepatol*. pp. 199-205 ISSN 0168-8278

Tilg, H.; Jalan, R.; Kaser, A.; Davies, N.A.; Offner, F.A.; Hodges, S.J.; Ludwiczek, O.; Shawcross, D.; Zoller, H.; Alisa, A.; Mookerjee, R.P.; Graziadei, I.; Datz, C.; Trauner, M.; Schuppan, D.; Obrist, P.; Vogel, W. & Williams, R. (2003). Anti-tumor necrosis factor-alpha monoclonal antibody therapy in severe alcoholic hepatitis. *J Hepatol.* Vol.38, No.4, pp. 419-425, ISSN 0168-8278

Tsung, A.; Sahai, R.; Tanaka, H.; Nakao, A.; Fink, M.P.; Lotze, M.T.; Yang, H.; Li, J.; Tracey, K.J.; Geller, D.A. & Billiar, T.R. (2005). The nuclear factor HMGB1 mediates hepatic injury after murine liver ischemia-reperfusion. *J Exp Med.* Vol.201, No.7, pp. 1135-1143, ISSN 0022-1007

Uesugi, T.; Froh, M.; Arteel, G.E.; Bradford, B.U. & Thurman, R.G. (2001). Toll-like receptor 4 is involved in the mechanism of early alcohol-induced liver injury in mice. *Hepatology.* Vol.34, No.1, pp. 101-108, ISSN 0270-9139

Uesugi, T.; Froh, M.; Arteel, G.E.; Bradford, B.U.; Wheeler, M.D.; Gabele, E.; Isayama, F. & Thurman, R.G. (2002). Role of lipopolysaccharide-binding protein in early alcohol-induced liver injury in mice. *J Immunol.* Vol.168, No.6, pp. 2963-2969, ISSN 0022-1767

Velayudham, A.; Dolganiuc, A.; Ellis, M.; Petrasek, J.; Kodys, K.; Mandrekar, P. & Szabo, G. (2009). VSL#3 probiotic treatment attenuates fibrosis without changes in steatohepatitis in a diet-induced nonalcoholic steatohepatitis model in mice. *Hepatology.* Vol.49, No.3, pp. 989-997, ISSN 1527-3350

Wasmuth, H.E.; Kunz, D.; Yagmur, E.; Timmer-Stranghoner, A.; Vidacek, D.; Siewert, E.; Bach, J.; Geier, A.; Purucker, E.A.; Gressner, A.M.; Matern, S. & Lammert, F. (2005). Patients with acute on chronic liver failure display "sepsis-like" immune paralysis. *J Hepatol.* Vol.42, No.2, pp. 195-201, ISSN 0168-8278

Weng, Y.I.; Aroor, A.R. & Shukla, S.D. (2008). Ethanol inhibition of angiotensin II-stimulated Tyr705 and Ser727 STAT3 phosphorylation in cultured rat hepatocytes: relevance to activation of p42/44 mitogen-activated protein kinase. *Alcohol.* Vol.42, No.5, pp. 397-406, ISSN 0741-8329

Yamada, Y.; Kirillova, I.; Peschon, J.J. & Fausto, N. (1997). Initiation of liver growth by tumor necrosis factor: deficient liver regeneration in mice lacking type I tumor necrosis factor receptor. *Proc Natl Acad Sci U S A.* Vol.94, No.4, pp. 1441-1446, ISSN 0027-8424

Yin, M.; Bradford, B.U.; Wheeler, M.D.; Uesugi, T.; Froh, M.; Goyert, S.M. & Thurman, R.G. (2001). Reduced early alcohol-induced liver injury in CD14-deficient mice. *J Immunol.* Vol.166, No.7, pp. 4737-4742, ISSN 0022-1767

Yin, M.; Wheeler, M.D.; Kono, H.; Bradford, B.U.; Gallucci, R.M.; Luster, M.I. & Thurman, R.G. (1999). Essential role of tumor necrosis factor alpha in alcohol-induced liver injury in mice. *Gastroenterology.* Vol.117, No.4, pp. 942-952, ISSN 0016-5085

You, M.; Matsumoto, M.; Pacold, C.M.; Cho, W.K. & Crabb, D.W. (2004). The role of AMP-activated protein kinase in the action of ethanol in the liver. *Gastroenterology.* Vol.127, No.6, pp. 1798-1808, ISSN 0016-5085

Zarember, K.A. & Godowski, P.J. (2002). Tissue expression of human Toll-like receptors and differential regulation of Toll-like receptor mRNAs in leukocytes in response to microbes, their products, and cytokines. *J Immunol.* Vol.168, No.2, pp. 554-561, ISSN 0022-1767

Zhang, H. & Meadows, G.G. (2009). Exogenous IL-15 in combination with IL-15R alpha rescues natural killer cells from apoptosis induced by chronic alcohol consumption. *Alcohol Clin Exp Res.* Vol.33, No.3, pp. 419-427, ISSN 1530-0277

Zhao, X.J.; Dong, Q.; Bindas, J.; Piganelli, J.D.; Magill, A.; Reiser, J. & Kolls, J.K. (2008). TRIF and IRF-3 binding to the TNF promoter results in macrophage TNF dysregulation and steatosis induced by chronic ethanol. *J Immunol.* Vol.181, No.5, pp. 3049-3056, ISSN 1550-6606

4

Endothelial Markers and Fibrosis in Alcoholic Hepatitis

Roxana Popescu[1], Doina Verdes[2], Nicoleta Filimon[3], Marioara Cornianu[4] and Despina Maria Bordean[5]
[1,2,4]University of Medicine and Pharmacy, Timisoara
[3]West University of Timisoara
[5]BUASVM Timisoara
Romania

1. Introduction

The alcohol, consumed in great quantities and for a long period of time determines, directly or by its metabolites, serious alterations of the hepatic function and structure. The causal mechanisms underlying this disease are not fully understood. Histological features of chronic alcoholic hepatitis include: hepatocellular injury, inflammation and repair of the damage with activation of Kupffer cells and hepatocellular regeneration.

The hepatic extracellular matrix (ECM) plays an important role in the stability of tissues and in regulating the growth and differentiation of cells. Liver fibrogenesis occurs by disrupting the balance between ECM compounds degradation and production, especially the synthesis and deposition of collagen (Wang et al., 2000). The ECM is made up of conjunctive - vascular structures which ensure the functional and nutritional support of the parenchyma. Liver injury like hepatitis and cirrhosis, caused by alcohol, initiates response from hepatic stellate cell (HSC) that gets activated by oxidative stress resulting in large amounts of collagen. After an acute liver injury parenchymal cells regenerate and replace the death hepatocytes. The depositions of ECM structures are initially limited and are associated with an inflammatory response. If the hepatic injury persists and then the liver regeneration fails, the hepatocytes are substituted with abundant fibrillar collagen (Bataller & Brenner, 2005).

The expression of endothelial cells markers CD31 and CD34 is heterogeneous, with a specific pattern for individual vessel types and different anatomic compartments of the same organ (Pusztaszeri et al., 2006).

CD31 is a transmembrane glycoprotein, member of the immunoglobulin superfamily, also designated as PECAM-1 (platelet endothelial cell adhesion molecule 1). CD31 is expressed on the surface of circulating platelets, monocytes, neutrophils and selected T cell subsets, but, with a few minor exceptions, PECAM-1 is not present on fibroblasts, epithelium, muscle, or other nonvascular cells. PECAM is a major constituent of the endothelial cell intercellular junction and a key participant in the adhesion cascade leading to transmigration of leukocytes during the inflammatory process (Newman, 1997). Also, several studies suggest that CD31 plays a major role in angiogenesis (DeLisser et al., 1997; Matsumura et al., 1997; Zhou et al., 1999).

CD34 is a 110-kDa transmembrane glycoprotein present on leukemic cells, endothelial cells and stem cells) (Pusztaszeri et al., 2006). CD34 is preferentially expressed on the surface of regenerating or migrating endothelial cells and is a marker of proliferating endothelial cells in the growing sprouts during angiogenesis (Poon et al., 2002). Usually, the liver sinusoids do not express CD34. But, pathological conditions can alter their phenotype and express this marker. Capillarization of hepatic sinusoids is a well-recognized phenomenon that occurs in long-standing liver disease and hepatic cirrhosis as well as in hepatocellular carcinoma (HCC) (Pusztaszeri et al., 2006).

The investigation of the expression of the endothelial cell markers CD31 and CD34 allow determining the degree of vascular distribution hepatic inflammation.

2. Histochemical and immunohistochemical diagnosis methods used for study of alcoholic hepatitis

2.1 Morphological diagnosis methods

The biological material harvesting by percutaneous liver biopsy or after a necropsy follows the same histological processing, involving fixing in formaldehyde 10%, inclusion in paraffin and making multiple serial sections. For routine diagnosis, deparaffinized sections from paraffin-embedded liver tissue were stained with hematoxylin-eosin technique (HE). For diagnostic purposes and to assess histopathological lesions, especially liver fibrosis, trichrome staining methods are applied in order to complement the data obtained on sections stained with HE. Gömori method highlights collagen in green, on red background of hepatocytes cytoplasm. By Masson method, the results are similar; the color obtained for fibrosis is green-blue on a red background of the cytoplasm. The lumen of the centrilobular vein - collapsed or difficult to distinguish on HE staining - can be easily observed on reticulin silver staining, following the shape and wall thickness, the presence of inflammation or fibrosis. Silver impregnation by Gordon-Sweet method to highlight reticulin fibers (type III collagen) applied in all cases with histological activity and fibrosis, has proved useful in diagnosis of piecemeal necrosis indicating the outline of portal spaces altered by piecemeal necrosis, in evaluation of focal necrosis area and to highlight reticulin fibers in nodular regeneration conditions. The silver staining for reticulin highlight the components of extracellular liver matrix from Disse space and centrilobular venules (Cornianu et al., 2007).

2.2 Additional immunohistochemical diagnosis methods

Using immunohistochemical methods (IHC) as special techniques is a next step in diagnosis after histological staining, allowing highlighting of new structures and functions. In order to perform immunohistochemical reactions, the staining techniques based on monoclonal antibodies which react with specific tissue antigens are applied. The immunohistochemical detection is performed on 5-µm thick, routinely formalin-fixed, paraffin-embedded specimens. Briefly, the sections are deparaffinied in xylene and rehydrated in serial solutions of ethanol and water. To block endogenous peroxidase activity the sections are incubated in 3% hydrogen peroxide in PBS (phosphate buffered saline). Immunostaining are performed with a monoclonal antibody diluted 1:50 in 1% bovine serum albumin in phosphate buffered saline. Antibody detection is usually performed using a horseradish peroxidase (HRP)-labeled goat anti-mouse secondary antibody followed by staining with a 3, 3′-diaminobenzidine chromogen (DAB) solution. Finally, slides are counterstained with hematoxylin. Positive staining is considered the cells with brown stain with a dotty, linear, semicircular or circular pattern.

3. Histopathological features in alcoholic chronic hepatitis

Alcohol hepatotoxicity is well known and generally related to the amount and duration of excessive consumption of alcohol. Alcoholic liver disease is characterized by a spectrum of clinical manifestations of liver, morphological modifications (Table 1)(Delladetsima et al., 1987; Kondili et al., 2005; Lefkowich, 2005; Lackner et al., 2008), as well associated injuries.

A. Alcoholic steatosis (fatty liver)	
	1. Macrovesicular steatosis
	2. Microvesicular steatosis
	3. Mixed variant of steatosis
	4. Lipogranulomas
	5. Foamy fatty degeneration
B. Alcoholic steatohepatitis	
	1. Ballooned hepatocytes (cell swelling)
	2. Steatosis
	3. Inflammation
	4. Perivenular fibrosis
	5. Vein occlusion
C. Cirrhosis	
	1. Micronodular cirrhosis that progress to macronodular cirrhosis
D. Hepatocellular carcinoma	

Table 1. Morphological features in alcoholic liver chronic disease.

To establish the chronic character of liver disease three types of lesions proved to be definitive: portal inflammation, hepatocyte necrosis and fibrosis. For stabilization and determining the degree of chronic hepatitis can be taken in consideration other histopathological aspects: steatosis; lesions of biliary canaliculi which translates by swelling of biliary epithelial cells; intralobular degeneration lesions evidenced by presence of apoptotic bodies.

3.1 Steatosis

Alcoholic steatosis is the most common histopatological feature of chronic alcoholic liver disease, is the first manifestation of excessive alcohol consumption. In terms of histology is translated by the accumulation of lipid droplets in the form of vacuoles of various sizes in the cytoplasm. Hepatic steatosis is present under three forms: microvesicular, macrovesicular a and mixed. In microvacuolar form the lipid inclusions have small dimensions and they are evenly distributed in cytoplasm without changing the nucleus position while the macrovacuolar form is characterized by the presence of a single large vacuole, occupying the entire cytoplasm of the hepatocyte pushing the nucleus to the periphery. Although histologically can be traced all three forms, in most cases is present the macrovacuolar steatosis (Figure 1). Some authors use the term steatosis and steatohepatitis to designate the same lesion while alcohol can induce a pure steatosis without inflammatory components. At other patients alcohol induces an acute hepatitis superposed steatosis. Zonal distribution of steatosis in alcoholic liver disease involves initially zone three and then the acinar part of zone two following that in severe steatosis the distribution to be diffuse involving the entire acinus (Cornianu et al., 2007).

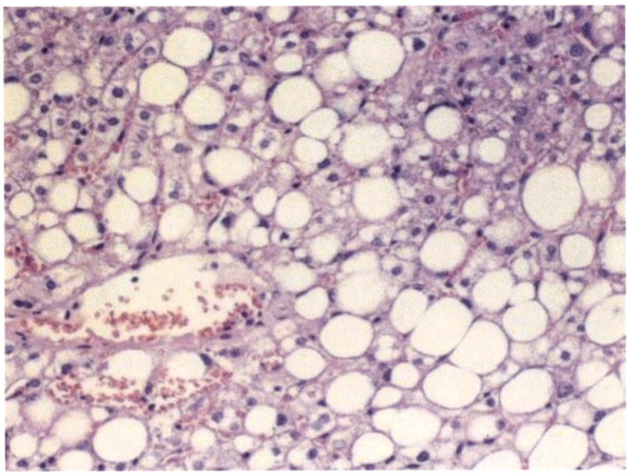

Fig. 1. Alcoholic chronic hepatitis, HE, x200 - panlobular macrovesicular steatosis with degenerative change.

3.2 Necroinflammatory process

The most important lesion in chronic hepatitis is "interface hepatitis" (piecemeal necrosis). Hepatocyte necrosis is with variable disposition and extension. It highlights coagulation necrosis of some isolated cells or Councilman acidophil bodies in periportal areas.

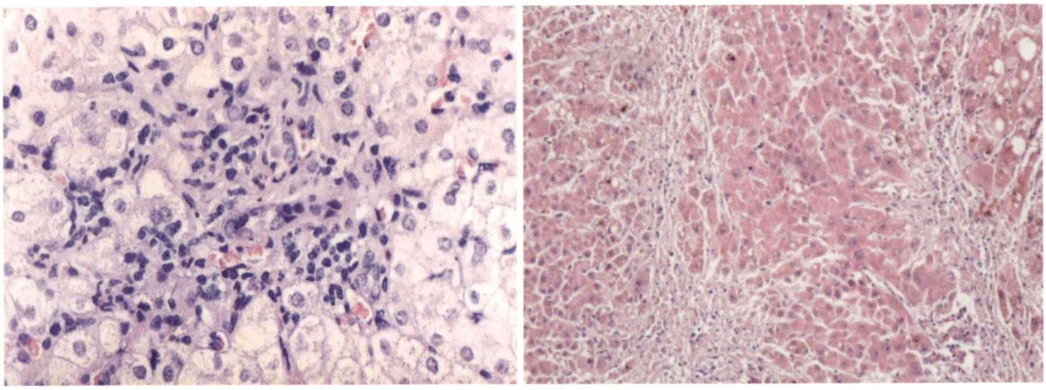

Fig. 2. Alcoholic chronic hepatitis. Focal necrosis, inflammatory infiltrate and acidophilic hepatocytes, HE, x200 (left). Bridging necrosis - large hepatocyte destruction (right).

Destruction of nearby group of hepatocytes located at the edge of liver parenchyma and portal connective structures, through cell-mediated immune mechanism, causes piecemeal necrosis. Unicellular necrosis located intralobular is betrayed by the presence of acidophil hepatocytes in an inflammatory outbreak. The infiltrative inflammatory process is made up of lymphocytes, plasmocytes but also of fibroblasts and fibrocytes (Figure 2). A more severe injury is confluent hepatic necrosis which forms porto-portal and porto-centrolobular bridges - bridging necrosis (Figure 2). Damaged hepatocytes place is taken by the collagen fibers and lymphocytes forming cords which linking the neighboring portal spaces and/or portal spaces and centrilobular veins. Association of periportal necrosis in bridges indicates a rapid progression to cirrhosis, in which the formed bridges become dense collagen septum which disorganizes the lobular architecture, forming hepatocyte nodules (Ishak, 2000).

3.3 Fibrosis

Fibrosis is an important element in chronic alcoholic hepatitis, being useful for the correct diagnosis, prognosis and the evolution of the disease. Toxic liver injury characterized by sinusoidal fibrosis, necrosis of pericentral hepatocytes, and narrowing and eventual fibrosis of central veins. The primary site of the toxic injury is represented by sinusoidal endothelial cells, followed by a circulatory compromise of centrilobular hepatocytes and fibrosis (De Leve et al., 2002). Liver cell necrosis is associated with varying degrees of perivenular, centrilobular, and pericellular fibrosis (Yip & Burt, 2006). Liver fibrosis is translated by a wide range of histopathological lesions:

- collagenization of the port areas (Figure 3)
- presence of bridging fibrosis porto-portal and porto-central fibrosis (as a consequence of disease progression) (Figure 3)
- perivenular fibrosis (Figure 4) (designated as a histological feature of alcoholic liver disease) – evidenced as a fibrous sleeve surrounding the terminal hepatic venula on at least two thirds of its circumference, being considered as a marker of progress to liver cirrhosis

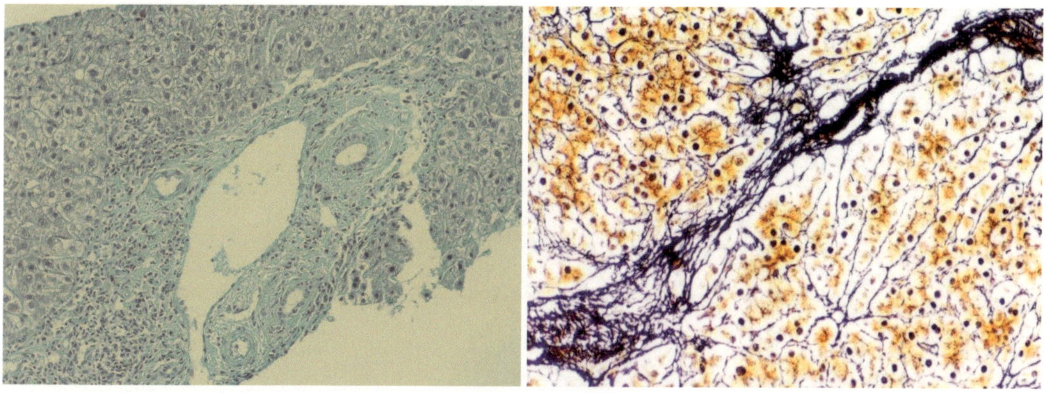

Fig. 3. Alcoholic chronic hepatitis. Portal fibrosis, Gömöri staining, x200 (left). Bridging fibrosis (porto-portal), silver staining, x200 (right).

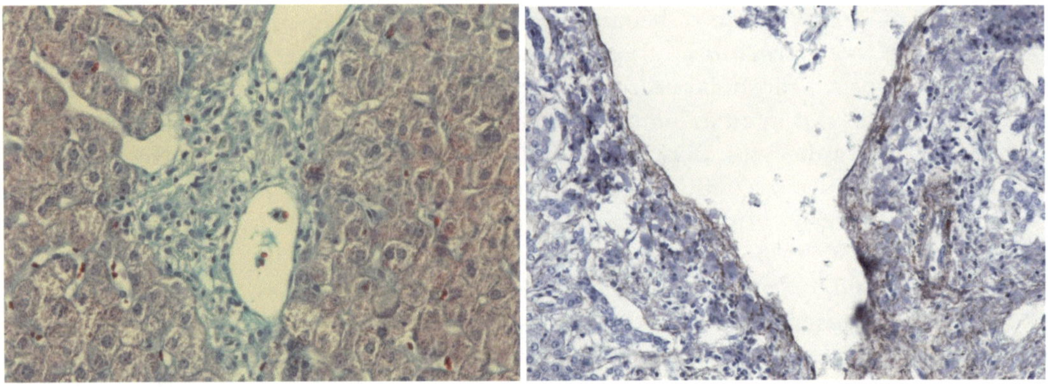

Fig. 4. Alcoholic chronic hepatitis - perivenular fibrosis. Gömöri staining, x400 (left) and Immunohistochemistry, collagen IV staining, x100 (right).

- collagenosis of the Disse space - capillarization of the hepatic sinusoids - accompanies progressive necroinflammation (Figure 5)
- regenerative nodules surrounded by fibrous connective septa (Figure 5)

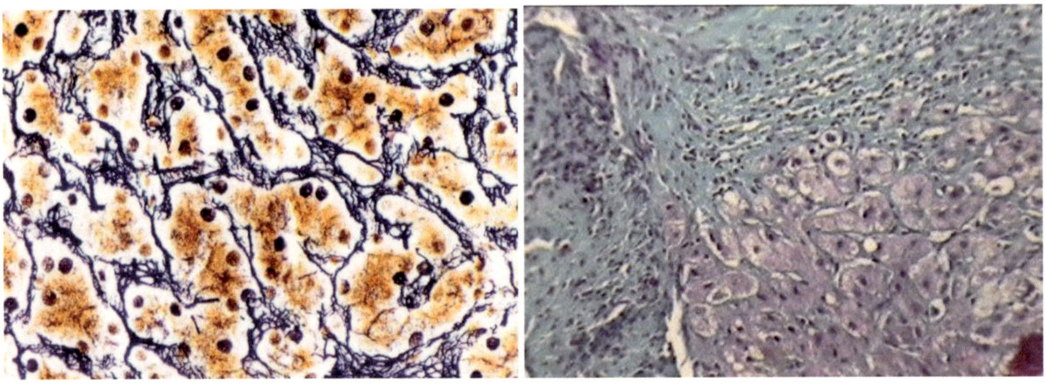

Fig. 5. Alcoholic hepatitis. Collagenization of the Diss space, silver staining, x400 (left) Fibrous connective septa, Gömöri staining, x400 (right).

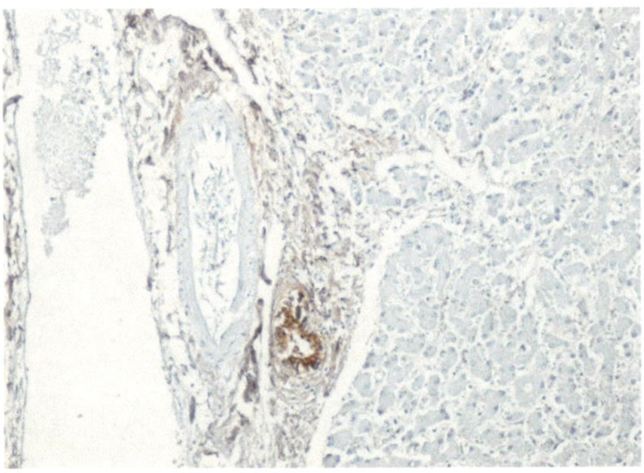

Fig. 6. Immunohistochemistry, collagen III positive staining at the portal area, x100.

In the fibrotic liver, the amounts of type III collagen (specific stroma) are increased not only in regions of portal fibrosis but also in the sinusoidal wall (Figure 6) (Sato et al., 2000). The first sign that the specific stroma participates in this liver injury is mirrored in the structure of the argyrophylic fibres. In the areas displaying of the hepatocytes necrosis, the process affects the argyrophylic fibres network of the specific stroma (Márcia Bersane et al., 2008). In an immunohistochemical study made on rat liver, Wei-Dong and collab., showed that in the normal liver, collagen I, III and IV is to be found at the level of the hepatic capsule, in the walls of blood vessels and in portal areas (Du et al., 1999). The hepatic sinusoids present positive reaction for collagen III and IV, but negative for collagen I (Marcia Bersane, 2008). Under pathological circumstances that engage the proliferation of the conjunctive tissue at hepatic level, numerous procollagen peptides-type IV and especially type III are formed in an excessive manner (Zhou et al., 2008). Collagen IV, being a constituent of the base membrane, accumulates in a precocious way both in viral hepatitis and in alcoholic hepatitis. Under conditions of viral or toxic aggression, collagen III and IV accumulates at the level of necrosis areas and along fibrous septa. In alcoholic hepatic fibrosis, increase the extracellular matrix protein expression of such as type III and IV collagen (Buck & Chojkier, 2003; Márcia Bersane, 2008; Bo et al., 2001; Fu et al., 2004). In the case of the alcoholic liver, in the fibroses areas, are detected an intensely positive reaction for collagen IV at the level of the portal tract and the central vein, but also at the level of Disse space, between the sinusoid cells and hepatocytes (Gorrellet al., 2003). After repeated injury, the extracellular matrix of basement membrane including type I, III, and IV collagen is over-deposited in perisinusoid (Li et al., 2005, Iwahashi et al., 2001).

4. Endothelial markers CD31 and CD34 expression and liver fibrosis

Under normal condition, the hepatic sinusoidal cells and the Kupffer cells express cell adhesion molecule like PECAM-1 (CD31) and ICAM-2 (intercellular cell adhesion molecule). Several studies were done to evaluate CD31 immunoreactions in liver disease, including alcoholic hepatitis. Ramadori et al. concluded that the expression pattern of CD31 is down regulated during inflammatory liver injury (Ramadori et al., 2008; Saile & Ramadori, 2007). In a study made on 103 patients with chronic viral and alcoholic hepatitis, Asanaza remarked that the pattern of the CD31 expression is negative in lymphocytes, in the bile epithelium cells, in the hepatocytes in the periportal area and in the central lobular area, but positive in sinusoidal endothelial cells, as well as at the level of the lobular and portal vessels, both in mild affections of the liver and in severe hepatic inflammation (Asanza et al., 1997; Garcia et al., 1998). Similar results were also emphasized in other studies, suggesting at the same time, that CD31 plays an essential part in the transendothelium migration of the leucocytes, and in livers may facilitate adhesion and transmigration of inflammatory cells (Chosay et al., 1998; Lalor et al., 2002; Neubauer et al., 2008). Chosay and colleagues investigate the role of PECAM-1in the pathophysiology of endotoxin-induced liver injury in a murine model. Their data showed that PECAM-1 is constitutively expressed on endothelial cells of large hepatic vessels, portal veins and arteries and hepatic veins, but not on sinusoidal endothelium (Chosay et al., 1998). The distribution of PECAM-1 in murine liver is similar to its distribution in human liver (Scoazec & Feldmann, 1991).

CD34 is preferentially expressed on the surface of regenerating or migrating endothelial cells and is a marker of proliferating endothelial cells in the growing sprouts during angiogenesis (Schlingemann et al., 1990). Microvessels stained by anti-CD34 are capillary-like, rather than having the appearance of sinusoids in normal liver (Poon et al., 2002). In nontumor liver tissues CD34 expression was mainly confined to small vessels in the portal area and also seen in sinusoids in the liver parenchyma near potral areas, with dotty, linear, semicircular and circular staining patterns. In tumor tissues, the characteristics of positive staining were similar to those in nontumor tissues. A study made on 324 patients with chronic alcoholic hepatitis, proved that the pattern of expression CD34 was moderately expressed in the periportal endothelium cells (Chedidi et. al., 2004). Some researchers have proved that CD34 is expresses in chronic hepatitis at the level the progenitor oval cells (Paku, 2001; Forbes et al., 2002; Weiss et. al., 2008).

In our recent study, we investigated the expression of the endothelial cell markers CD31 and CD34 to determine the degree of vascular distribution in alcoholic chronic hepatitis and compare it with liver fibrosis. The immunohistochemical technique was made in order to complete the histological study and in order to highlight certain particular aspects of the liver when under aggression of toxic agents.

We noticed an unspecific lesion pattern, with variable histological aspects both at the level of the parenchyma and at the level of the extracellular matrix. At the lobular level we noticed areas with apparently unaltered architectonics but also some altered areas caused by the enlargement of the port spaces as a result of the inflammatory processes and/or fibrosis. At the port level, we signaled inflammation of varied intensity. The infiltrative inflammatory process is made up of lymphocytes, plasmocytes but also of fibroblasts and fibrocytes. The perilobular inflammatory process turns into an interlobular one on some preparations, the inflammatory infiltrate having the same structure as the one present at the level of the port area. The capacity of the immune system cells to infiltrate the liver represent a consequence of the hepatic toxic injury and has been characterized in alcoholic hepatitis. Leukocyte infiltration into the liver parenchyma of immune cells includes monocytes, lymphocytes and neutrophils (Thiele et. al., 2004). At the cell level, especially at the cells in the peripheral lobule area, thus in the proximity of the portal areas, we identified hepatocytes which displayed alterations of degenerative type: micro- and macro-vesicular steatosis and balloon cell degeneration (Le Bousse-Kerdilès et al., 2008).

By means of the trichromic colorations applied in all the study cases, we were able to identify the collagenization of the port areas, the collagenosis of the Disse spaces, perivenular fibrosis, and the extension of the fibrosis under the form of real fibrosis bridges. Through this the hepatic lesions were grouped in: minimum, mild, moderate and severe; while for fibrosis was obtained a valor scale from 1 to 4. Conform to fibrosis scoring methods the pathologic grading of fibrosis may be grouped in four categories (Table 2) (Brunt, 2000).

Score	Description
0	No fibrosis
1	Stellate enlargement of portal tract but without septa formation
2	Enlargement of portal tract with rare septa formation
3	Numerous septa without cirrhosis
4	Cirrhosis

Table 2. Fibrosis Scoring.

Histological examination revealed no fibrosis (F0) in 8 patients (19,51%), stage 1 fibrosis (F1) in 6 patients (14,6%), stage 2 (F2) in 12 patients (29,2%), stage 3 (F3) in 12 patients (29,2%) and stage 4 (F4) in 3 patients (7,3%)(Figure 7).

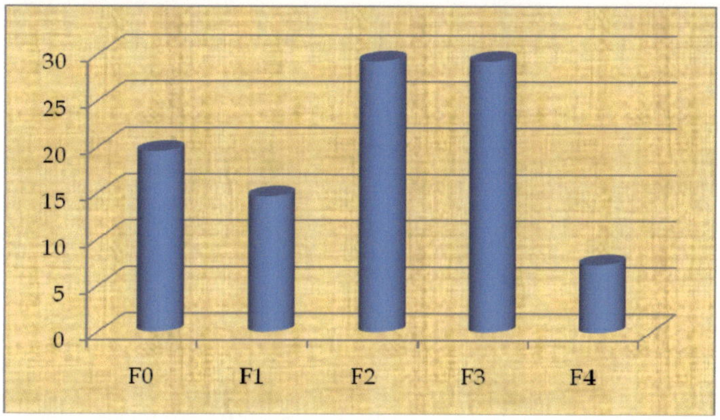

Fig. 7. The stage of fibrosis in patient with alcoholic liver disease.

In our study, all the cases with normal liver histology were CD31 and CD34 negative. By analyzing the immunohistochemical reaction for CD31 we have noticed that this one is negative for the central lobular area, but CD31-positive cells were observed in vessels of the portal area and in the sinusoids of the hepatic parenchyma near the portal area (Figure 8).

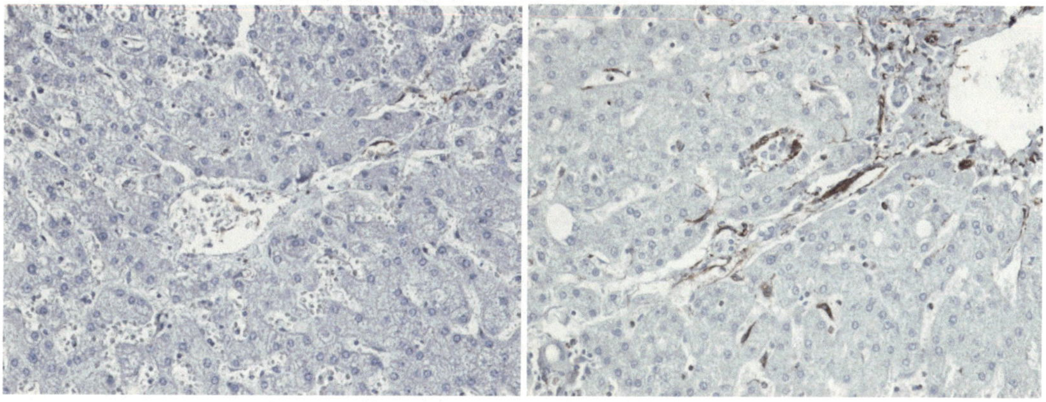

Fig. 8. Immunohistochemistry, anti CD31 staining, x100. Negative immunoexpression in central area (left) and positive expression in periportal space (right).

CD34 displays positive immunoreactions at the level of endothelium cells in the hepatic sinusoid in the periportal area, at the level of the central lobular vein as well as at the level of the venules and arterioles in the portal area (Figure 9) (Popescu et al., 2009).

CD34 pozitive reaction was found in 27,7% patients with F1 and F2 fibrosis and 73,3% patients with F3 and F4 fibrosis (Table 3). Additionally, the CD31 expression in all cases was mainly restricted to portal vessels and sinusoidal cells, in close relation with the periportal histological features or with inflammatory injury degree. CD31 pattern was positively expressed in 22,2% of cases with F1-F2 fibrosis and in 77,7% with F3-F4 of cases (Table 4).

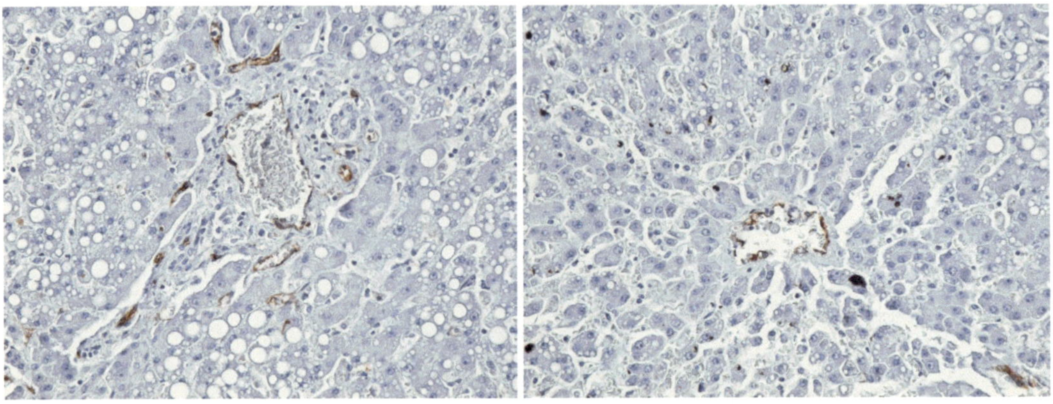

Fig. 9. Immunohistochemistry, anti CD34 staining, x100. CD34 expression in portal area (left) and central area (right).

CD 34	Stage F1 and F2	Stage F3 and F4
CD 34 positives cells	27.7%	73.3%

Table 3. Expression of CD34 in alcoholic liver.

CD 31	Stage F1 and F2	Stage F3 and F4
CD 31 positives cells	22.2%	77.7%

Table 4. Expression of CD31 in alcoholic liver.

Regarding correlation between stage of fibrosis and endolthelial cells markers, similar studies was done in liver disease. Akyol et al. investigate the relationships between the histopathological features of nonalcoholic fatty liver disease (NAFLD) and CD31 expression to identify hepatic stellate cell activation and capillarization. Their results showed a correlation between the fibrotic stage and CD31 expression, the highest staining scores of CD31 in zone 3, while the portal/septal area was the dominant zone for control groups (Akyol et al., 2005). On the other hand, angiogenesis plays an important role in chronic inflammation, accumulation of inflammatory infiltrate and fibrosis. In liver, angiogenesis is characterized by capillarization of the sinusoid. Also, Amarapurkar and colleague evaluate the expression of CD34, vascular endothelial growth factor (VEGF) and fibrosis in chronic liver disease (Amarapurkar et al., 2007). They report that none of patient with normal liver histology expressed the CD34 or VEGF positives cells. The capillarization and the histological change at the sinusoidal level occur with inflammation and fibrosis (Park et al., 1998). The degree of positivity increases with the stage of fibrosis. Also, they found significantly high expression of CD34 in hepatocellular carcinoma as compared to chronic disease. Increased vascular proliferation and pathological angiogenesis in hepatocellular carcinoma was reported in a comparison with chronic hepatitis and cirrhosis. The extracellular matrix affects the phenotype of the endothelial cells. The sinusoidal capillarization has the consequence the loss of endothelial fenestration and formation of variable amounts of basal membrane (Ichida et al., 1990; Semela & Dufour, 2004). Endothelial cells become positive for CD31 and CD34 and are used as indirect markers to detect microvascular density in liver carcinogenesis (Frachon et al., 2001).

5. Conclusion

To sum up, a direct correlation existed between endothelial cell markers CD31 and CD34 epression and the progression of fibrosis in alcoholic liver disease. The immunohistochemical methods of this molecule can be an important clue in future prognostic strategies.

6. References

Akyol, G; Erdem, O. & Yilmaz, G. (2005). Nonalcoholic fatty liver disease. Correlation with histology and viral hepatitis. *Saudi Medical Journal*, Vol.26, No.12, pp. 1904-1910, ISSN 0379-5284

Amarapurkar, A.D.; Amarapurkar, D.N.; Vibhav, S. & Patel, N.D. (2007). Angiogenesis in chronic liver disease. *Annals of Hepatology*, Vol.6, No.3, pp. 170-173, ISSN 1665-2681

Asanza, C.G.; Garcia-Monzon, C.; Clemente G.; Salcedo, M.; Garcia-Buey, L.; Garcia-Iglesias, C.; Ares, B.R.; Alvarez, E. & Moreno-Otero, R. (1997). Immunohistochemical Evidence of Immunopathogenetic Mechanisms in Chronic Hepatitis C Recurrence After Liver Transplantation. *Hepatology*, Vol.26, pp. 755-763, ISSN 0270-9139

Bataller, R. & Brenner, D.A. (2005). Liver fibrosis. *Journal of Clinical Investigation*, Vol.115, pp. 209-218, ISSN 0021-9738

Bo, A.H.; Tian, C.S.; Xue, G.P.; Du, J.H. & Xu, Y.L. (2001). Morphology of immune and alcoholic liver diseases in rats. *Shijie Huaren Xiaohua Zazhi*, Vol.9, pp. 157-160, ISSN 1007-9139

Brunt, E.M. (2000). Grading and staging the histopathological lesions of chronic hepatitis: The Knodell histology activity index and beyond. *Hepatology*, Vol.31, No.1, pp. 241-246, ISSN 0270-9139

Buck, M. & Chojkier, M. (2003). Signal transduction in the liver: C/EBPbeta modulates cell proliferation and survival. *Hepatology*, Vol.37, No.4, pp. 731-738, ISSN 0270-9139, Chedidi, A.; Arain, S.; Snyder, A.; Mathurin, P.; Capron, F. & Naveau, S. (2004). The Immunology of Fibrogenesis in Alcoholic Liver Disease. *Archives of Pathology & Laboratory Medicine*, Vol.128, pp. 1230-1238, ISSN 0003-9985

Chosay, J.G.; Fisher, M.A.; Farhood, A.; Ready, K.A.; Dunn, C.J. & Jaeschke, H. (1998). Role of PECAM-1 (CD31) in neutrophil transmigration in murine models of liver and peritoneal inflammation. *American Journal Physiology Gastrointestinal Liver Physiology*, Vol.274, pp. 776-782, ISSN 0193-1857

Cornianu, M.; Lazar, E.; Dema, A.; Taban, S. & Lazar, D. (2007). *Interpretarea biopsiei hepatice*, Edit. Eurobit, ISBN 978-973-620-335-0, Timisoara, Romania

Delladetsima, J.K.; Horn, T. & Poulsen, H. (1987). Portal tract lipogranulomas in liver biopsies. *Liver International*. Vol.7, No.1, pp. 9-17, ISSN 1478-3223

DeLeve, L.; Shulman, H.M. & McDonald, G.B. (2002). Toxic injury to hepatic sinusoids: sinusoidal obstruction syndrome (veno-occlusive disease). *Seminars in Liver Disease*, Vol.22, No.1, pp. 27-38, ISSN 0272-8087

DeLisser, H.M.; Christofidou-Solomidou, M.; Strieter, R.M.; Burdick, M.D.; Robinson, C.S.; Wexler, R.S.; Kerr, J.S.; Garlanda, C.; Merwin, J.R.; Madri, J.A. & Albelda, S. M. (1997). Involvement of endothelial PECAM-1/CD31 in angiogenesis. *American Journal of Pathology*, Vol.151, No.3, pp. 671-677, ISSN 0002-9440

Du, W.D.; Zhang, Y.E.; Zhai, W.R. & Zhou, X.M. (1999). Dynamic changes of type I, III and IV collagen synthesis and distribution of collagen-producing cells in carbon tetrachloride-induced rat liver fibrosis. *World Journal of Gastroenterology,* Vol. 5, pp. 397-403, ISSN 1007-9327

Forbes, S.; Vig, P. & Poulsom, R. (2002). Hepatic stem cells. *Journal Pathology,* Vol.197, pp. 510-518, ISSN 0022-3417

Frachon, S.; Gouysse, G.; Dumortier, J.; Couvelard, A.; Nejjari, M.; Mion, F.; Berger, F.; Paliard, P.; Boillot, O. & Scoazec, J.-Y. (2001). Endothelial cell marker expression in dysplastic lesions of the liver: an immunohistochemical study. *Journal of Hepatology,* Vol.34, No.6, pp. 850–857, ISSN 0168-8278

Fu Xu, G.; Wang, X.Y.; Ge, G.L.; Li, P.T.; Jia, X.; Tian, D.L.; Jiang, L.D. & Yang, J.X. (2004). Dynamic changes of capillarization and peri-sinusoid fibrosis in alcoholic liver diseases. *World Journal Gastroenterology,* Vol.10, No.2, pp. 238-243, ISSN 1007-9327

Garcia-Monzon, C.; Jara, P.; Fernandez-Bermejo, M.; Hierro, L.; Frauca, E.; Camarena, C.; Diaz, C.; De La Vega, A.; Larrauri, J.; Garcia-Iglesias, C.; Borque, M.J.; Sanz. P.; Garcia-Buey, L.; Moreno-Monteagudo, J.A. & Moreno-Otero, R. (1998). Chronic Hepatitis C in Children: A Clinical and Immunohistochemical Comparative Study With Adult Patients. *Hepatology,* Vol.28, No.6, pp. 1691-1701, ISSN 0270-9139

Gorrell, M.D.; Wang, X.M.; Levy, M.T.; Kable, E.; Marinos, G.; Cox, G. & McCaughan, G.W. (2003). Intrahepatic expression of collagen and fibroblast activation protein (FAP) in hepatitis C virus infection. *Advances in Experimental Medicine and Biology,* Vol.524, pp. 235-243, ISSN 0065-2598

Ichida, T.; Hata, K.; Yamada, S.; Hatano, T.; Miyagiwa, M.; Miyabayashi, C.; Matsui, S. & Wisse, E. (1990). Subcellular abnormalities of liver sinusoidal lesions in human hepatocellular carcinoma. *Journal of submicroscopic cytology and pathology,* Vol.22, No.2, pp.221–229, ISSN 1122-9497

Ishak, K.M. (2000). Pathologic Features of Chronic Hepatitis, *American Journal of Clinical Pathology,* Vol.113, pp. 40-55, ISSN 0002-9173

Iwahashi, M.; Muragaki, Y.; Ooshima, A. & Nakano, R. (2001). Overexpression of Type IV Collagen in Chorionic Villi in Hydatidiform Mole. *The Journal of Clinical Endocrinology & Metabolism,* Vol.86, No.6, pp. 2649-2652, ISSN 0021-972X

Kondili, L.A.; Taliani, G.; Cerga, G.; Tosti, M.E.; Babameto, A. & Resuli, B. (2005). Correlation of alcohol consumption with liver histological features in non-cirrhotic patients. *European Journal of Gastroenterology and Hepatology,* Vol.17, No.2, pp. 155-159, ISSN 0954-691X

Lalor, P.F.; Edwards, S.; McNab, G.; Salmi, M.; Jalkanen, S. & Adams, D.H. (2002). Vascular Adhesion Protein-1 Mediates Adhesion and Transmigration of Lymphocytes on Human Hepatic Endothelial Cells. *Journal of Immunology,* Vol.169, pp. 983-992, ISSN 0022-1767

Lackner, C.; Gogg-Kamerer, M.; Zatloukal, K.; Stumptner, C.; Brunt, E.M. & Denk, H. (2008). Ballooned hepatocytes in steatohepatitis: the value of keratin immunohistochemistry for diagnosis. *Journal Hepatology.* Vol.48, No.5, pp. 821-828, ISSN 0168-8278

Lefkowitch, J.H. (2005). Morphology of alcoholic liver disease. Clinics in Liver Disease. Vol.9, No.1, pp. 37-53, ISSN 1089-3261

Le Bousse-Kerdilès, M.C.; Martyré, M.C. & Samson, M. (2008). Cellular and molecular mechanisms underlying bone marrow and liver fibrosis: a review. *European Cytokine Network*, Vol.19, No.2, pp. 69-80, ISSN 1148-5493

Li, J.; Niu, J.Z.; Wang, J.F.; Li, Y. & Tao, X.H. (2005). Pathological mechanisms of alcohol-induced hepatic portal hypertension in early stage fi brosis rat model. *World Journal of Gastroenterology*, Vol.11, No.41, pp. 6483-6488, ISSN 1007-9327

Márcia Bersane, A.M.; Torres, I. & Coelho, K.I.R. (2008). Experimental poisoning by Senecio brasiliensis in calves: quantitative and semi-quantitative study on changes in the hepatic extracellular matrix and sinusoidal cells. *Pesq. Vet. Bras.*, Vol.28, No.1, pp. 43-50, ISSN 0100-736X

Matsumura, T.; Wol, K. & Petzelbauer, P. (1997). Endothelial cell tube formation depends on cadherin 5 and CD31 interactions with filamentous actin. *Journal of Immunology*, Vol.158, pp.3408-3416, ISSN 0022-1767

Neubauer, K.; Lindhorst, A.; Tron, K.; Ramadori, G. & Saile B. (2008). Decrease of PECAM-1-gene-expression induced by proinflammatory cytokines IFN-γ and IFN-α is reversed by TGF-β in sinusoidal endothelial cells and hepatic mononuclear phagocytes. *BMC Physiology*, Vol.8, pp. 9, ISSN 1472-6793

Newman, P.J. (1997). The biology of PECAM-1. *Journal of Clinical Investigation*, Vol.100, pp.25-29, ISSN 0021-9738

Park, Y.N.; Yang, C.P.; Fernandez, G.J.; Cubukcu, O.; Thung, S.N. & Theise, N.D. (1998). Neoangiogenesis and sinusoidal "capilarization" in dysplastic nodules of the liver. *American Journal of Surgical Pathology*, Vol.22, pp. 656-662, ISSN 0147-5185

Paku, S.; Schnur, J. & Nagy, P. (2001). Origin and structural evolution of the early proliferating oval cells in rat liver. *American Journal of Pathology*, Vol.158, pp.1313-1323, ISSN 0002-9440

Popescu, R.; Verdes, D.; Muntean, I.; Gotia, S.R. & Filimon, N. (2009). Alcoholic hepatitis histological and immunohistochemical study, *Annals of RSCB*, Vol. XIV, No.2, pp. 215-219, ISSN 1583-6258

Pusztaszeri, M.P.; Seelentag, W. & Fred, T. (2006). Bosman. Immunohistochemical Expression of Endothelial Markers CD31, CD34, von Willebrand Factor, and Fli-1 in Normal Human Tissues. *Journal of Histochemistry & Cytochemistry*, Vol.54, No.4, pp. 385-395, ISSN 0022-1554

Ramadori, G.; Moriconi, F.; Malik, I. & Dudas, J. (2008). Physiology and pathophysiology of liver inflammation, damage and repair. *Journal of Physiology and Pharmacology*, Vol.59, No.1, pp. 107-117, ISSN 0867-5910

Saile, B. & Ramadori, G. (2007). Inflammation, damage, repair and liver fibrosis-role of cytokines and different cell types. *Z. Gastroenterology*, Vol.45, pp. 77-86, ISSN 0016-5085

Sato, S.; Adachi, A.; Wakamatsu, K.; Sasaki, Y.; Satomura, K. & Asano, G. (2000). Abnormal elastic system fibers in fibrotic human liver. *Medical Electron Microscopy*,Vol.33, No.3, pp. 135-142, ISSN 0918-4287

Semela, D. & Dufour, J.F. (2004). Angiogenesis and hepatocellular carcinoma. *Journal of Hepatology*, Vol.41, pp. 864-880, ISSN 0168-8278

Scoazec, J. Y. & Feldmann, G. (1991). In situ immunophenotyping st udy of endothelial cells of the human hepatic sinusoid: results and functional implications. *Hepatology*, Vol.14, pp. 789-797, ISSN 0270-9139

Schlingemann, R.O.; Rietveld, F.J.; de-Waal, R.M.; Bradley, N.J.; Skene, A.I.; Davies, A.J.; Greaves, M.F.; Denekamp, J. & Ruiter, D.J. (1990). Leukocyte antigen CD34 is expressed by a subset of cultured endothelial cells and on endothelial abluminal microprocesses in the tumor stroma. *Lab. Invest.*, Vol.62, No. 6, pp. 690-696, ISSN 0023-6837

Thiele, G.M.; Duryeei, M.J.; Willisi, M.S.; Sorrelli, M.F.; Freemani, T.L.; Tumai, D.J. & Klasseni, L.W. (2004). Malondialdehyde-acetaldehyde (MAA) modified proteins induce pro-inflammatory and pro-fibrotic responses by liver endothelial cells. *Comparative Hepatology*, Vol.3, No.1, pp. 25, ISSN 1476-5926

Poon, T.N.R.; Oi-Lin Ng, I.; Lau, C.; Yu, W.C.; Yang, Z-F.; Fan, S.T. & Wong, J. (2002). Tumor Microvessel Density as a Predictor of Recurrence After Resection of Hepatocellular Carcinoma: A Prospective Study, *Journal of Clinical Oncology*, Vol.20, No.7, pp. 1775-1785, ISSN 0732-183X

Yip, W.W. & Burt, A.D. (2006). Alcoholic liver disease. *Semin Diagn Pathol.* Vol.23, No.3-4, pp. 149-60, ISSN 0740-2570

Zhou, Z.; Christofidou-Solomidou, M.; Garlanda, C. & DeLisser, H.M. (1999). Antibody against murine PECAM-1 inhibits tumor angiogenesis in mice. *Angiogenesis*, Vol.3, No.2, pp.181-188, ISSN 0969-6970

Zhou, Y.J.; Yao, H.Q.; Wang, J.; Wang, H. & Chen, Y.C. (2008). Influence of spleen-firming therapeutics on collagen fibers of hepatic fibrosis rat. *Journal of Chinese Clinical Medicine*, Vol.3, No.2, pp. 82-86, ISSN 1562-9023

Wang, L.T.; Zhang, B. & Chen, J.J. (2000). Effect of anti-fibrosis compound on collagen expression of hepatic cells in experimental liver fibrosis of rats. *World Journal Gastroenterology*, Vol.6, No.6, pp. 877-880, ISSN 1007-9327

Weiss, T.S.; Lichtenauer, M.; Kirchner, S.; Stock, P.; Aurich, H.; Christ, B.; Brockhoff, G.; Kunz-Schughart, L.A.; Jauch, K.W.; Schlitt, H.J. & Thasler, W.E. (2008). Hepatic progenitor cells from adult human livers for cell transplantation. *Gut*, Vol.57, pp. 1129-1138, ISSN 0017-5749

5

Ethanol-Induced Mitochondrial Induction of Cell Death-Pathways Explored

Harish Chinna Konda Chandramoorthy,
Karthik Mallilankaraman and Muniswamy Madesh
Department of Biochemistry, Temple University School of Medicine, Philadelphia, PA, USA

1. Introduction

Alcohol consumption is one of the major source for chronic liver diseases. It is striking that women are more susceptible to the toxic effects of alcohol although alcoholic liver disease (ALD) is common in men (*1*). In recent times, global burden on ALD has prompted researchers to investigate this disease based on age, gender, social status and race. However, in all these conditions and known variable severities of ALD, the basic pathophysiological condition is oxidative stress, which leads to liver damage (*1, 2*). In an overview, ALD leads to hepatocyte death, liver cirrhosis and organ dysfunction through production of reactive oxygen species (ROS), inflammatory cytokines and mitochondrial impairment. ROS are important mediators of apoptosis in liver diseases and are produced in response to paracrine factors such as ethanol (EtOH) (*2*). This chapter focuses on the role of EtOH induced ROS mediated cell death.

Over two decades, several pathways have been proposed in ALD. Recent studies have educated our understanding on these pathways, most of which work as cohort induced by direct/indirect effects of alcohol metabolism and clearance. Majority of cell death pathways (apoptosis, necrosis and the recently described necroptosis) converge at cellular damage associated with excessive production of ROS (superoxide ($O_2^{\bullet-}$) and hydrogen peroxide (H_2O_2)) that results in oxidative stress (*3, 4*). Under pathophysiological conditions, NAD(P)H oxidase, xanthine oxidase (XO) and the mitochondrial respiratory chain are the major sources of ROS. Normally, 5% of the metabolized cellular oxygen is converted into ROS which are effectively detoxified by endogenous antioxidants such as superoxide dismutase (SOD), glutathione peroxidase (GPx) and catalase (Cat). ROS overproduction resulting from acute and chronic exposure to alcohol can exceed the capacity of endogenous antioxidants (*5, 6*). Excessive ROS triggers various cellular signaling pathways leading to cell death in both vascular and epithelial cells. Although ROS is known to elicit liver damage, the signaling pathways operative in alcohol induced ROS overproduction in liver cells remain elusive.

Mitochondrial respiratory chain is the second major source of cellular ROS. However, mitochondria itself is an important target for cellular ROS resulting in mitochondrial dysfunction and permeabilization of outer mitochondrial membrane (OMM) (*7, 8*). In addition, studies have demonstrated that inhibition of mitochondrial electron transport results in ROS production leading to alteration in mitochondrial morphology and bioenergetics (*9*). Furthermore, OMM permeabilization leads to cytochrome *c* release and mitochondrial dysfunction (*10*).

Multidomain proapoptotic Bcl-2 family proteins are suggested to play a role in $O_2^{\bullet -}$ induced mitochondrial dysfunction (*11, 12*). Studies have shown that chronic EtOH consumption increases the expression of anti-apoptotic Bcl-2 and Bcl-x_L proteins by an interleukin-6-dependent mechanism (*13, 14*). Though, up regulation of proapoptotic Bax protein is observed in patients with ALD, the roles of Bax and Bak in initiating mitochondrial apoptotic events are poorly understood. Our previous studies have shown that $O_2^{\bullet -}$-mediated mitochondrial phase of apoptosis is mainly dependent on Bid but not Bax (*15, 16*).

Enhanced circulation of TNF-α and other cytokines have been reported in both ALD patients and animal models (*17*). In ALD, alcohol-induced $O_2^{\bullet -}$ elicits production of proinflammatory cytokine such as TNF-α which subsequently sensitizes hepatocyte cell death through gangliosides (*18-23*). Interestingly, in hepatocytes, TNF-α binds to either TNFR1 (type1 tumor necrosis factor receptor) or TNFR2 (type 2 tumor necrosis factor receptor) to initiate cell death. TNF-α mediated activation of apoptosis requires two adaptor molecules such as TNF receptor associated death domain protein (TRADD) and Fas – activated death domain protein (FADD). These in turn activate caspase 8 which further proteolytically cleaves downstream caspases and pro apoptotic bcl-2 family protein Bid. The active form of Bid (t-Bid) facilitates OMM permeabilization (*15*). On the other hand, ligation of TNF-α–TNFR1 recruits receptor-interacting protein 1 kinase (RIP1), TNFR death domain serine-theronine kinase 2 (TRAF2) which generates ceramide via activation of sphingomyelinases. Ceramide induces mitochondrial permeability transition pore (MPTP) opening, mitochondrial matrix swelling and membrane permeabilization, in concert with pro-apoptotic Bcl-2 family protein Bad (*24*). Recently our study has shown that TNF-α-induced necroptosis, the alternate form of cell death, requires TNFR adaptor protein FADD and NFκB downstream signaling molecule NEMO. FADD mediates the formation of necrosome consisting of RIP1-RIP3 kinases. The necrosome induced mitochondrial dysfunction in necroptosis requires Bax and Bak (*25*). TNFR1 mediated cell death is an extensively studied model and has been associated in many disease conditions including ALD.

Ca^{2+} has been known as an important intracellular second messenger that plays a dual role in cell survival and death. In liver, Ca^{2+} signaling is known to regulate a variety of cellular functions ranging from proliferation to apoptosis. Under pathological conditions, elevation in intracellular calcium ($[Ca^{2+}]_i$) facilitates cell death (*26, 27*) via inositol 1,4,5-triphosphate ($InsP_3$) (*28, 29*) and oxidation of STIM1(*30*). Inositol 1,4,5-triphosphate receptor ($InsP_3R$) mediated $[Ca^{2+}]_i$ changes leads to rapid Ca^{2+} release from ER and the subsequent Ca^{2+} entry through slow-activating plasma membrane store operated channels (SOC) (*31-33*). In hepatocytes, the Type II InsP3 R is known to trigger Ca^{2+} waves that can transmit through intercellular junctions throughout the liver (*34*). ER-mitochondria link and the mitochondrial Ca^{2+} ($[Ca^{2+}]_m$) uptake through uniporter is known to promote $[Ca^{2+}]_m$ overload which subsequently leads to mitochondrial depolarization and increased mROS production (*10, 28, 35, 36*). The aberrant Ca^{2+} homeostasis has been linked with ALD (*37, 38*). Despite the vast knowledge, the actual intricacies on the mechanism of Ca^{2+} induced mitochondrial dysfunction remain largely unexplored. In addition to the functional damage, the structural damage to the mitochondrion is known to play a very important role in accelerating EtOH induced apoptosis in hepatocytes. In support, a recent study has evidenced the mitochondrial structural changes (fig.1) in an animal model for ALD (39).

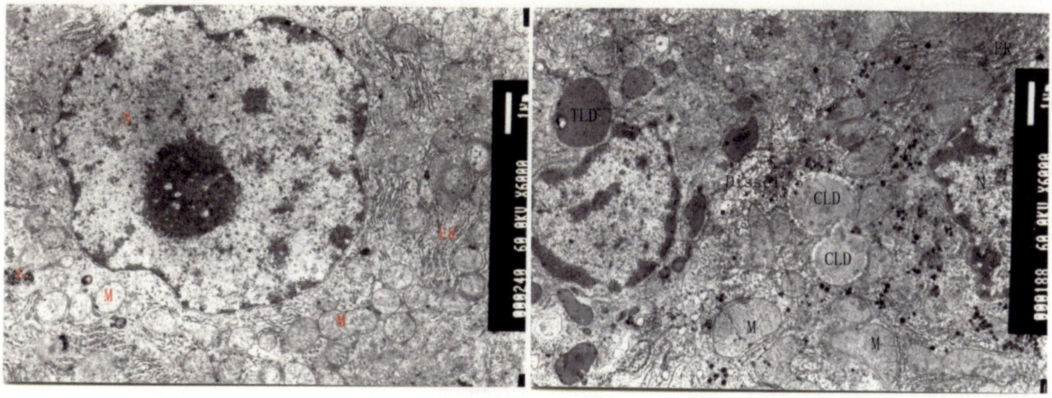

Fig. 1. Mitochondria appearance under electron microscope (EM × 6000); **A**: Mitochondria in normal group; **B**: Mitochondria in model group. M: mitochondria, G: glycogen, N nucleus, ER: endoplasmic reticulum, LD: lipid droplet. The long arrow shows abnormally distributed chromatin in nuclei, the short one is megamitochondrion and the arrow head is U-type mitochondria (Electron micrograph reproduced with permission from © 2007 Yan, M *et al.* Originally published in World J Gastroenterology 2007April 28;13(16): 2352-2356).

2. Role of ethanol in ROS production

Oxidative stress has been implicated to play a major role in ALD. The formation of reactive oxygen species (ROS) and reactive nitrogen species (RNS) represent an important cause of oxidative injury associated with free radical formation. ROS is known to damage and degrade lipids, proteins and DNA by which it affects the structure and function of the cell. Using animal models and samples from subjects with ALD, studies have shown the role of ROS in EtOH induced tissue damage (*40, 41*). Modification of mitochondrial proteins by ROS to disulphide, sulphenic, sulphinic and sulphonic residues and RNS to nitration products of tyrosine residues and nitrosation products of thiols have been well documented to occur in membrane and matrix proteins within mitochondria (*42, 43*). This section describes in detail the role of ROS in ALD. Oxygen is foremost common chemical frequently involved in the formation of free radical. Molecular oxygen is oxidized to generate two molecules of water by accepting four electrons and protons at one time. During this process several intermediary state of reactants exist like superoxide ($O_2^{\bullet-}$); peroxide (O_2^{2-}), which normally exists in cells as hydrogen peroxide (H_2O_2); and the hydroxyl radical ($OH^{\bullet}$). Superoxide, peroxide, and the hydroxyl radical are considered the primary free radicals. It has been estimated that only about 3 to 5 percent of the O_2 consumed by the mitochondrial respiratory chain is converted to ROS. Nevertheless, the toxic effects of oxygen in biological systems—such as oxidation of lipids, inactivation of enzymes, nucleic acid mutations and destruction of cell membranes are attributed to the reduction of O_2 to free radicals. The first and foremost effect of alcohol metabolism in the cellular milieu is the loss of NAD^+/NADH ratio that affects mitochondrial respiratory chain and subsequent generation of superoxide anion (*44*). In respect to EtOH induced ROS production, our laboratory has demonstrated that EtOH induced mROS production lead to mitochondrial morphology changes and functional alterations (Fig. 2). Briefly, (1) Acute delivery of EtOH (50mM) resulted in mitochondrial fragmentation (filamentous to globular morphology - fig.2A). (2) EtOH-fragmented mitochondria exhibit exaggerated $O_2^{\bullet -}$ production (fig.2B &C). (3) EtOH treatment induced elevated mROS, altered mitochondrial Ca^{2+} handling and mitochondrial dysfunction (fig.2D&E). (4) $O_2^{\bullet -}$ induced mitochondrial membrane potential ($\Delta\Psi_m$) loss and cytochrome *c* release was abrogated by the antiapoptotic Bcl-2 protein Bcl-xL and (5) Bax/Bak double knockout cells are resistant to $O_2^{\bullet -}$-mediated $\Delta\Psi_m$ loss and cytochrome *c* release, however, Bak but not Bax is essential for $O_2^{\bullet -}$-induced $\Delta\Psi_m$ loss and cytochrome *c* release (fig 3A-D).

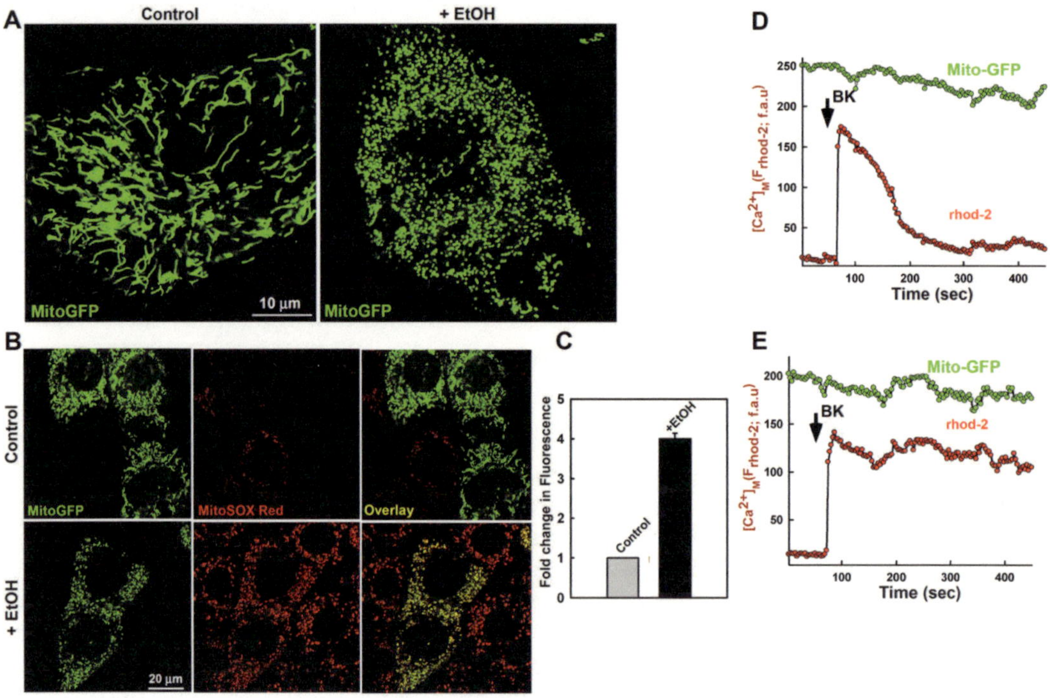

Fig. 2. EtOH augments alterations of mitochondrial morphology, $O_2^{\bullet -}$ production, and mitochondrial Ca^{2+} uptake in live cells. (A) Mito-eGFP (enhanced GFP)-expressing vascular endothelial cells (left panel) were exposed to 50 mM EtOH for 30 h (right panel). EtOH treatment resulted in short, globular mitochondrial tubules. (B) Mito-eGFP-expressing cells either left untreated (top) or exposed for 30 h to 50 mM EtOH (bottom) were loaded with the mitochondrion-derived $O_2^{\cdot -}$ indicator MitoSOX Red and imaged by confocal microscopy. EtOH-treated cells, but not control cells, displayed enhanced mitochondrial $O_2^{\bullet -}$ production. (C) Quantitation of mitochondrial ROS production in live cells. Following treatment, cells were loaded with the mitochondrial Ca^{2+} indicator rhod-2 for 45 min and stimulated with bradykinin (BK; 10 nM). Representative traces of mitochondrial Ca^{2+} uptake in response to bradykinin in (D) control and (E) EtOH-treated cells. EtOH-treated cells, but not control cells, displayed sustained mitochondrial Ca^{2+} elevation. f.a.u., fluorescence arbitrary units. (Reproduced with permission from © 2009 Madesh *et al*. Originally published in *Mol Cell Biol*. **2009** Jun;29(11):3099-112).

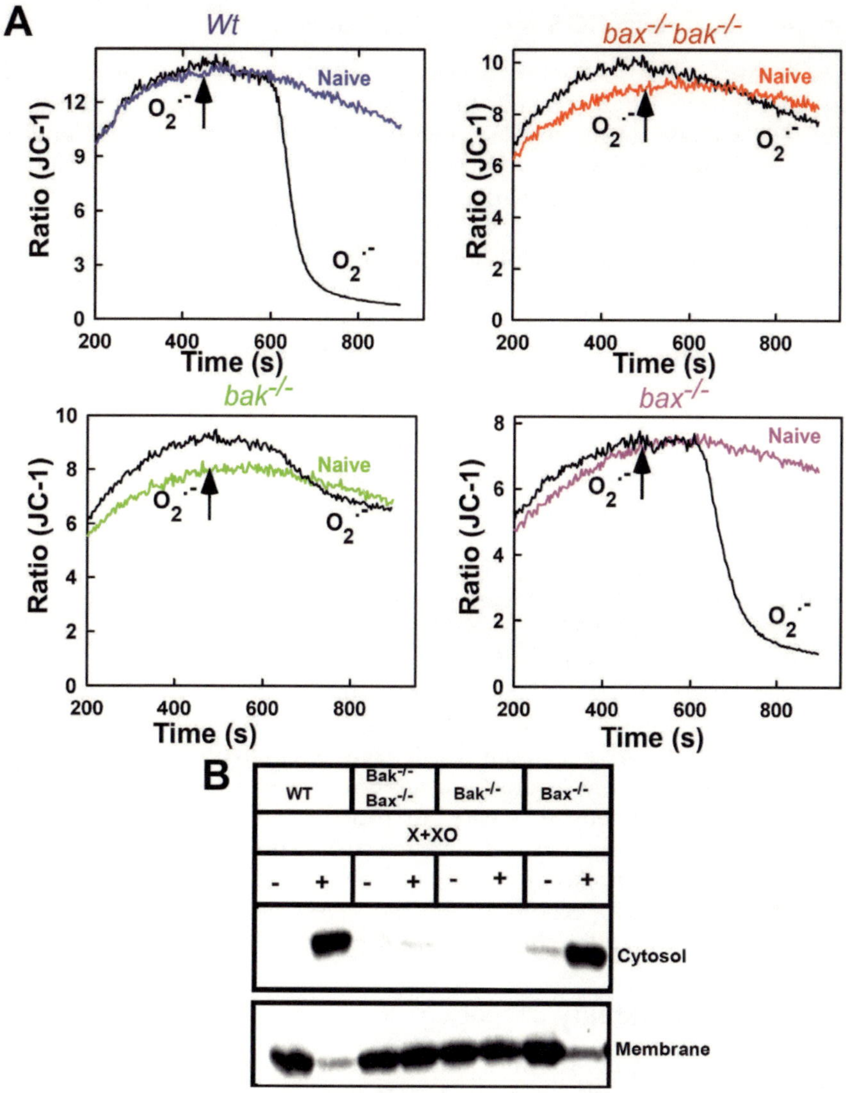

Fig. 3. (A) Wild type, *bax-/- bak-/-* double knockout, *bax-/-* and *bak-/-* MEFs were probed for cytochrome *c* in $O_2^{\bullet -}$-generating system. $\Delta\Psi_m$ was measured after $O_2^{\bullet -}$ treatment in permeabilized, TMRE-loaded *bax-/- bak-/-* MEFs expressing (B) GFP alone or together with (C) Bak or (D) Bax. Cells were exposed to the $O_2^{\bullet -}$-generating system or FCCP as indicated. (Reproduced with permission from © 2009 Madesh *et al*. Originally published in *Mol Cell Biol.* **2009** Jun;29(11):3099-112).

Taken together it is evident that $O_2^{\bullet -}$-evokes mitochondrial phase of apoptosis during chronic EtOH exposure. In addition, $O_2^{\bullet -}$ mediated tBid generation induces selective activation of mitochondrial Bak, triggering cytochrome *c* release and $\Delta\Psi_m$ loss that lead to apoptosis (*15*). Though mitochondria is known to play a crucial role in EtOH induced cell death, the upstream signaling molecules other than $O_2^{\bullet -}$ that target mitochondria is a open area of research in ALD.

3. Calcium and its role in ROS mediated apoptosis

$[Ca^{2+}]_m$ signals are known to control variety of responses in liver including apoptosis. Chronic EtOH exposure in rats leads to sustained Ca^{2+} elevation that triggers MPTP opening. MPTP opening leads to Ca^{2+} overload in the mitochondria and results in mitochondrial swelling a phenomenon observed in EtOH fed rats but not in control rats (*45*). Cells at basal metabolic rate tightly regulate free Ca^{2+} in the range of 100 to 200 nM in both cytosol and mitochondria through NCX (Na^+/Ca^{2+} exchanger), PMCA (Plasma membrane Ca^{2+}-ATPase) and SERCA (Sarcoendoplasmic reticulum Ca^{2+}-ATPase) pumps. Mitochondria play an important role in rapid uptake of Ca^{2+} through a uniporter and is then released slowly back into the cytosol (*46-48*). EtOH is known to induce elevated $[Ca^{2+}]_i$ by altering the $[Ca^{2+}]_m$ buffering capacity. Endothelial cells lining the capillaries and veins are first to encounter ethanol. Ethanol exposure activates the endothelial cells which are known to signal the immune cells. Our studies have previously shown ROS generation by activated macrophages evoked an $[Ca^{2+}]_i$ transient in endothelial cells (*28*). However sustained increase in $[Ca^{2+}]_i$ coupled with altered mitochondrial Ca^{2+} handling capacity leads to irreversible cell injury (*16, 28, 49*). Though, the exact source of increased cellular Ca^{2+} in ALD is poorly understood, several pathways have been proposed for the increased calcium flux. Receptor mediated pathways (G Protein-Coupled Receptor and tyrosine kinase receptor) that generate second messengers like $InsP_3$ which binds to $InsP_3R$ on endoplasmic reticulum trigger Ca^{2+} release (*50*). Further the $[Ca^{2+}]_m$ uptake was directly proportional to the magnitude of $[Ca^{2+}]_c$. Under pathophysiological conditions, the GPCR (G Protein-Coupled Receptor) Ca^{2+} linked mROS is essential for leukocyte/endothelial cell adhesion (*50*). EtOH exposure in HepG2 cells induces $[Ca^{2+}]_m$ overload that triggers mROS (fig 2D & E). In the cellular milieu, Ca^{2+} is compartmentalized as gradients in different organelles in the range of μM to nM (Ca^{2+}=ER>mitochondria>lysosomes>cytosol=nucleus). During ALD the alterations in Ca^{2+} homeostasis leads to $[Ca^{2+}]_m$ overload. Under pathological or physiological conditions $[Ca^{2+}]_m$ levels dictate the cells to program either towards cell death or survival signals in the liver. Accumulation of Ca^{2+} in mitochondria beyond the transition threshold opens the MPTP, resulting in $\Delta\psi_m$ loss, mitochondrial swelling, mROS overproduction and finally leading to cell death (*51*).

4. Mitochondrial permeability transition

Ca^{2+}-linked cell death program in ALD may be either apoptotic or necrotic phenomenon determined by OMM permeabilization and MPTP opening respectively. Ca^{2+} overload leads to oxidative stress that permanently leads to MPTP opening exposing the mitochondrial inner membrane permeable to all solutes of molecular weight up to 1.5Kd (39). Furthermore, the persistent MPTP opening leads to irreversible mitochondrial depolarization. Mitochondrial depolarization, in conjunction with mROS overproduction and subsequent inner mitochondrial membrane (IMM) damage sets the stage for apoptosis (*52*). A major pathway that leads to mitochondrial damage in a broad spectrum of inflammatory or ischemia-related conditions results from the amplification of mitochondrial and cytosolic $O_2^{\bullet-}$ production (*53*). ROS mediated cell death, in particular $O_2^{\bullet-}$-mediated apoptosis, begins with rupture of the outer mitochondrial membrane (OMM) and cytochrome *c* release that subsequently trigger MPTP opening resulting in mitochondrial swelling. MPTP opening is also known to be involved in initiation of the apoptotic machinery without damage to the OMM. ROS and $[Ca^{2+}]_m$ overload acts synergistically to trigger MPTP opening, and evokes cytochrome *c* release and subsequent activation of caspases (10).

$O_2^{\bullet-}$ or H_2O_2 exposure amplifies the Ca^{2+}-induced MPTP opening in a permeabilized cell system which in turn could be attenuated with either $O_2^{\bullet-}$ scavengers SOD or SOD mimetic, MnTBAP, or H_2O_2 scavenger catalase (fig 4A & B). However, $O_2^{\bullet-}$ -induced cytochrome *c* release was insensitive to inhibitors of MPTP (*16*). Thus, MPTP opening is not essential for $O_2^{\bullet-}$-induced cytochrome c release. In addition, exogenous delivery of cytochrome *c* eliminated the $O_2^{\bullet-}$ -induced $\Delta\Psi_m$ loss. These data suggest that integrity of the IMM and matrix space was preserved during $O_2^{\bullet-}$-induced cytochrome *c* release *(15, 16)*.

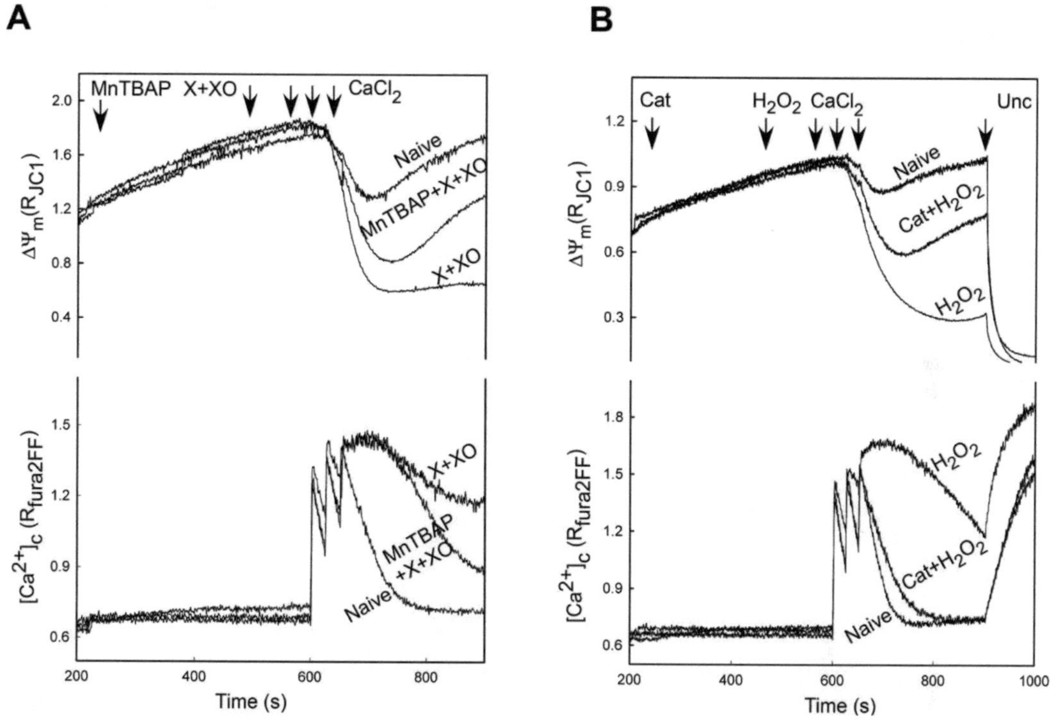

Fig. 4. Effect of ROS on Ca^{2+}-induced PTP opening and Cytochrome *c* release in permeabilized HepG2 cells. (A) $O_2^{\bullet-}$-generating system (xanthine [0.1mM] plus xanthine oxidase [20 mU/ml]) and (B) H_2O_2 (90 mM) augmented Ca^{2+}-induced depolarization (three pulses, 30 M $CaCl_2$ each) and decreased mitochondrial Ca^{2+} uptake. These effects were inhibited by an $O_2^{\bullet-}$-scavenger, MnTBAP (20 μM; 68 ±4.5% decrease in depolarization and 78 ±13% decrease in $[Ca^{2+}]_c$ rise at 900 s; n= 3), and catalase (Cat; 2500U/ml), respectively. At the end of the measurements, cells were exposed to FCCP (Unc; 1μM), a protonophore that caused rapid and complete dissipation of $\Delta\Psi_m$. (Reproduced with permission from © 2001 Madesh and Hajnóczky. Originally published in *J. Cell Biol.* 155:1003-1015).

5. Role of Bcl-2 family proteins in ROS-induced $\Delta\psi_m$ loss

Although ROS-induced Ca^{2+} dependent MPTP opening is associated with cytochrome *c* release, in particular, superoxide selectively triggers OMM permeabilization and cytochrome *c* release independent of Ca^{2+} dependant MPTP opening. $O_2^{\bullet-}$ produced by the mitochondrial respiratory chain has been reported to cause cardiolipid destruction in the IMM and dissipation of the $\Delta\Psi_m$ (*54, 55*). However, $O_2^{\bullet-}$ produced under various pathophysiological conditions including ALD, causes OMM permeabilization in a Bax/Bak dependant manner. Antiapoptotic Bcl-2 family protein Bcl-x_L prevents $O_2^{\bullet-}$-induced $\Delta\Psi_m$ loss and cytochrome *c* release, implying a role for proapoptotic Bcl-2 proteins Bax and Bak. Despite their high homology, Bax and Bak have distinct subcellular localization and functional regulation. Bax is largely a cytosolic protein that undergoes conformational change that is prerequisite for mitochondrial phase of apoptosis. In contrast, Bak is a mitochondrial integral membrane protein which undergoes oligomerization upon activation by proapoptotic BH3-only proteins (tBid). $O_2^{\bullet-}$-induced mitochondrial functional changes require either Bax or Bak. BH3 which constitute a subset of pro-apoptotic members of the Bcl-2 protein family are necessary to induce apoptosis (*10, 56*). $O_2^{\bullet-}$-mediated $\Delta\Psi_m$ loss and cytochrome *c* release is absent in Bax/Bak (*bax-/- bak-/-*) doubly deficient cells. Interestingly, Bak is necessary and sufficient for $O_2^{\bullet-}$-induced $\Delta\Psi_m$ loss and cytochrome *c* release. Mitochondria isolated from heart of *bak-/-* mice are resistant to $O_2^{\bullet-}$-induced mitochondrial depolarization. Further, *bid-/-* deficient MEFs are also insensitive to $O_2^{\bullet-}$-induced mitochondrial phase of apoptosis. Conversely, mitochondria from Bax-deficient mice display $O_2^{\bullet-}$-induced mitochondrial depolarization. Upon TNF, Fas ligand or $O_2^{\bullet-}$ challenge, the cytosolic BH3-only protein Bid undergoes proteolytic processing (caspase 8 and caspase 2) to generate active form of Bid-tBid. tBid elicited $O_2^{\bullet-}$-induced mitochondrial depolarization and cytochrome *c* release requires Bak. Taken together, these findings

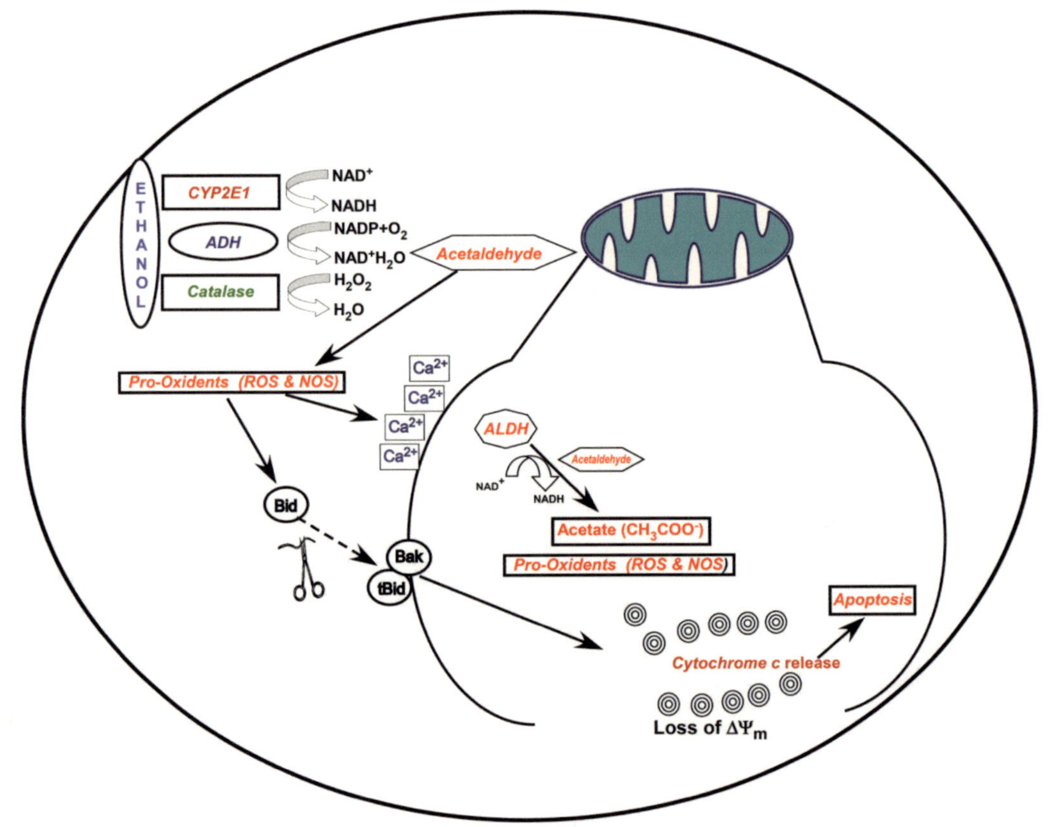

Fig. 5. Mitochondria are prime target for EtOH-induced cell death-Scheme.

implicate the requirement of Bak and Bid for $O_2^{\bullet -}$-induced $\Delta\Psi_m$ loss and cytochrome *c* release (*15, 16, 24, 10, 57*).

6. Conclusion

The aberrant rate of cell death is a hallmark of ALD. It is evident that ethanol induced ROS mediated oxidative stress is responsible for induction of apoptosis. The sequential events such as changes in redox status, increase in cytosolic ROS, sustained $[Ca^{2+}]_m$ elevation and translocation of pro-apoptotic proteins from cytosol to mitochondria are intimately linked with ethanol metabolism (fig 5). Major cell death pathways such as apoptosis, necrosis and the recently described necroptosis are associated with oxidative stress. Though, ROS production is proposed as a major factor in ethanol induced cell death little is known about the downstream mechanisms of the multimode cell death. In conclusion, mitochondria are prime target where multiple stress signaling pathways converge to induce cell death in the context of ALD.

7. Acknowledgements

This work was supported by the National Institutes of Health grant (R01 HL086699, HL086699-01A2S1, 1S10RR027327-01) to MM. We thank Yanling Zheng, Temple University for her great help in literature search.

8. References

[1] World Health Organization. *Global status report on alcohol and health*, World Health Organization, Geneva.
[2] Wu, D., and Cederbaum, A. I. (2003) Alcohol, oxidative stress, and free radical damage, *Alcohol Res Health 27*, 277-284.
[3] Shaw, S., Jayatilleke, E., Ross, W. A., Gordon, E. R., and Leiber, C. S. (1981) Ethanol-induced lipid peroxidation: potentiation by long-term alcohol feeding and attenuation by methionine, *J Lab Clin Med 98*, 417-424.
[4] Wheeler, M. D., Kono, H., Yin, M., Rusyn, I., Froh, M., Connor, H. D., Mason, R. P., Samulski, R. J., and Thurman, R. G. (2001) Delivery of the Cu/Zn-superoxide dismutase gene with adenovirus reduces early alcohol-induced liver injury in rats, *Gastroenterology 120*, 1241-1250.
[5] Finkel, T., and Holbrook, N. J. (2000) Oxidants, oxidative stress and the biology of ageing, *Nature 408*, 239-247.
[6] Thannickal, V. J., and Fanburg, B. L. (2000) Reactive oxygen species in cell signaling, *Am J Physiol Lung Cell Mol Physiol 279*, L1005-1028.
[7] Adrain, C., Creagh, E. M., and Martin, S. J. (2001) Apoptosis-associated release of Smac/DIABLO from mitochondria requires active caspases and is blocked by Bcl-2, *EMBO J 20*, 6627-6636.
[8] Vaughn, A. E., and Deshmukh, M. (2008) Glucose metabolism inhibits apoptosis in neurons and cancer cells by redox inactivation of cytochrome c, *Nat Cell Biol 10*, 1477-1483.
[9] Gonzalez-Flecha, B., Cutrin, J. C., and Boveris, A. (1993) Time course and mechanism of oxidative stress and tissue damage in rat liver subjected to in vivo ischemia-reperfusion, *J Clin Invest 91*, 456-464.

[10] Madesh, M., Zong, W. X., Hawkins, B. J., Ramasamy, S., Venkatachalam, T., Mukhopadhyay, P., Doonan, P. J., Irrinki, K. M., Rajesh, M., Pacher, P., and Thompson, C. B. (2009) Execution of superoxide-induced cell death by the proapoptotic Bcl-2-related proteins Bid and Bak, *Mol Cell Biol 29*, 3099-3112.
[11] Du, C., Fang, M., Li, Y., Li, L., and Wang, X. (2000) Smac, a mitochondrial protein that promotes cytochrome c-dependent caspase activation by eliminating IAP inhibition, *Cell 102*, 33-42.
[12] Mikhailov, V., Mikhailova, M., Degenhardt, K., Venkatachalam, M. A., White, E., and Saikumar, P. (2003) Association of Bax and Bak homo-oligomers in mitochondria. Bax requirement for Bak reorganization and cytochrome c release, *J Biol Chem 278*, 5367-5376.
[13] Kendrick, S. F., O'Boyle, G., Mann, J., Zeybel, M., Palmer, J., Jones, D. E., and Day, C. P. Acetate, the key modulator of inflammatory responses in acute alcoholic hepatitis, *Hepatology 51*, 1988-1997.
[14] Hong, F., Kim, W. H., Tian, Z., Jaruga, B., Ishac, E., Shen, X., and Gao, B. (2002) Elevated interleukin-6 during ethanol consumption acts as a potential endogenous protective cytokine against ethanol-induced apoptosis in the liver: involvement of induction of Bcl-2 and Bcl-x(L) proteins, *Oncogene 21*, 32-43.
[15] Madesh, M., Antonsson, B., Srinivasula, S. M., Alnemri, E. S., and Hajnoczky, G. (2002) Rapid kinetics of tBid-induced cytochrome c and Smac/DIABLO release and mitochondrial depolarization, *J Biol Chem 277*, 5651-5659.
[16] Madesh, M., and Hajnoczky, G. (2001) VDAC-dependent permeabilization of the outer mitochondrial membrane by superoxide induces rapid and massive cytochrome c release, *J Cell Biol 155*, 1003-1015.
[17] Hoek, J. B., and Pastorino, J. G. (2002) Ethanol, oxidative stress, and cytokine-induced liver cell injury, *Alcohol 27*, 63-68.
[18] Niemela, O., Parkkila, S., Pasanen, M., Iimuro, Y., Bradford, B., and Thurman, R. G. (1998) Early alcoholic liver injury: formation of protein adducts with acetaldehyde and lipid peroxidation products, and expression of CYP2E1 and CYP3A, *Alcohol Clin Exp Res 22*, 2118-2124.
[19] Thurman, R. G. (1998) II. Alcoholic liver injury involves activation of Kupffer cells by endotoxin, *Am J Physiol 275*, G605-611.
[20] Kishore, R., Hill, J. R., McMullen, M. R., Frenkel, J., and Nagy, L. E. (2002) ERK1/2 and Egr-1 contribute to increased TNF-alpha production in rat Kupffer cells after chronic ethanol feeding, *Am J Physiol Gastrointest Liver Physiol 282*, G6-15.
[21] Lemasters, J. J., Nieminen, A. L., Qian, T., Trost, L. C., Elmore, S. P., Nishimura, Y., Crowe, R. A., Cascio, W. E., Bradham, C. A., Brenner, D. A., and Herman, B. (1998) The mitochondrial permeability transition in cell death: a common mechanism in necrosis, apoptosis and autophagy, *Biochim Biophys Acta 1366*, 177-196.
[22] Hatano, E., Bradham, C. A., Stark, A., Iimuro, Y., Lemasters, J. J., and Brenner, D. A. (2000) The mitochondrial permeability transition augments Fas-induced apoptosis in mouse hepatocytes, *J Biol Chem 275*, 11814-11823.
[23] Hoek, J. B., Cahill, A., and Pastorino, J. G. (2002) Alcohol and mitochondria: a dysfunctional relationship, *Gastroenterology 122*, 2049-2063.
[24] Roy, S. S., Madesh, M., Davies, E., Antonsson, B., Danial, N., and Hajnoczky, G. (2009) Bad targets the permeability transition pore independent of Bax or Bak to switch between Ca2+-dependent cell survival and death, *Mol Cell 33*, 377-388.
[25] Irrinki, K. M., Mallilankaraman, K., Thapa, R. J., Chandramoorthy, H. C., Smith, F. J., Jog, N. R., Gandhirajan, R. K., Kelsen, S. G., Houser, S. R., May, M. J., Balachandran,

S., and Madesh, M. (2011) Requirement of FADD, NEMO and BAX/BAK for Aberrant Mitochondrial Function in TNF{alpha}-Induced Necrosis, *Mol Cell Biol.*

[26] Hajnoczky, G., Davies, E., and Madesh, M. (2003) Calcium signaling and apoptosis, *Biochem Biophys Res Commun 304*, 445-454.

[27] Orrenius, S., Zhivotovsky, B., and Nicotera, P. (2003) Regulation of cell death: the calcium-apoptosis link, *Nat Rev Mol Cell Biol 4*, 552-565.

[28] Madesh, M., Hawkins, B. J., Milovanova, T., Bhanumathy, C. D., Joseph, S. K., Ramachandrarao, S. P., Sharma, K., Kurosaki, T., and Fisher, A. B. (2005) Selective role for superoxide in InsP3 receptor-mediated mitochondrial dysfunction and endothelial apoptosis, *J Cell Biol 170*, 1079-1090.

[29] Szalai, G., Krishnamurthy, R., and Hajnoczky, G. (1999) Apoptosis driven by IP(3)-linked mitochondrial calcium signals, *EMBO J 18*, 6349-6361.

[30] Hawkins, B. J., Irrinki, K. M., Mallilankaraman, K., Lien, Y. C., Wang, Y., Bhanumathy, C. D., Subbiah, R., Ritchie, M. F., Soboloff, J., Baba, Y., Kurosaki, T., Joseph, S. K., Gill, D. L., and Madesh, M. S-glutathionylation activates STIM1 and alters mitochondrial homeostasis, *J Cell Biol 190*, 391-405.

[31] Putney, J. W., Jr., and Bird, G. S. (1993) The signal for capacitative calcium entry, *Cell 75*, 199-201.

[32] Parekh, A. B., and Penner, R. (1997) Store depletion and calcium influx, *Physiol Rev 77*, 901-930.

[33] Berridge, M. J., Bootman, M. D., and Lipp, P. (1998) Calcium--a life and death signal, *Nature 395*, 645-648.

[34] Hirata, K., Pusl, T., O'Neill, A. F., Dranoff, J. A., and Nathanson, M. H. (2002) The type II inositol 1,4,5-trisphosphate receptor can trigger Ca2+ waves in rat hepatocytes, *Gastroenterology 122*, 1088-1100.

[35] Pinton, P., Giorgi, C., Siviero, R., Zecchini, E., and Rizzuto, R. (2008) Calcium and apoptosis: ER-mitochondria Ca2+ transfer in the control of apoptosis, *Oncogene 27*, 6407-6418.

[36] Albano, E. (2006) Alcohol, oxidative stress and free radical damage, *Proc Nutr Soc 65*, 278-290.

[37] Pacher, P., and Hajnoczky, G. (2001) Propagation of the apoptotic signal by mitochondrial waves, *EMBO J 20*, 4107-4121.

[38] King, A. L., Swain, T. M., Dickinson, D. A., Lesort, M. J., and Bailey, S. M. Chronic ethanol consumption enhances sensitivity to Ca(2+)-mediated opening of the mitochondrial permeability transition pore and increases cyclophilin D in liver, *Am J Physiol Gastrointest Liver Physiol 299*, G954-966.

[39] Yan, M., Zhu, P., Liu, H. M., Zhang, H. T., and Liu, L. (2007) Ethanol induced mitochondria injury and permeability transition pore opening: role of mitochondria in alcoholic liver disease, *World J Gastroenterol 13*, 2352-2356.

[40] Arteel, G. E. (2003) Oxidants and antioxidants in alcohol-induced liver disease, *Gastroenterology 124*, 778-790.

[41] Chen, Y. L., Chen, L. J., Bair, M. J., Yao, M. L., Peng, H. C., Yang, S. S., and Yang, S. C. Antioxidative status of patients with alcoholic liver disease in southeastern Taiwan, *World J Gastroenterol 17*, 1063-1070.

[42] Bailey, S. M., Landar, A., and Darley-Usmar, V. (2005) Mitochondrial proteomics in free radical research, *Free Radic Biol Med 38*, 175-188.

[43] D'Autreaux, B., and Toledano, M. B. (2007) ROS as signalling molecules: mechanisms that generate specificity in ROS homeostasis, *Nat Rev Mol Cell Biol 8*, 813-824.

[44] Wu, D., and Cederbaum, A. I. (2009) Oxidative stress and alcoholic liver disease, *Semin Liver Dis 29*, 141-154.
[45] King, A. L., Swain, T. M., Dickinson, D. A., Lesort, M. J., and Bailey, S. M. (2010) Chronic ethanol consumption enhances sensitivity to Ca(2+)-mediated opening of the mitochondrial permeability transition pore and increases cyclophilin D in liver, *Am J Physiol Gastrointest Liver Physiol 299*, G954-966.
[46] Csordas, G., Varnai, P., Golenar, T., Roy, S., Purkins, G., Schneider, T. G., Balla, T., and Hajnoczky, G. Imaging interorganelle contacts and local calcium dynamics at the ER-mitochondrial interface, *Mol Cell 39*, 121-132.
[47] Berridge, M. J., Bootman, M. D., and Roderick, H. L. (2003) Calcium signalling: dynamics, homeostasis and remodelling, *Nat Rev Mol Cell Biol 4*, 517-529.
[48] Hajnoczky, G., Csordas, G., Madesh, M., and Pacher, P. (2000) The machinery of local Ca2+ signalling between sarco-endoplasmic reticulum and mitochondria, *J Physiol 529 Pt 1*, 69-81.
[49] Shi, Y., Inoue, S., Shinozaki, R., Fukue, K., and Kougo, T. (1998) Release of cytokines from human umbilical vein endothelial cells treated with platinum compounds in vitro, *Jpn J Cancer Res 89*, 757-767.
[50] Hawkins, B. J., Solt, L. A., Chowdhury, I., Kazi, A. S., Abid, M. R., Aird, W. C., May, M. J., Foskett, J. K., and Madesh, M. (2007) G protein-coupled receptor Ca2+-linked mitochondrial reactive oxygen species are essential for endothelial/leukocyte adherence, *Mol Cell Biol 27*, 7582-7593.
[51] Hawkins, B. J., Solt, L. A., Chowdhury, I., Kazi, A. S., Abid, M. R., Aird, W. C., May, M. J., Foskett, J. K., and Madesh, M. (2007) G protein-coupled receptor Ca2+-linked mitochondrial reactive oxygen species are essential for endothelial/leukocyte adherence, *Mol Cell Biol 27*, 7582-7593.
[52] Smaili, S. S., Hsu, Y. T., Carvalho, A. C., Rosenstock, T. R., Sharpe, J. C., and Youle, R. J. (2003) Mitochondria, calcium and pro-apoptotic proteins as mediators in cell death signaling, *Braz J Med Biol Res 36*, 183-190.
[53] Green, D. R., and Kroemer, G. (2004) The pathophysiology of mitochondrial cell death, *Science 305*, 626-629.
[54] Cohen, J. I., Chen, X., and Nagy, L. E. Redox signaling and the innate immune system in alcoholic liver disease, *Antioxid Redox Signal 15*, 523-534.
[55] Zamzami, N., Marchetti, P., Castedo, M., Decaudin, D., Macho, A., Hirsch, T., Susin, S. A., Petit, P. X., Mignotte, B., and Kroemer, G. (1995) Sequential reduction of mitochondrial transmembrane potential and generation of reactive oxygen species in early programmed cell death, *J Exp Med 182*, 367-377.
[56] Zamzami, N., Marchetti, P., Castedo, M., Zanin, C., Vayssiere, J. L., Petit, P. X., and Kroemer, G. (1995) Reduction in mitochondrial potential constitutes an early irreversible step of programmed lymphocyte death in vivo, *J Exp Med 181*, 1661-1672.
[57] Kim, H., Rafiuddin-Shah, M., Tu, H. C., Jeffers, J. R., Zambetti, G. P., Hsieh, J. J., and Cheng, E. H. (2006) Hierarchical regulation of mitochondrion-dependent apoptosis by BCL-2 subfamilies, *Nat Cell Biol 8*, 1348-1358.
[58] Wei, M. C., Lindsten, T., Mootha, V. K., Weiler, S., Gross, A., Ashiya, M., Thompson, C. B., and Korsmeyer, S. J. (2000) tBID, a membrane-targeted death ligand, oligomerizes BAK to release cytochrome c, *Genes Dev 14*, 2060-2071.

6

Cellular Signaling Pathways in Alcoholic Liver Disease

Pranoti Mandrekar and Aditya Ambade
University of Massachusetts Medical School, Department of Medicine, Worcester, USA

1. Introduction

The pathogenesis of acute and chronic alcohol consumption is complex with diverse consequences in different tissues. Alcohol abuse is associated with a continuum of liver abnormalities ranging from steatosis or fat deposition, steatohepatitis or fat plus inflammation to cirrhosis and hepatocellular carcinoma. The progression of alcohol-induced liver damage involves both parenchymal and non-parenchymal cells of the liver. The signaling pathways affected by direct or indirect alcohol exposure range from oxidative stress mechanims, metabolism related effects, inflammation, and apoptosis. Understanding the interactions of inter- and intra-cellular signaling pathways in the liver during alcohol exposure will aid in identification of new integrative approaches as it relates to alcoholic liver disease and provide potential new directions to develop therapeutic target intervention. The goal of this chapter is to review signaling pathways related to oxidative stress and inflammatory responses modulated by alcohol in parenchymal and non-parenchymal cells of the liver important to ALD. Here, we will first review liver cell types involved in alcohol-induced oxidative stress and inflammation resulting in hepatic injury and then discuss the signaling pathways identified in ALD.

2. Cell types involved in ALD

Research done, so far, on the effects of cellular stress pathways and immune cell activation during ALD indicates involvement of different liver cell types. Liver cells such as hepatocytes, Kupffer cells, endothelial cells, etc., are directly or indirectly affected by alcohol. Alcohol-induced oxidative stress in the liver microenvironment affects not only the resident liver cells but also circulating immune cells such as dendritic cells, neutrophils, T cells and bone-marrow derived stem cells that migrate to the liver, contributing to inflammatory responses and thus propagating alcoholic liver injury.

2.1 Hepatocytes

Hepatocytes make up 70-80% of the total mass of the liver and are involved in protein synthesis, protein storage and transformation of carbohydrates, synthesis of cholesterol, bile salts and phospholipids, and detoxification, modification and excretion of exogenous and endogenous substances. Chronic alcohol consumption has long been associated with progressive liver disease towards the development of hepatic cirrhosis and subsequent increased risk for developing hepatocellular carcinomas. Many of the deleterious effects of alcohol can be attributed to its metabolism primarily occurring in hepatocytes (Lu & Cederbaum, 2008).

Acute and chronic alcohol exposure increases the production of reactive oxygen species (ROS), lowers cellular antioxidant levels, and enhances oxidative stress in the liver (Cederbaum et al., 2009). Ethanol-induced oxidative stress plays a major role in the mechanisms by which ethanol sensitizes to liver injury (Cederbaum et al., 2009). In isolated hepatocytes, this damaging effect of chronic ethanol is evident in that a greater sensitivity to proapoptotic challenges is observed, more specifically, to the cytotoxic actions of tumor necrosis factor α (TNFα) (Hoek & Pastorino, 2004). The presence of alcohol results in an oxidative environment and TNFα mediated hepatocyte death (Pastorino & Hoek, 2000). Ethanol administration also facilitates apoptosis by increasing the amount of Fas protein expression on hepatocytes (McVicker et al., 2006). Besides ROS, reactive nitrogen species (RNS) generated in response to inducible nitric oxide synthase (iNOS) activation in hepatocytes during chronic alcohol exposure also contributes to liver injury (McKim et al., 2003). iNOS knock-out mice were protected from ALD (McKim et al., 2003). Ethanol promotes oxidative stress, not only by increased formation of ROS but also depletion of anti-oxidative defenses in hepatocytes. For instance, depletion of glutathione from mitochondria leads to increased accumulation of ROS (Fernandez-Checa et al., 1997).

The induction of mitochondrial dysfunction is also linked to the metabolism of alcohol by cytochrome P4502E1 (CYP2E1) and increased oxidative stress (Cederbaum et al., 2009). Primary hepatocytes and rat hepatoma cells when treated with ethanol led to an increase in ROS/RNS and loss of mitochondrial function due to damaged mitochondrial DNA and ribosomes and subsequent inhibition of mitochondrial protein synthesis (Mantena et al., 2007). These studies suggest that alcohol induced oxidative stress pathways in hepatocytes set the stage for proinflammatory cytokine induced cell death and alcoholic liver injury.

2.2 Kupffer cells or liver resident macrophages

Kupffer cells, non-parenchymal cells of the liver, are specialized macrophages located in the liver and their activation plays a central role in early ethanol-induced liver injury. In the universally accepted "two-hit" model of alcoholic liver injury, recognition of gut-derived endotoxin by the Kupffer cells is the first step leading to induction of pro-inflammatory responses (Thurman et al., 1999). Engagement of endotoxin with the Toll-like receptor 4 (TLR4) and CD14 receptor on Kupffer cells activates the down-stream kinases, interleukin-1 receptor associated kinase (IRAK) and I-kappa-B kinase (IKK) and transcription factor nuclear factor-κB (NFκB) and induction of pro-inflammatory cytokines such as TNFα (Takeda & Akira, 2005). Kupffer cells produce reactive oxygen species (ROS) in response to chronic alcohol exposure as well as endotoxin (Kono et al., 2000). Alcohol-induced sensitization to lipopolysaccharide (LPS) has been attributed to ROS production (Thakur et al., 2006a). Previous studies from Nagy and colleagues (Nagy, 2003) show that chronic ethanol feeding increases the sensitivity of Kupffer cells to LPS, leading to increased TNFα expression. This sensitization can be reversed by treatment of primary cultures of alcohol-exposed Kupffer cells with adiponectin, an anti-inflammatory adipokine (Thakur et al.,

2006b). Globular adiponectin prevents LPS-stimulated TNFα expression in Kupffer cells through the activation of the interleukin (IL)-10/STAT3/HO-1 (heme oxygenase-1) pathway (Mandal et al., 2010). In vivo pretreatment with diphenyliodonium (DPI), an inhibitor of NADPH oxidase, in alcohol-fed rats, normalized ROS production, decreased LPS-induced extracellular signal-regulated kinase (ERK1/2) phosphorylation and inhibited TNFα production in Kupffer cells (Kono et al., 2000; Thakur et al., 2006b). The importance of toll-like receptors (TLR) particularly TLR4 expressed on Kupffer cells plays a major part in ALD. Based on studies so far, it is perceivable that increased sensitization of Kupffer cells to endotoxin/LPS resulting in enhanced inflammatory responses contributes to alcoholic liver disease.

2.3 Dendritic cells

Dendritic cells (DCs) are central mediators of immune regulation, yet little is known about liver DCs. Myeloid DCs (mDCs), one of the most potent antigen-presenting cells (APC) in vivo, represent a terminally differentiated stage of monocytes (Palucka et al., 1998). Myeloid dendritic cells (mDCs) capture antigens in the periphery and then migrate to the lymphoid organs to initiate immunity (Steinman & Inaba, 1999). Alcohol-treated mDCs show reduced IL-12, increased IL-10 production, and a decrease in expression of the costimulatory molecules CD80 and CD86 (Mandrekar et al., 2004). Cytokine profiles of mDCs isolated from ethanol-fed mice indicate enhanced interleukin (IL)-1β and IL-10 and decreased TNFα, IL-12, interferon gamma (IFNγ), and IL-6 secretion (Aloman et al., 2007; Eken et al., 2011). Altered DC function is one of the major changes induced by long-term alcohol consumption, which subsequently impairs the cellular immune response. Chronic alcoholism in the absence of liver disease in patients is associated with an increased secretion of inflammatory cytokines by peripheral blood dendritic cells (Laso et al., 2007). Hepatic DCs from chronic alcohol-fed mice are less affected than splenic DCs, which exhibit impaired functional maturation following CpG stimulation (Lau et al., 2006). Thus, alcohol exerts a negative influence on innate and adaptive immunity leading to severe immunosupression (Lau et al., 2009). Inflammatory responses mediated by increased TNFα in liver fibrosis were associated with altered dendritic cell function (Connolly et al., 2009). Future studies are needed to identify signaling mechanisms contributing to DC dysfunction during chronic alcohol exposure.

2.4 Neutrophils

Neutrophils, the most abundant phagocyte constitutes 50% to 60% of the total circulating white blood cells and can secrete products that stimulate monocytes and macrophages. Neutrophil secretions increase phagocytosis and the formation of reactive oxygen compounds involved in intracellular killing (Soehnlein et al., 2008). In the alcoholic liver, damage by neutrophils can contribute to injury in response to the release of endotoxins produced by bacteria (Ricevuti, 1997). Neutrophil dysfunction in alcoholic hepatitis is associated with endotoxemia, increased expression of TLR2, 4, and 9 as well as energy depletion leading to increased incidence of infection (Stadlbauer et al., 2009). Augmentation of TLR 2, 4, and 9 did not improve phagocytic function of neutrophils, indicating that TLR overexpression may be the result and not the cause of neutrophil activation (Stadlbauer et al., 2009). Neutrophil contact with hepatocytes mediates oxidative killing of hepatocytes by initiation of oxidative-stress mediated respiratory burst and neutrophil degranulation leading to hepatocellular necrosis (Ramaiah & Jaeschke, 2007). Induction of osteopontin (OPN), an important mediator of inflammation regulated by oxidative stress pathways (Maziere et al., 2010) is the likely contributing factor for higher neutrophil recruitment to the liver in female rats during alcoholic steatohepatitis (Banerjee et al., 2006). Hepatic neutrophil infiltration can be largely inhibited in vivo by a neutralizing OPN antibody (Banerjee et al., 2006).

2.5 T cells

In alcoholic liver disease, the number of lymphocytes in the liver increases and the type and distribution of these infiltrating cells determines the nature of inflammation. Steatohepatitis is associated with a T helper (Th)1 cytokine response characterized by IFNγ and TNFα elevation, that reflects involvement of T lymphocytes, in particular $CD4^+$ T cells (Tiegs, 2007). In the liver, IL-17 secreting cells contribute to inflammatory infiltrates in alcoholic cirrhosis, and alcoholic hepatitis foci show many Th17 cells, including T lymphocytes and neutrophils (Lemmers et al., 2009). Chronic alcohol consumption significantly induces peripheral T cell lymphopenia in female C57BL/6 mice, up-regulates expression of CD43 on $CD8^+$ T cells, increases the percentage of interferon-γ-producing T cells; decreases the percentage of $CD8^+CD28^+$ T cells; and down-regulates the expression of CD28 on $CD4^+$ T cells (Gurung et al., 2009; Laso et al., 2000). In vivo bromodeoxyuridine incorporation in the same experiments demonstrated that chronic alcohol consumption increases proliferation of memory T cells, and accelerates peripheral T cell turnover (Zhang & Meadows, 2005). Patients with advanced ALD show a high prevalence of circulating IgG and T-lymphocytes towards epitopes derived from protein modification by hydroxyethyl free radicals (HER) and end-products of lipid peroxidation. In both chronic alcohol-fed rats and heavy drinkers the elevation of IgG against lipid peroxidation-derived antigens is associated with an increased production of pro-inflammatory cytokines/chemokines and severity of histological signs of liver inflammation (Albano & Vidali, 2009).

2.6 Natural killer (NK) and natural killer T (NKT) cells

Although a variety of cell populations infiltrate the liver during inflammation, it is generally assumed that CD8+ T lymphocytes promote while natural killer (NK) cells inhibit liver fibrosis (Park et al., 2009). NK cells inhibited liver fibrosis by directly killing activated hepatic stellate cells and production of gamma-interferon (IFNγ) (Jeong & Gao, 2008). In a chronic alcohol exposure model, poly I:C activation of NK cell cytotoxicity against hepatic stellate cells was attenuated in ethanol-fed mice compared with pair-fed mice, which was due to reduced natural killer group 2 member D (NKG2D), tumor necrosis factor-related apoptosis-inducing ligand (TRAIL), and IFNγ expression on NK cells from ethanol-fed mice (Jeong et al., 2008).

On the other hand, natural killer T cells (NKT) are an important subset of T lymphocytes and are unique in their ability to produce both Th1 and Th2 associated cytokines, thus being capable of steering the immune system into either inflammation or tolerance. Disruption of NKT cell numbers or function results in severe deficits in immune surveillance against pathogens and tumor cells. Experimental evidence suggests that hepatosteatosis may increase resident hepatic as well as peripheral NKT cells. The change in NKT cell numbers in animal models of alcohol-related hepatosteatosis are associated with a disruption of cytokine homeostasis, resulting in a more pronounced release of proinflammatory cytokines which renders the steatotic liver highly susceptible to secondary insults (Minagawa et al., 2004). In alcohol-fed animals, liver NKT cells increase, and further activation by alpha-galactosylceramide causes lethal liver injury (Minagawa et al., 2004). This can be explained by alcohol-induced hepatocyte sensitization to cell-mediated lysis, which develops concomitant to increased cytolytic activity of natural killer T cells. Alcohol-fed natural killer T cell-deficient mice exhibit a delay in alcohol-induced liver injury (Minagawa et al., 2004). In general, based on the tissue microenvironment, NK and NKT cells can accelerate early liver injury by producing proinflammatory cytokines and killing hepatocytes in an oxidative milieu.

2.7 Bone-marrow derived stem cells (BMSCs)

While maturation, activation, and proliferation of lymphoid cells occurs in secondary lymphoid organs (spleen, thymus, and lymph nodes), generation of these cells occurs from progenitor cells termed as bone marrow derived stem cells. Bone marrow derived stem cells were originally thought to contribute to liver repair based on the environmental insult but recent evidence suggests these cells may contribute to liver injury and fibrosis (Dalakas et al., 2010). Alcoholic hepatitis patients show increased CD34+ cell counts in liver tissue and in blood as compared with matched controls. Alcohol induced liver injury mobilizes CD34+ stem cells into circulation and recruits them into the liver. These bone marrow derived stem cells contribute to the hepatic myofibroblast population but not to parenchymal lineages and do not promote hepatocyte repair (Dalakas et al., 2010). Bone marrow stem cells generally reside in a hypoxic environment and increased reactive oxygen species (ROS) modulates their cell cycle allowing them to escape the bone marrow and affecting their self-renewal (Iwasaki & Suda, 2009). Recent studies show that acute alcohol exposure affects the hematopoeitic stem cell response to bacterial infections by inhibiting differentiation and impairing host defense in alcohol abusers (Raasch et al., 2010). Further Inokuchi et. al. (Inokuchi et al., 2011) indicate the importance of bone marrow derived cells in alcohol induced liver injury. Whether the effect of alcohol on stem cells links to alteration in immune and hepatocyte injury during ALD is unclear.

3. Signaling pathways and inflammation

3.1 Toll like receptors in ALD

Toll-like receptors (TLRs) are membrane-associated or endosomal and recognize distinct microbial components activating different signaling pathways by selective utilization of adaptor molecules (Takeda & Akira, 2005). TLRs mediate responses to a number of danger signals including extracellular pathogens and intracellular mediators such as ROS, high mobility group protein (HMGB)1, fibrinogen and heat shock proteins (hsps) (Lotze et al., 2007). The role of toll-like receptors (TLRs) and particularly TLR4 has been investigated in alcoholic tissue injury (Hritz et al., 2008; Uesugi et al., 2001; Inokuchi et al., 2011). Increasing evidence suggests that various TLRs, signaling components activated by TLRs play an important role in the pathogenesis of ALD. Figure 1 shows signaling adapters and kinases down-stream of TLRs, some of which have been directly or indirectly altered by alcohol exposure and implicated in liver injury. The cross-talk of stress regulated intracellular molecules with TLRs, intracellular kinases and transcription factors resulting in alterations in cytokines/chemokines in ALD are of great importance and need further investigation.

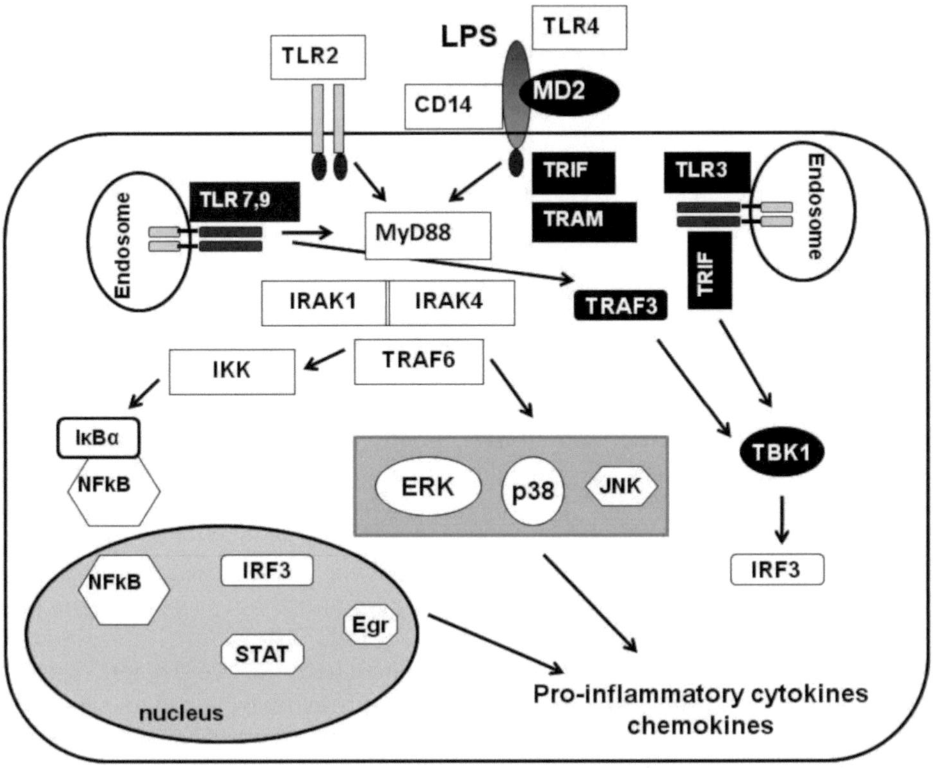

Fig. 1. Innate immune signaling in ALD. Toll like receptors particularly TLR4, in ALD, activate down-stream signaling adaptors, kinases and transcription factors to induce pro-inflammatory cytokines and chemokines. All signaling molecules that have been studied in ALD are identified by black color font whereas molecules not studied in ALD yet are seen in white color font.

Pattern recognition receptors (PRRs) are expressed on liver non-parenchymal and parenchymal cells and function as sensors of microbial danger signals enabling the vertebrate host to initiate an immune response. The complexity of cellular expression of PRRs in the liver provides unique aspects to pathogen recognition and tissue damage in the liver (Szabo et al., 2006). It is now well accepted that the innate immune system recognizes both damage (or danger)- and pathogen-associated molecular patterns (DAMPs and PAMPs, respectively) through pattern recognition receptors, such as Toll-like receptors (TLRs) and/or Nod-like receptors (NLRs). TLRs such as TLR4 and TLR2 that detect PAMPs for instance LPS and lipoproteins are located on the cell surface whereas TLRs such as TLR3, TLR7 and TLR9 that detect viral RNA and DNA are located in the endosome (Takeda & Akira, 2005). Engagement of LPS and activation of the CD14/TLR4 complex activates down-stream signaling molecules such as IRAK1/4, TRAF6 leading to activation of MAP kinases and NFκB in the liver (Mandrekar & Szabo, 2009). Recent studies by (Hritz et al., 2008; Inokuchi et al., 2011) indicate the requirement for TLR4 in alcohol induced steatosis. Oxidative stress also contributes to TLR4 signaling in macrophages and various other cell types in the liver via NADPH oxidase (Park et al., 2004). A pivotal role for NADPH oxidase in TLR4 mediated alcoholic liver injury has been recently shown (Hritz et al., 2008; Thakur et al., 2006a). Gustot et. al. (Gustot et al., 2006) also showed that oxidative stress regulates TLR 2, 4, 6 and 9 mRNA induction in alcoholic liver injury. In vivo alcohol exposure activates oxidative stress pathways and increases sensitization to TLR ligands, particularly TLR4, in alcoholic liver disease (Hritz et al., 2008; Gustot et al., 2006). TLR2 deficiency did not seem to have a significant effect on alcoholic liver injury (Hritz et. al., 2008).

The role of DAMPs in chronic liver diseases has been reported previously. Amongst the well characterized DAMPs, HMGB1, S100 proteins, hyaluronan and heat shock protein 60 (hsp60) are known to be recognized by TLR2 and TLR4 (Lotze et al., 2007) . In addition, necrotic or apoptotic cells are also recognized as DAMPs by TLRs (Sloane et al., 2010). In alcoholic liver injury, apoptotic bodies generated due to alcohol-induced oxidative stress could be recognized by DAMPs (McVicker et al., 2007) and thus play an important role in inflammatory responses in the liver.

3.2 IKK and MAPK signaling

Activation of TLR4 recruits IRAK-1 to the TLR4 complex via interaction with MyD88 and IRAK-4 (Takeda & Akira, 2005). The role of MyD88, the common TLR4 adaptor molecule was recently evaluated in a mouse model of alcoholic liver injury (Hritz et al., 2008). These studies showed that MyD88 knock-out mice were highly susceptible to alcohol-induced fatty liver (Hritz et al., 2008). While alcohol feeding in TLR4 deficient mice prevented liver injury, alcohol-fed MyD88 deficient mice showed increased oxidative stress and liver injury (Hritz et al., 2008). TLR4-induced MyD88-dependent and independent pathways lead to IKK kinase activation resulting in pro-inflammatory cytokine production (Takeda & Akira, 2005). Chronic alcohol exposure induces LPS-mediated IRAK-1 kinase activation in murine macrophages (Mandrekar et al., 2009).

Members of the mitogen-activated protein kinase (MAPK) family including extracellular receptor activated kinases 1/2 (ERK1/2), p38 and c-jun-N-terminal kinase (JNK) are activated down-stream of TLRs resulting in pro-inflammatory cytokine TNFα production (Weinstein et al., 1992). Chronic alcohol increases LPS-induced ERK1/2 activation and subsequent transcription of Egr-1, an immediate early gene transcription factor, contributing to expression of TNFα in murine hepatic macrophages (Kishore et al., 2002; Shi et al., 2002). LPS stimulation of Kupffer cells in vitro exposed to chronic alcohol in vivo exhibited increased p38 activity and decreased JNK activity (Kishore et al., 2001). Inhibition of p38 activation completely abrogated alcohol-mediated stabilization of TNFα mRNA likely via interaction with tristetraprolin (TTP) (Mahtani et al., 2001). Conversely, ERK1/2 inhibition did not alter TNFα mRNA stability but affected mRNA transcription in chronic alcohol exposed macrophages (Kishore et al., 2002).

3.3 Transcription factors and alcohol

TLR4-induced MyD88-independent signaling leads to activation of NFκB and/or interferon regulatory factor 3 (IRF3) resulting in induction of pro-inflammatory cytokines or Type I

IFN (Fig 1) (Kawai et al., 2001; Fitzgerald et al., 2003). Studies so far have shown that chronic alcohol exposure induces LPS/TLR4 mediated NFκB activation in human monocytes and macrophages contributing to production of pro-inflammatory cytokine, TNFα (Mandrekar et al., 2009). Other investigators found that activated IRF3 binds to the TNFα promoter in macrophages after chronic alcohol administration (Zhao et al., 2008) and induces TNFα production. While IRF3 in myeloid cells contributes to alcoholic liver injury, IRF3 and Type I interferons in parenchymal cells appears to be protective (Petrasek et. al., 2010). Whether NFκB and IRF3 in myeloid cells act in concert with each other to increase pro-inflammatory cytokines and liver injury is not yet clear. LPS stimulation of JNK leads to phosphorylation of c-jun and subsequent binding of c-jun to CRE/activator protein (AP)-1 site in the TNFα promoter (Diaz & Lopez-Berestein, 2000). Although chronic alcohol feeding decreased JNK activity without any effect on TNFα mRNA, short-term alcohol exposure increased JNK phosphorylation as well as AP-1 binding in the presence of combined TLR4 plus TLR2 stimulation (Oak et al., 2006) in human monocytes. Recent studies indicate a role for AP-1 in RANTES expression during alcohol mediated inflammation (Yeligar et al., 2009).

Alcoholic steatosis is associated with increased expression of genes regulating fatty acid synthesis and suppression of genes involved in fatty acid oxidation (Crabb & Liangpunsakul, 2006). Transcription factors like sterol regulatory element binding protein (SREBP) and peroxisome proliferator activated receptor (PPAR)α play a pivotal role in early alcoholic liver injury and rodent models as well as in vitro treatment with alcohol show downregulation of PPARα mRNA (Wan et al., 1995). Further, DNA binding activity of PPARα is significantly reduced resulting in decreased target gene expression after alcohol exposure (Galli et al., 2001). Decreased PPARα activity was accompanied by increased oxidative stress in the liver resulting in increased sensitization of TNFα induced liver injury (Crabb & Liangpunsakul, 2006). Further studies are needed to establish a direct relationship between oxidative stress, cytokines and hepatic fatty acid metabolism in alcoholic liver disease.

The role of STAT3, another transcription factor in alcoholic liver injury has been investigated (Gao, 2005). Compared with wild-type mice, Kupffer cells from alcohol-fed hepatocyte-specific STAT3KO mice produced similar amounts of ROS and hepatic proinflammatory cytokines compared to control mice. On the other hand, Kupffer cells from M/N-STAT3KO mice produced higher ROS and TNFα compared with wild-type controls. These results suggest that STAT3 in hepatocytes promotes ROS production and inflammation whereas myeloid cell STAT3 reduces ROS and hepatic inflammation during alcoholic liver injury (Horiguchi et al., 2008). Endothelial STAT3 seems to play an important dual role of attenuating hepatic inflammation and sinusoidal endothelial cell death during alcoholic liver injury (Miller et al., 2010). Thus, STAT3 may regulate liver injury during alcohol exposure in a cell-type dependent manner.

3.4 Anti-inflammatory pathways in ALD

Diminution of inflammatory gene expression to curb the inflammatory response during ALD is pivotal to development of injury. Various anti-inflammatory mediators such as IL-10, prostaglandins, transforming growth factor (TGF)-β (Schmidt-Weber & Blaser, 2004; Asadullah et al., 2003) have been identified to control the inflammatory response. In addition, intracellular signaling molecules such as IRAK-M, ST2, phosphoinositide (PI)3-

kinase (K), suppressor of cytokine signaling (SOCS) 1, A20 and single immunoglobulin IL-1R-related molecule (SIGIRR) (Han & Ulevitch, 2005) also contribute to the anti-inflammatory pathway. While chronic alcohol did not significantly affect IL-10 during alcohol exposure in wild-type mice (Hill et al., 2002), IL-10 deficient mice showed greater susceptibility to alcoholic liver injury due to increase in pro-inflammatory cytokines (Hill et al., 2002). These results suggest that anti-inflammatory cytokine IL-10 is unable to counter-regulate the sustained pro-inflammatory activation in the chronic alcoholic liver. Recent studies show that IL-10 was decreased in alcohol exposed Type-I IFN receptor deficient mice, indicating a role for Type I IFNs in induction of anti-inflammatory responses during ALD (Petrasek et al., 2011). Other immunoinhibitory molecules such as SOCS1 and SOCS3 and adiponectin appear to induce anti-inflammatory responses during ALD. Adiponectin is decreased after chronic alcohol feeding and treatment of mice with adiponectin (Thakur et al., 2006b) prevents alcohol-induced liver injury. This protective effect of adiponectin has been attributed to decreased LPS-induced ERK1/2 signaling resulting in normalization of TNFα production by Kupffer cells after chronic alcohol exposure (Thakur et al., 2006b). Additional studies to understand anti-inflammatory mechanisms will provide a better understanding of the contribution of these molecules in alcohol-induced liver injury.

4. Signaling pathways and hepatocyte injury

Alcohol-induced liver disease is linked to a state of "oxidative stress" and induction of cell death. Alcohol exposure, whether acute or chronic increases production of ROS, lowers the anti-oxidant systems, and results in enhancement of oxidative stress. The consequences of ROS generation in the alcoholic liver are widespread. Some ROS related effects of alcohol include oxidative stress induced by metabolizing enzymes such as CYP2E1, formation of adducts, stress at the level of the endoplasmic reticulum, stress-induced heat shock proteins, regulation of nuclear receptors, all leading to sensitization of hepatocytes to cellular injury and death.

4.1 Alcohol metabolism and oxidative stress

The classical pathway of alcohol metabolism involves enzymatic breakdown of alcohol by the enzyme, alcohol dehydrogenase and its subsequent conversion to acetaldehyde and formation of free radicals. In addition, the microsomal electron transport system also oxidizes ethanol via catalysis by the cytochrome P450 enzymes. The 2E1 isoform of the cytochrome P450 system is induced during chronic alcohol consumption and results in formation of ROS and increased generation of hydroxyl radicals (Cederbaum, 2001). The role of CYP2E1 in hepatocyte injury has been elucidated using HEPG2 cells expressing CYP2E1 (Wu & Cederbaum, 1996). Increased oxidative stress from induction of CYP2E1 in vivo sensitizes hepatocytes to LPS and TNF toxicity (Wu & Cederbaum, 1996). Oxidants, such as peroxynitrite, activation of p38 and JNK MAP kinases and mitochondrial dysfunction are downstream mediators of the CYP2E1-LPS/TNF potentiated hepatotoxicity (Lu & Cederbaum, 2009). Further, studies indicate that oral alcohol feeding of CYP2E1 knock-out mice prevents alcoholic liver injury and this may be due to inhibition of oxidative stress and up-regulation of PPARα (Lu et al., 2008). Oxidation of ethanol by alcohol dehydrogenase and subsequent metabolism of acetaldehyde results in increased NADH/NAD+ ratio in the cytoplasm and mitochondria. The increase in NADH results in inhibition of mitochondrial β-oxidation and accumulation of intracellular lipids leading to steatosis (Polavarapu et al., 1998; Wu & Cederbaum, 2003). Future studies on pathways activated by alcohol metabolism in various cell types of the liver would provide additional information to identify strategies to alleviate alcoholic liver injury.

4.2 Alcohol and protein adducts

Alcohol metabolism and oxidative stress results in the formation of reactive aldehydes such as acetaldehyde, malondialdehyde (MDA) and 4-hydroxy-2-nonenal (HNE) that can bind to proteins to form adducts. In vivo models of chronic alcohol consumption have shown that acetaldehyde, MDA and HNE adduct formation is increased in various organs including the liver. Acetaldehyde and MDA react with proteins synergistically to form hybrid protein adducts called malondialdehyde- acetaldehyde (MAA) adducts (Niemela et al., 1994). Recognition of MAA-adducts by Kupffer cells, endothelial and stellate cells via the scavenger receptor leads to upregulation of cytokine and chemokine production, and increased expression of adhesion molecules (Thiele et al., 2004; Duryee et al., 2005). Circulating antibodies to MAA-adducts were detected in patients with alcoholic hepatitis and cirrhosis and correlated with the severity of liver injury (Rolla, 2000). Although evidence suggests the existence of protein adducts during chronic alcohol consumption, their identification in animal models has been challenging and limits their role in pathogenesis of ALD.

4.3 ER stress and ALD

The unfolded protein response (UPR) that is a protective response of the cell is referred to as the ER stress response during pathological conditions. In alcoholic liver disease increased expression of GRP78, GRP94, CHOP and caspase-12 indicated a UPR/ER stress response (Kaplowitz & Ji, 2006). Up-regulation of ER-localized transcription factors and activation such as SREBP-1c and SREBP-2 was associated with increased lipid accumulation and induction of fatty liver during chronic alcohol (Ji et al., 2006). Another important inducer of ER stress, homocysteine, was increased in alcoholic human subjects leading to hyperhomocystenemia, also observed in alcohol feeding models (Ji & Kaplowitz, 2003). The role of ER stress in triglyceride accumulation and fatty liver comes from studies showing that betaine increases an enzyme, betaine homocysteine methyltransferase (BHMT) and reduces homocysteine levels to inhibit lipid accumulation (Ji & Kaplowitz, 2003). Although several studies suggests a pivotal role for ER stress in alcoholic liver disease, the alcohol-mediated mechanisms that trigger ER stress are not fully understood.

4.4 Alcohol and heat shock proteins

Stress or heat shock proteins (hsps) are ubiquitious, highly conserved proteins and originally identified for their cytoprotective function and assistance in the correct folding of nascent and stress-accumulated misfolded proteins. Oxidative stress induces heat shock proteins via activation of the heat shock transcription factor (HSF) (Finkel & Holbrook, 2000). Earlier studies on the effects of ethanol on the heat shock proteins in neuronal cells (Miles et al., 1991) showed that chronic alcohol increases Hsc 70 mRNA transcription and this may be important in neuronal adaptation and development of tolerance and dependence in alcoholics. Male Wistar rats fed with acute as well as chronic ethanol feeding (for 12 weeks) showed induction of hsp70 in the various regions of the brain and the liver (Calabrese et al., 1996; Calabrese et al., 1998). Hsp90 levels were also increased in cultured rat hepatocytes exposed to acute alcohol (Ikeyama et al., 2001). Studies have also shown that acute and chronic alcohol induces HSF activation and differentially induces hsp70 and hsp90 to affect inflammatory cytokine production in macrophages (Mandrekar et al., 2008). Comprehensive studies on the role of heat shock proteins and their chaperone function in the liver will provide further information to develop therapeutic strategies in ALD.

4.5 Alcohol and nuclear receptors

Nuclear receptors are a class of unique intracellular transcription factors that are activated by their ligands and can directly bind to DNA to regulate transcription of target genes that play key roles in development and cellular homeostasis (Wang & Wan, 2008). Three groups of nuclear receptors exist: the first is the classic steroid or thyroid hormone receptors such as glucocorticoid reeptor (GR) and thyroid receptor (TR), the second is the nuclear orphan receptors such as the nuclear receptor related-1 (Nurr-1) and neuron derived orphan receptor-1 (NOR1), the third class receptors that include the retinoid X receptor (RXR), peroxisome proliferators activated receptors (PPARs) and liver X receptor (LXR). It is the third class of nuclear receptors, particularly PPARs that are implicated in hepatic lipid metabolism and inflammatory processes and have been the main area of interest in alcohol-induced steatosis. Among various PPARs, the importance of PPARα in lipid metabolism and PPARγ in inflammatory processes is being investigated in alcoholic liver disease (Crabb & Liangpunsakul, 2006). PPARα dimerizes with another nuclear receptor, RXR to control transcription of target genes involved in free fatty acid transport and oxidation (Issemann & Green, 1990; Bocos et al., 1995). Whereas PPARγ is an essential regulator for adipocyte differentiation and lipid storage in mature adipocytes (Rosen & Spiegelman, 2001; Tsai & Maeda, 2005), both PPARα and PPARγ exert anti-inflammatory effects (Wang & Wan, 2008). Ethanol feeding of mice induced fatty liver injury and was accompanied by inhibition of transcriptional and DNA binding activity of PPARα, resulting in decreased expression of target genes such as carnitine palmitoyl transferase-1 (CPT-1) (Galli et al., 2001; Nakajima et al., 2004). Ethanol seemed to down-regulate RXR expression and PPARα levels to influence PPRE binding (Wan et al., 1995; Beigneux et al., 2000). Like hepatocyte-specific RXRα deficient mice, PPARα-null mice are more susceptible to alcohol-induced liver injury (Nakajima et al., 2004; Gyamfi et al., 2008). Treatment with PPARα agonists WY14643 resulted in increased expression of genes related to fatty acid oxidation and hence amelioration of alcoholic liver disease (Fischer et al., 2003). Thus, it appears that impaired activation of PPARα during ethanol consumption contributes to alcoholic fatty liver induction. Recent studies show that PPARα and γ agonists can reduce severity of chronic alcohol induced liver injury even in the context of continued alcohol consumption (de la Monte et al., 2011). Thus, nuclear localization of PPARs and their DNA binding partners, RXRs seem to play an important role in alcohol induced fatty liver injury.

4.6 Death receptor pathways: intrinsic and extrinsic

Chronic alcohol-induced hepatocyte apoptosis is a multifactorial process and involves interactions of oxidative stress and cytokines that activate death receptors and mitochondrial death pathways (Fig 2). Studies show that chronic alcohol-induced hepatocyte apoptosis occurs via the receptor-mediated pathway: TNFα and Fas receptors, and the intrinsic pathway: mitochondrial apoptotic pathway (Hoek & Pastorino, 2002). Activation of the death receptor pathways, Fas/FasL and TNFα/TNFR1 is strongly implicated in alcoholic liver disease (Hoek & Pastorino, 2002). Increased TNFα and TNF-R1 levels in animal models and humans with alcohol steatohepatitis have suggested an involvement of the TNFα/TNF-R1 pathway in hepatocyte killing (Pastorino et al., 2003; Pianko et al., 2000). Increased oxidative stress in chronic alcohol exposed rats promotes hepatocyte apoptosis and necrosis and is implicated in the alcohol-induced sensitization to the pro-apoptotic action of TNFα (Pastorino et al., 2003; Pastorino & Hoek, 2000). Additionally, TNFR1 knock-out mice, but not TNFR2 knock-out mice, were resistant to alcoholic liver injury (Yin et al., 2008) further strengthening a role for the TNFα/TNFR1

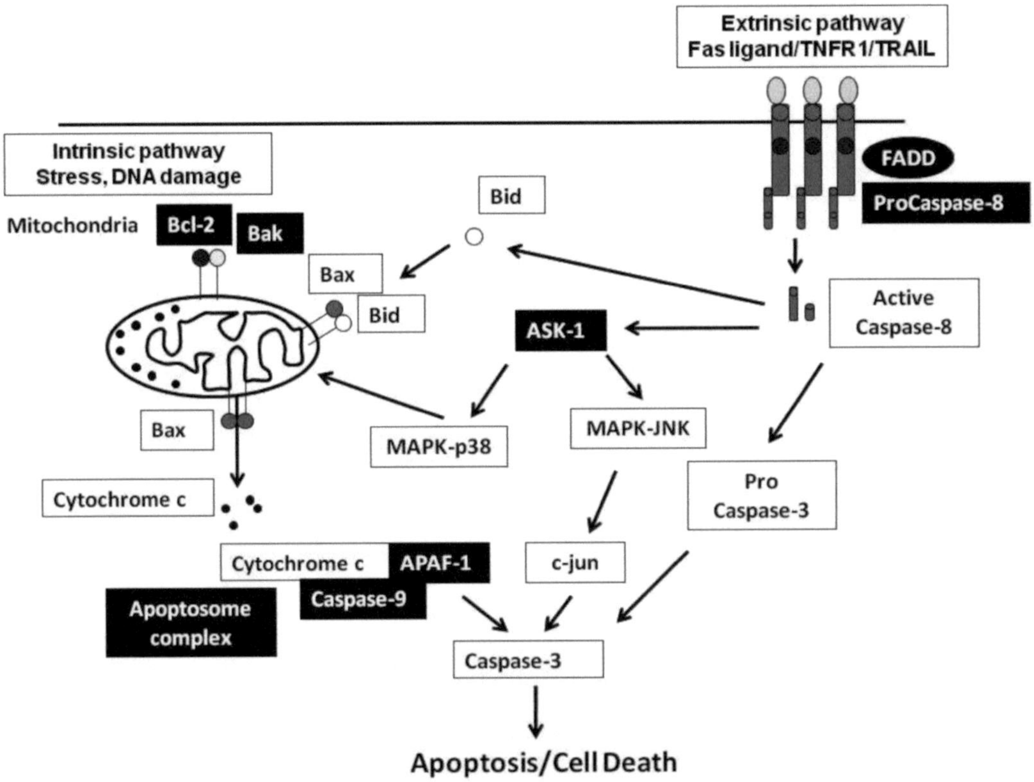

Fig. 2. Apoptotic signaling pathways in ALD. Two major apoptotic pathways are illustrated: one activated via death receptor activation ('extrinsic') and the other by stress-inducing stimuli ('intrinsic'). Triggering of cell surface death receptors of the tumour necrosis factor (TNF) receptor superfamily, including CD95 (Fas) and TNF-related apoptosis-inducing ligand (TRAIL)-R results in rapid activation of the initiator caspase 8 through the adaptor molecule Fas-associated death domain protein (FADD). In the intrinsic pathway, stress-induced apoptosis results in perturbation of mitochondria, release of cytochrome *c* and cell death. All signaling molecules that have been studied in ALD are identified by black color font whereas molecules not studied in ALD yet are seen in white color font.

pathway in alcoholic liver disease. Besides TNFα, FasL and Fas receptor expression were increased in livers of alcohol-fed mice (Deaciuc et al., 1999) leading to Fas-mediated cell killing, suggesting a significant role for the Fas/FasL pathway. Expression of Fas receptor also increased in human hepatocytes during alcoholic liver disease (Taieb et al., 1998).

Studies have shown that alcohol induced ROS generation leads to alteration in mitochondrial membrane permeability and membrane potential that in turn initiates the release of proapoptotic factors such as cytochrome c (Hoek & Pastorino, 2002; Hoek, 2002). Transition of mitochondrial permeability then results in increased caspase-3 activation in hepatocytes and this depends on p38 MAPK activation but is independent of caspase-8 (Pastorino et al., 2003; Pastorino & Hoek, 2000). Studies also implicate a role for MAP kinase, JNK2, independent of caspase-8, in TNF-induced mitochondrial death pathways (Schattenberg et al., 2006). The exposure of hepatocytes to ethanol induces ROS-mediated JNK activation, c-jun phosphorylation, Bid fragmentation, cytochrome c release and pro-caspase 3 cleavage (Cabrales-Romero Mdel et al., 2006). Whether alcohol affects JNK2 activation is not clear. But recent studies indicate a role for JNK1, but not JNK2, in CYP2E1 and TNFα mediated hepatoxicity (Wang et al., 2011). Chronic ethanol feeding also decreases ATP concentration associated with decreased viability in hepatocytes isolated from rats fed either high- or low-fat, ethanol-containing diets (Bailey & Cunningham, 1999). Various studies now show that decreased ATP synthesis accompanied by reduced mitochondrial protein synthesis, inhibition of the oxidative phosphorylation system (OxPhos) and damage to mitochondrial DNA leads to dysfunctional mitochondria in alcoholic liver disease (Bailey & Cunningham, 2002). Detailed studies of death receptors and mitochondrial sensitization mechanisms leading to hepatocyte death by alcohol will improve our understanding of ALD.

5. Therapeutic targets in ALD

While mechanistic studies have pointed to various therapeutic targets, abstinence from alcohol appears to be most effective in resolution of ALD. However, motivating patients to maintain sobriety, follow their compliance and prevent relapse are major obstacles in treatment of ALD. Pharmacotherapy using naltrexone and disulfuram assist in reducing or eliminating alcohol intake (Bouza et al., 2004; Williams, 2005). Nutritional therapy with supplementation of minerals like Zn (Kang & Zhou, 2005) and vitamins have been used to improve and attenuate alcoholic hepatitis. While multiple clinical trials have supported the use of glucocorticosteroids in patients with alcoholic hepatitis (McCullogh & O'Connor, 1998), their benefit still remains in question (Christensen, 2002). Considering the dysregulated inflammatory response in alcoholic hepatitis, various studies used specific anti-TNFα antibody therapy (Tilg et al., 2003) with little or no success. Complete neutralization of TNFα led to increased complications such as tuberculosis infections limiting its clinical utility. Future therapeutic interventions will thus have to be focused on partial attenuation of TNFα with lower infectious complications. Recent studies show that treatment with IL-22 ameliorates alcoholic liver injury in a mouse model of ALD (Ki et al., 2010). Based on induction of oxidative stress by alcohol, a combined regimen of anti-oxidant therapies including N-acetylsysteine and vitamins has been tested without significant differences in improvement rates of ALD (Stewart et al., 2007). Other alternative therapies using silymarin, S-adenosylmethionine and betaine have been suggested for future clinical trials (Frazier et al., 2011). While liver transplantation offers the most effective treatment, limited organ availability and post-transplant drinking dampen long-term outcomes. Future research combining biologics and anti-oxidant therapies may offer lasting therapeutic efficacies in ALD patients.

6. Conclusions and future directions

Alcoholic liver disease is a very complex and multifactorial disorder. Alcohol exerts its effects at many levels; individual signaling molecules, cells and finally the entire organ. Integrative approaches providing a comprehensive picture of how alcohol affects intracellular signaling pathways in tissues at different levels (Guo & Zhakari, 2008) is needed. A multidimensional analysis of inflammation and death signaling pathways in immune and non-immune cells of the liver to identify molecular targets in the host leading to systemic and organ inflammation will enhance our understanding of the pathogenesis of alcoholic liver disease. Until now various key signaling cascades triggered in the innate immune response such as toll-like receptor, interferon, NFκB and stress pathways such as ROS mediated activation of transcription factors, heat shock proteins or chaperones, mitochondrial damage and ER stress, have been viewed as separate entities rather than an integrated network of molecular interactions in alcoholic liver injury. A pathway diagram map which attempts to integrate these pathways will present a powerful aid for interpreting pathway interactions and highlight the valuable contributions of molecular interactions contributing to initiation and perpetuation of ALD. Future approaches to enable comprehensive analysis of these interactions could offer a powerful tool to understand diagnosis, prognosis, and treatment of ALD.

7. Acknowledgements

This work was supported by PHS grant # AA017545 (to PM) and AA017986 (to PM) from the National Institute of Alcohol Abuse and Alcoholism, NIH and and its contents are solely the responsibility of the authors and do not necessarily represent the views of the NIAAA.

8. References

Albano, E., & Vidali, M. (2009). Immune mechanisms in alcoholic liver disease. *Genes & Nutrition, 5(2),* 141-147.

Aloman, C., Gehring, S., Wintermeyer, P., Kuzushita, N., & Wands, J. R. (2007). Chronic ethanol consumption impairs cellular immune responses against HCV NS5 protein due to dendritic cell dysfunction. *Gastroenterology, 132*(2), 698-708.

Asadullah, K., Sterry, W., & Volk, H. D. (2003). Interleukin-10 therapy--review of a new approach. *Pharmacological Reviews, 55*(2), 241-269.

Bailey, S. M., & Cunningham, C. C. (2002). Contribution of mitochondria to oxidative stress associated with alcoholic liver disease. *Free Radical Biology & Medicine, 32*(1), 11-16.

Bailey, S. M., & Cunningham, C. C. (1999). Effect of dietary fat on chronic ethanol-induced oxidative stress in hepatocytes. *Alcoholism, Clinical and Experimental Research, 23*(7), 1210-1218.

Banerjee, A., Apte, U. M., Smith, R., & Ramaiah, S. K. (2006). Higher neutrophil infiltration mediated by osteopontin is a likely contributing factor to the increased

susceptibility of females to alcoholic liver disease. *The Journal of Pathology, 208*(4), 473-485.
Beigneux, A. P., Moser, A. H., Shigenaga, J. K., Grunfeld, C., & Feingold, K. R. (2000). The acute phase response is associated with retinoid X receptor repression in rodent liver. *The Journal of Biological Chemistry, 275*(21), 16390-16399.
Bocos, C., Gottlicher, M., Gearing, K., Banner, C., Enmark, E., Teboul, M., et al. (1995). Fatty acid activation of peroxisome proliferator-activated receptor (PPAR). *The Journal of Steroid Biochemistry and Molecular Biology, 53*(1-6), 467-473.
Bouza, C., Angeles, M., Munoz, A., & Amate, J. M. (2004). Efficacy and safety of naltrexone and acamprosate in the treatment of alcohol dependence: A systematic review. *Addiction (Abingdon, England), 99*(7), 811-828.
Cabrales-Romero Mdel, P., Marquez-Rosado, L., Fattel-Fazenda, S., Trejo-Solis, C., Arce-Popoca, E., Aleman-Lazarini, L., et al. (2006). S-adenosyl-methionine decreases ethanol-induced apoptosis in primary hepatocyte cultures by a c-jun N-terminal kinase activity-independent mechanism. *World Journal of Gastroenterology : WJG, 12*(12), 1895-1904.
Calabrese, V., Renis, M., Calderone, A., Russo, A., Barcellona, M. L., & Rizza, V. (1996). Stress proteins and SH-groups in oxidant-induced cell damage after acute ethanol administration in rat. *Free Radical Biology & Medicine, 20*(3), 391-397.
Calabrese, V., Renis, M., Calderone, A., Russo, A., Reale, S., Barcellona, M. L., et al. (1998). Stress proteins and SH-groups in oxidant-induced cellular injury after chronic ethanol administration in rat. *Free Radical Biology & Medicine, 24*(7-8), 1159-1167.
Cederbaum, A. I. (2001). Introduction-serial review: Alcohol, oxidative stress and cell injury. *Free Radical Biology & Medicine, 31*(12), 1524-1526.
Cederbaum, A. I., Lu, Y., & Wu, D. (2009). Role of oxidative stress in alcohol-induced liver injury. *Archives of Toxicology, 83*(6), 519-548.
Christensen, E. (2002). Alcoholic hepatitis--glucocorticosteroids or not? *Journal of Hepatology, 36*(4), 547-548.
Connolly, M. K., Bedrosian, A. S., Mallen-St Clair, J., Mitchell, A. P., Ibrahim, J., Stroud, A., et al. (2009). In liver fibrosis, dendritic cells govern hepatic inflammation in mice via TNF-alpha. *The Journal of Clinical Investigation, 119*(11), 3213-3225.
Crabb, D. W., & Liangpunsakul, S. (2006). Alcohol and lipid metabolism. *Journal of Gastroenterology and Hepatology, 21 Suppl 3*, S56-60.
Dalakas, E., Newsome, P. N., Boyle, S., Brown, R., Pryde, A., McCall, S., et al. (2010). Bone marrow stem cells contribute to alcohol liver fibrosis in humans. *Stem Cells and Development, 19*(9), 1417-1425.
de la Monte, S. M., Pang, M., Chaudhry, R., Duan, K., Longato, L., Carter, J., et al. (2011). Peroxisome proliferator-activated receptor agonist treatment of alcohol-induced hepatic insulin resistance. *Hepatology Research : The Official Journal of the Japan Society of Hepatology, 41*(4), 386-398.
Deaciuc, I. V., Fortunato, F., D'Souza, N. B., Hill, D. B., Schmidt, J., Lee, E. Y., et al. (1999). Modulation of caspase-3 activity and fas ligand mRNA expression in rat liver cells in vivo by alcohol and lipopolysaccharide. *Alcoholism, Clinical and Experimental Research, 23*(2), 349-356.
Diaz, B., & Lopez-Berestein, G. (2000). A distinct element involved in lipopolysaccharide activation of the tumor necrosis factor-alpha promoter in monocytes. *Journal of Interferon & Cytokine Research : The Official Journal of the International Society for Interferon and Cytokine Research, 20*(8), 741-748.

Duryee, M. J., Freeman, T. L., Willis, M. S., Hunter, C. D., Hamilton, B. C.,3rd, Suzuki, H., et al. (2005). Scavenger receptors on sinusoidal liver endothelial cells are involved in the uptake of aldehyde-modified proteins. *Molecular Pharmacology, 68*(5), 1423-1430.

Eken, A., Ortiz, V., & Wands, J. R. (2011). Ethanol inhibits antigen presentation by dendritic cells. *Clinical and Vaccine Immunology : CVI, 18*(7), 1157-1166.

Fernandez-Checa, J. C., Kaplowitz, N., Garcia-Ruiz, C., Colell, A., Miranda, M., Mari, M., et al. (1997). GSH transport in mitochondria: Defense against TNF-induced oxidative stress and alcohol-induced defect. *The American Journal of Physiology, 273*(1 Pt 1), G7-17.

Finkel, T., & Holbrook, N. J. (2000). Oxidants, oxidative stress and the biology of ageing. *Nature, 408*(6809), 239-247.

Fischer, M., You, M., Matsumoto, M., & Crabb, D. W. (2003). Peroxisome proliferator-activated receptor alpha (PPARalpha) agonist treatment reverses PPARalpha dysfunction and abnormalities in hepatic lipid metabolism in ethanol-fed mice. *The Journal of Biological Chemistry, 278*(30), 27997-28004.

Fitzgerald, K. A., Rowe, D. C., Barnes, B. J., Caffrey, D. R., Visintin, A., Latz, E., et al. (2003). LPS-TLR4 signaling to IRF-3/7 and NF-kappaB involves the toll adapters TRAM and TRIF. *The Journal of Experimental Medicine, 198*(7), 1043-1055.

Frazier, T. H., Stocker, A. M., Kershner, N. A., Marsano, L. S., & McClain, C. J. (2011). Treatment of alcoholic liver disease. *Therapeutic Advances in Gastroenterology, 4*(1), 63-81.

Galli, A., Pinaire, J., Fischer, M., Dorris, R., & Crabb, D. W. (2001). The transcriptional and DNA binding activity of peroxisome proliferator-activated receptor alpha is inhibited by ethanol metabolism. A novel mechanism for the development of ethanol-induced fatty liver. *The Journal of Biological Chemistry, 276*(1), 68-75.

Gao, B. (2005). Cytokines, STATs and liver disease. *Cellular & Molecular Immunology, 2*(2), 92-100.

Guo, M., Zakhari, S. (2008). Commentary: Systems Biology and its Relevance to Alcohol Research. *Alcohol Research and Health, 31*(1), 5-11.

Gurung, P., Young, B. M., Coleman, R. A., Wiechert, S., Turner, L. E., Ray, N. B., et al. (2009). Chronic ethanol induces inhibition of antigen-specific CD8+ but not CD4+ immunodominant T cell responses following listeria monocytogenes inoculation. *Journal of Leukocyte Biology, 85*(1), 34-43.

Gustot, T., Lemmers, A., Moreno, C., Nagy, N., Quertinmont, E., Nicaise, C., et al. (2006). Differential liver sensitization to toll-like receptor pathways in mice with alcoholic fatty liver. *Hepatology (Baltimore, Md.), 43*(5), 989-1000.

Gyamfi, M. A., He, L., French, S. W., Damjanov, I., & Wan, Y. J. (2008). Hepatocyte retinoid X receptor alpha-dependent regulation of lipid homeostasis and inflammatory cytokine expression contributes to alcohol-induced liver injury. *The Journal of Pharmacology and Experimental Therapeutics, 324*(2), 443-453.

Han, J., & Ulevitch, R. J. (2005). Limiting inflammatory responses during activation of innate immunity. *Nature Immunology, 6*(12), 1198-1205.

Hill, D. B., D'Souza, N. B., Lee, E. Y., Burikhanov, R., Deaciuc, I. V., & de Villiers, W. J. (2002). A role for interleukin-10 in alcohol-induced liver sensitization to bacterial lipopolysaccharide. *Alcoholism, Clinical and Experimental Research, 26*(1), 74-82.

Hoek, J. B., Cahill, A., & Pastorino, J. G. (2002). Alcohol and mitochondria: A dysfunctional relationship. *Gastroenterology, 122*(7), 2049-2063.

Hoek, J. B., & Pastorino, J. G. (2004). Cellular signaling mechanisms in alcohol-induced liver damage. *Seminars in Liver Disease, 24*(3), 257-272.

Hoek, J. B., & Pastorino, J. G. (2002). Ethanol, oxidative stress, and cytokine-induced liver cell injury. *Alcohol (Fayetteville, N.Y.), 27*(1), 63-68.

Horiguchi, N., Wang, L., Mukhopadhyay, P., Park, O., Jeong, W. I., Lafdil, F., et al. (2008). Cell type-dependent pro- and anti-inflammatory role of signal transducer and activator of transcription 3 in alcoholic liver injury. *Gastroenterology, 134*(4), 1148-1158.

Hritz, I., Mandrekar, P., Velayudham, A., Catalano, D., Dolganiuc, A., Kodys, K., et al. (2008). The critical role of toll-like receptor (TLR) 4 in alcoholic liver disease is independent of the common TLR adapter MyD88. *Hepatology (Baltimore, Md.), 48*(4), 1224-1231.

Ikeyama, S., Kusumoto, K., Miyake, H., Rokutan, K., & Tashiro, S. (2001). A non-toxic heat shock protein 70 inducer, geranylgeranylacetone, suppresses apoptosis of cultured rat hepatocytes caused by hydrogen peroxide and ethanol. *Journal of Hepatology, 35*(1), 53-61.

Inokuchi, S., Tsukamoto, H., Park, E., Liu, Z. X., Brenner, D. A., & Seki, E. (2011). Toll-like receptor 4 mediates alcohol-induced steatohepatitis through bone marrow-derived and endogenous liver cells in mice. *Alcoholism, Clinical and Experimental Research, 35*(8), 1509-1518.

Issemann, I., & Green, S. (1990). Activation of a member of the steroid hormone receptor superfamily by peroxisome proliferators. *Nature, 347*(6294), 645-650.

Iwasaki, H., & Suda, T. (2009). Cancer stem cells and their niche. *Cancer Science, 100*(7), 1166-1172.

Jeong, W. I., & Gao, B. (2008). Innate immunity and alcoholic liver fibrosis. *Journal of Gastroenterology and Hepatology, 23 Suppl 1*, S112-8.

Jeong, W. I., Park, O., & Gao, B. (2008). Abrogation of the antifibrotic effects of natural killer cells/interferon-gamma contributes to alcohol acceleration of liver fibrosis. *Gastroenterology, 134*(1), 248-258.

Ji, C., Chan, C., & Kaplowitz, N. (2006). Predominant role of sterol response element binding proteins (SREBP) lipogenic pathways in hepatic steatosis in the murine intragastric ethanol feeding model. *Journal of Hepatology, 45*(5), 717-724.

Ji, C., & Kaplowitz, N. (2003). Betaine decreases hyperhomocysteinemia, endoplasmic reticulum stress, and liver injury in alcohol-fed mice. *Gastroenterology, 124*(5), 1488-1499.

Kang, Y. J., & Zhou, Z. (2005). Zinc prevention and treatment of alcoholic liver disease. *Molecular Aspects of Medicine, 26*(4-5), 391-404.

Kaplowitz, N., Ji, C. (2006). Unfolding new mechanisms of alcoholic liver disease in the endoplasmic reticulum. *J Gastroenterol Hepatol, Oct*(21), 3:S7-9.

Kawai, T., Takeuchi, O., Fujita, T., Inoue, J., Muhlradt, P. F., Sato, S., et al. (2001). Lipopolysaccharide stimulates the MyD88-independent pathway and results in activation of IFN-regulatory factor 3 and the expression of a subset of lipopolysaccharide-inducible genes. *Journal of Immunology (Baltimore, Md.: 1950), 167*(10), 5887-5894.

Ki, S. H., Park, O., Zheng, M., Morales-Ibanez, O., Kolls, J. K., Bataller, R., et al. (2010). Interleukin-22 treatment ameliorates alcoholic liver injury in a murine model of chronic-binge ethanol feeding: Role of signal transducer and activator of transcription 3. *Hepatology (Baltimore, Md.), 52*(4), 1291-1300.

Kishore, R., Hill, J. R., McMullen, M. R., Frenkel, J., & Nagy, L. E. (2002). ERK1/2 and egr-1 contribute to increased TNF-alpha production in rat kupffer cells after chronic ethanol feeding. *American Journal of Physiology.Gastrointestinal and Liver Physiology, 282*(1), G6-15.

Kishore, R., McMullen, M. R., & Nagy, L. E. (2001). Stabilization of tumor necrosis factor alpha mRNA by chronic ethanol: Role of A + U-rich elements and p38 mitogen-activated protein kinase signaling pathway. *The Journal of Biological Chemistry, 276*(45), 41930-41937.

Kono, H., Rusyn, I., Yin, M., Gabele, E., Yamashina, S., Dikalova, A., et al. (2000). NADPH oxidase-derived free radicals are key oxidants in alcohol-induced liver disease. *The Journal of Clinical Investigation, 106*(7), 867-872.

Laso, F. J., Iglesias-Osma, C., Ciudad, J., Lopez, A., Pastor, I., Torres, E., et al. (2000). Alcoholic liver cirrhosis is associated with a decreased expression of the CD28 costimulatory molecule, a lower ability of T cells to bind exogenous IL-2, and increased soluble CD8 levels. *Cytometry, 42*(5), 290-295.

Laso, F. J., Vaquero, J. M., Almeida, J., Marcos, M., & Orfao, A. (2007). Chronic alcohol consumption is associated with changes in the distribution, immunophenotype, and the inflammatory cytokine secretion profile of circulating dendritic cells. *Alcoholism, Clinical and Experimental Research, 31*(5), 846-854.

Lau, A. H., Abe, M., & Thomson, A. W. (2006). Ethanol affects the generation, cosignaling molecule expression, and function of plasmacytoid and myeloid dendritic cell subsets in vitro and in vivo. *Journal of Leukocyte Biology, 79*(5), 941-953.

Lau, A. H., Szabo, G., & Thomson, A. W. (2009). Antigen-presenting cells under the influence of alcohol. *Trends in Immunology, 30*(1), 13-22.

Lemmers, A., Moreno, C., Gustot, T., Marechal, R., Degre, D., Demetter, P., et al. (2009). The interleukin-17 pathway is involved in human alcoholic liver disease. *Hepatology (Baltimore, Md.), 49*(2), 646-657.

Lotze, M.T., Zeh, H.J., Rubartelli, A., Sparvero, L.J., Amoscato, A.A., Washburn, N.R., Devera, M.E., Liang, X., Tor, M., Billiar, T. (2007). The grateful dead: damage-associated molecular pattern molecules and reduction/oxidation regulate immunity. *Immunol Rev, Dec* (220), 60-81.

Lu, Y., & Cederbaum, A. I. (2009). CYP2E1 potentiation of LPS and TNFalpha-induced hepatotoxicity by mechanisms involving enhanced oxidative and nitrosative stress, activation of MAP kinases, and mitochondrial dysfunction. *Genes & Nutrition,*

Lu, Y., & Cederbaum, A. I. (2008). CYP2E1 and oxidative liver injury by alcohol. *Free Radical Biology & Medicine, 44*(5), 723-738.

Lu, Y., Zhuge, J., Wang, X., Bai, J., & Cederbaum, A. I. (2008). Cytochrome P450 2E1 contributes to ethanol-induced fatty liver in mice. *Hepatology (Baltimore, Md.), 47*(5), 1483-1494.

Mahtani, K. R., Brook, M., Dean, J. L., Sully, G., Saklatvala, J., & Clark, A. R. (2001). Mitogen-activated protein kinase p38 controls the expression and posttranslational modification of tristetraprolin, a regulator of tumor necrosis factor alpha mRNA stability. *Molecular and Cellular Biology, 21*(19), 6461-6469.

Mandal, P., Park, P. H., McMullen, M. R., Pratt, B. T., & Nagy, L. E. (2010). The anti-inflammatory effects of adiponectin are mediated via a heme oxygenase-1-dependent pathway in rat Kupffer cells. *Hepatology (Baltimore, Md.), 51*(4), 1420-1429.

Mandrekar, P., Bala, S., Catalano, D., Kodys, K., & Szabo, G. (2009). The opposite effects of acute and chronic alcohol on lipopolysaccharide-induced inflammation are linked to IRAK-M in human monocytes. *Journal of Immunology (Baltimore, Md.: 1950), 183*(2), 1320-1327.

Mandrekar, P., Catalano, D., Dolganiuc, A., Kodys, K., & Szabo, G. (2004). Inhibition of myeloid dendritic cell accessory cell function and induction of T cell anergy by alcohol correlates with decreased IL-12 production. *Journal of Immunology (Baltimore, Md.: 1950), 173*(5), 3398-3407.

Mandrekar, P., Catalano, D., Jeliazkova, V., & Kodys, K. (2008). Alcohol exposure regulates heat shock transcription factor binding and heat shock proteins 70 and 90 in monocytes and macrophages: Implication for TNF-alpha regulation. *Journal of Leukocyte Biology, 84*(5), 1335-1345.

Mandrekar, P., & Szabo, G. (2009). Signalling pathways in alcohol-induced liver inflammation. *Journal of Hepatology, 50*(6), 1258-1266.

Mantena, S. K., King, A. L., Andringa, K. K., Landar, A., Darley-Usmar, V., & Bailey, S. M. (2007). Novel interactions of mitochondria and reactive oxygen/nitrogen species in alcohol mediated liver disease. *World Journal of Gastroenterology : WJG, 13*(37), 4967-4973.

Maziere, C., Gomila, C., & Maziere, J. C. (2010). Oxidized low-density lipoprotein increases osteopontin expression by generation of oxidative stress. *Free Radical Biology & Medicine, 48*(10), 1382-1387.

McCullough, A. J., & O'Connor, J. F. (1998). Alcoholic liver disease: Proposed recommendations for the american college of gastroenterology. *The American Journal of Gastroenterology, 93*(11), 2022-2036.

McKim, S. E., Gabele, E., Isayama, F., Lambert, J. C., Tucker, L. M., Wheeler, M. D., et al. (2003). Inducible nitric oxide synthase is required in alcohol-induced liver injury: Studies with knockout mice. *Gastroenterology, 125*(6), 1834-1844.

McVicker, B. L., Tuma, D. J., Kharbanda, K. K., Kubik, J. L., & Casey, C. A. (2007). Effect of chronic ethanol administration on the in vitro production of proinflammatory cytokines by rat Kupffer cells in the presence of apoptotic cells. *Alcoholism, Clinical and Experimental Research, 31*(1), 122-129.

McVicker, B. L., Tuma, D. J., Kubik, J. L., Tuma, P. L., & Casey, C. A. (2006). Ethanol-induced apoptosis in polarized hepatic cells possibly through regulation of the fas pathway. *Alcoholism, Clinical and Experimental Research, 30*(11), 1906-1915.

Miles, M. F., Diaz, J. E., & DeGuzman, V. S. (1991). Mechanisms of neuronal adaptation to ethanol induces Hsc70 gene transcription in NG108-15 neuroblastoma x glioma cells. *The Journal of Biological Chemistry, 266*(4), 2409-2414.

Miller, A. M., Wang, H., Park, O., Horiguchi, N., Lafdil, F., Mukhopadhyay, P., et al. (2010). Anti-inflammatory and anti-apoptotic roles of endothelial cell STAT3 in alcoholic liver injury. *Alcoholism, Clinical and Experimental Research, 34*(4), 719-725.

Minagawa, M., Deng, Q., Liu, Z. X., Tsukamoto, H., & Dennert, G. (2004). Activated natural killer T cells induce liver injury by fas and tumor necrosis factor-alpha during alcohol consumption. *Gastroenterology, 126*(5), 1387-1399.

Nagy, L. E. (2003). Recent insights into the role of the innate immune system in the development of alcoholic liver disease. *Experimental Biology and Medicine (Maywood, N.J.), 228*(8), 882-890.

Nakajima, T., Kamijo, Y., Tanaka, N., Sugiyama, E., Tanaka, E., Kiyosawa, K., et al. (2004). Peroxisome proliferator-activated receptor alpha protects against alcohol-induced liver damage. *Hepatology (Baltimore, Md.), 40*(4), 972-980.

Niemela, O., Parkkila, S., Yla-Herttuala, S., Halsted, C., Witztum, J. L., Lanca, A., et al. (1994). Covalent protein adducts in the liver as a result of ethanol metabolism and lipid peroxidation. *Laboratory Investigation; a Journal of Technical Methods and Pathology, 70*(4), 537-546.

Oak, S., Mandrekar, P., Catalano, D., Kodys, K., & Szabo, G. (2006). TLR2- and TLR4-mediated signals determine attenuation or augmentation of inflammation by acute alcohol in monocytes. *Journal of Immunology (Baltimore, Md.: 1950), 176*(12), 7628-7635.

Palucka, K. A., Taquet, N., Sanchez-Chapuis, F., & Gluckman, J. C. (1998). Dendritic cells as the terminal stage of monocyte differentiation. *Journal of Immunology (Baltimore, Md.: 1950), 160*(9), 4587-4595.

Park, H. S., Jung, H. Y., Park, E. Y., Kim, J., Lee, W. J., & Bae, Y. S. (2004). Cutting edge: Direct interaction of TLR4 with NAD(P)H oxidase 4 isozyme is essential for lipopolysaccharide-induced production of reactive oxygen species and activation of NF-kappa B. *Journal of Immunology (Baltimore, Md.: 1950), 173*(6), 3589-3593.

Park, O., Jeong, W. I., Wang, L., Wang, H., Lian, Z. X., Gershwin, M. E., et al. (2009). Diverse roles of invariant natural killer T cells in liver injury and fibrosis induced by carbon tetrachloride. *Hepatology (Baltimore, Md.), 49*(5), 1683-1694.

Pastorino, J. G., & Hoek, J. B. (2000). Ethanol potentiates tumor necrosis factor-alpha cytotoxicity in hepatoma cells and primary rat hepatocytes by promoting induction of the mitochondrial permeability transition. *Hepatology (Baltimore, Md.), 31*(5), 1141-1152.

Pastorino, J. G., Shulga, N., & Hoek, J. B. (2003). TNF-alpha-induced cell death in ethanol-exposed cells depends on p38 MAPK signaling but is independent of bid and caspase-8. *American Journal of Physiology.Gastrointestinal and Liver Physiology, 285*(3), G503-16.

Petrasek, J., Dolganiuc, A., Csak, T., Nath, B., Hritz, I., Kodys, K., et al. (2011). Interferon regulatory factor 3 and type I interferons are protective in alcoholic liver injury in mice by way of crosstalk of parenchymal and myeloid cells. *Hepatology (Baltimore, Md.), 53*(2), 649-660.

Pianko, S., Patella, S., & Sievert, W. (2000). Alcohol consumption induces hepatocyte apoptosis in patients with chronic hepatitis C infection. *Journal of Gastroenterology and Hepatology, 15*(7), 798-805.

Polavarapu, R., Spitz, D. R., Sim, J. E., Follansbee, M. H., Oberley, L. W., Rahemtulla, A., et al. (1998). Increased lipid peroxidation and impaired antioxidant enzyme function is associated with pathological liver injury in experimental alcoholic liver disease in rats fed diets high in corn oil and fish oil. *Hepatology (Baltimore, Md.), 27*(5), 1317-1323.

Raasch, C. E., Zhang, P., Siggins, R. W.,2nd, LaMotte, L. R., Nelson, S., & Bagby, G. J. (2010). Acute alcohol intoxication impairs the hematopoietic precursor cell response to pneumococcal pneumonia. *Alcoholism, Clinical and Experimental Research, 34*(12), 2035-2043.

Ramaiah, S. K., & Jaeschke, H. (2007). Hepatic neutrophil infiltration in the pathogenesis of alcohol-induced liver injury. *Toxicology Mechanisms and Methods, 17*(7), 431-440.

Ricevuti, G. (1997). Host tissue damage by phagocytes. *Annals of the New York Academy of Sciences, 832*, 426-448.

Rolla, R., Vay, D., Mottaran, E., Parodi, M., Traverso, N., Arico, S., et al. (2000). Detection of circulating antibodies against malondialdehyde-acetaldehyde adducts in patients with alcohol-induced liver disease. *Hepatology (Baltimore, Md.), 31*(4), 878-884.

Rosen, E. D., & Spiegelman, B. M. (2001). PPARgamma : A nuclear regulator of metabolism, differentiation, and cell growth. *The Journal of Biological Chemistry, 276*(41), 37731-37734.

Schattenberg, J. M., Singh, R., Wang, Y., Lefkowitch, J. H., Rigoli, R. M., Scherer, P. E., et al. (2006). JNK1 but not JNK2 promotes the development of steatohepatitis in mice. *Hepatology (Baltimore, Md.), 43*(1), 163-172.

Schmidt-Weber, C. B., & Blaser, K. (2004). Regulation and role of transforming growth factor-beta in immune tolerance induction and inflammation. *Current Opinion in Immunology, 16*(6), 709-716.

Shi, L., Kishore, R., McMullen, M. R., & Nagy, L. E. (2002). Chronic ethanol increases lipopolysaccharide-stimulated egr-1 expression in RAW 264.7 macrophages: Contribution to enhanced tumor necrosis factor alpha production. *The Journal of Biological Chemistry, 277*(17), 14777-14785.

Sloane, J. A., Blitz, D., Margolin, Z., & Vartanian, T. (2010). A clear and present danger: Endogenous ligands of toll-like receptors. *Neuromolecular Medicine, 12*(2), 149-163.

Soehnlein, O., Kenne, E., Rotzius, P., Eriksson, E. E., & Lindbom, L. (2008). Neutrophil secretion products regulate anti-bacterial activity in monocytes and macrophages. *Clinical and Experimental Immunology, 151*(1), 139-145.

Stadlbauer, V., Mookerjee, R. P., Wright, G. A., Davies, N. A., Jurgens, G., Hallstrom, S., et al. (2009). Role of toll-like receptors 2, 4, and 9 in mediating neutrophil dysfunction in alcoholic hepatitis. *American Journal of Physiology.Gastrointestinal and Liver Physiology, 296*(1), G15-22.

Steinman, R. M., & Inaba, K. (1999). Myeloid dendritic cells. *Journal of Leukocyte Biology, 66*(2), 205-208.

Stewart, S., Prince, M., Bassendine, M., Hudson, M., James, O., Jones, D., et al. (2007). A randomized trial of antioxidant therapy alone or with corticosteroids in acute alcoholic hepatitis. *Journal of Hepatology, 47*(2), 277-283.

Szabo, G., Dolganiuc, A., & Mandrekar, P. (2006). Pattern recognition receptors: A contemporary view on liver diseases. *Hepatology (Baltimore, Md.), 44*(2), 287-298.

Taieb, J., Mathurin, P., Poynard, T., Gougerot-Pocidalo, M. A., & Chollet-Martin, S. (1998). Raised plasma soluble fas and fas-ligand in alcoholic liver disease. *Lancet, 351*(9120), 1930-1931.

Takeda, K., & Akira, S. (2005). Toll-like receptors in innate immunity. *International Immunology, 17*(1), 1-14.

Thakur, V., Pritchard, M. T., McMullen, M. R., Wang, Q., & Nagy, L. E. (2006a). Chronic ethanol feeding increases activation of NADPH oxidase by lipopolysaccharide in rat Kupffer cells: Role of increased reactive oxygen in LPS-stimulated ERK1/2 activation and TNF-alpha production. *Journal of Leukocyte Biology, 79*(6), 1348-1356.

Thakur, V., Pritchard, M. T., McMullen, M. R., & Nagy, L. E. (2006b). Adiponectin normalizes LPS-stimulated TNF-alpha production by rat Kupffer cells after chronic ethanol feeding. *American Journal of Physiology.Gastrointestinal and Liver Physiology, 290*(5), G998-1007.

Thiele, G. M., Duryee, M. J., Willis, M. S., Sorrell, M. F., Freeman, T. L., Tuma, D. J., et al. (2004). Malondialdehyde-acetaldehyde (MAA) modified proteins induce pro-inflammatory and pro-fibrotic responses by liver endothelial cells. *Comparative Hepatology, 3 Suppl 1*, S25.

Thurman, R. G., Bradford, B. U., Iimuro, Y., Frankenberg, M. V., Knecht, K. T., Connor, H. D., et al. (1999). Mechanisms of alcohol-induced hepatotoxicity: Studies in rats. *Frontiers in Bioscience : A Journal and Virtual Library, 4*, e42-6.

Tiegs, G. (2007). Cellular and cytokine-mediated mechanisms of inflammation and its modulation in immune-mediated liver injury. *Zeitschrift Fur Gastroenterologie, 45*(1), 63-70.

Tilg, H., Jalan, R., Kaser, A., Davies, N. A., Offner, F. A., Hodges, S. J., et al. (2003). Anti-tumor necrosis factor-alpha monoclonal antibody therapy in severe alcoholic hepatitis. *Journal of Hepatology, 38*(4), 419-425.

Tsai, Y. S., & Maeda, N. (2005). PPARgamma: A critical determinant of body fat distribution in humans and mice. *Trends in Cardiovascular Medicine, 15*(3), 81-85.

Uesugi, T., Froh, M., Arteel, G. E., Bradford, B. U., & Thurman, R. G. (2001). Toll-like receptor 4 is involved in the mechanism of early alcohol-induced liver injury in mice. *Hepatology (Baltimore, Md.), 34*(1), 101-108.

Wan, Y. J., Morimoto, M., Thurman, R. G., Bojes, H. K., & French, S. W. (1995). Expression of the peroxisome proliferator-activated receptor gene is decreased in experimental alcoholic liver disease. *Life Sciences, 56*(5), 307-317.

Wang, K., & Wan, Y. J. (2008). Nuclear receptors and inflammatory diseases. *Experimental Biology and Medicine (Maywood, N.J.), 233*(5), 496-506.

Wang, X., Wu, D., Yang, L., & Cederbaum, A. I. (2011). Hepatotoxicity mediated by pyrazole (CYP2E1) plus TNF-alpha treatment occurs in jnk2(-/-) but not in jnk1(-/-) mice. *Hepatology (Baltimore, Md.),*

Weinstein, S. L., Sanghera, J. S., Lemke, K., DeFranco, A. L., & Pelech, S. L. (1992). Bacterial lipopolysaccharide induces tyrosine phosphorylation and activation of mitogen-activated protein kinases in macrophages. *The Journal of Biological Chemistry, 267*(21), 14955-14962.

Williams, S. H. (2005). Medications for treating alcohol dependence. *American Family Physician, 72*(9), 1775-1780.

Wu, D., & Cederbaum, A. I. (2003). Alcohol, oxidative stress, and free radical damage. *Alcohol Research & Health : The Journal of the National Institute on Alcohol Abuse and Alcoholism, 27*(4), 277-284.

Wu, D., & Cederbaum, A. I. (1996). Ethanol cytotoxicity to a transfected HepG2 cell line expressing human cytochrome P4502E1. *The Journal of Biological Chemistry, 271*(39), 23914-23919.

Yeligar, S. M., Machida, K., Tsukamoto, H., & Kalra, V. K. (2009). Ethanol augments RANTES/CCL5 expression in rat liver sinusoidal endothelial cells and human endothelial cells via activation of NF-kappa B, HIF-1 alpha, and AP-1. *Journal of Immunology (Baltimore, Md.: 1950), 183*(9), 5964-5976.

Yin, X. M., Ding, W. X., & Gao, W. (2008). Autophagy in the liver. *Hepatology (Baltimore, Md.), 47*(5), 1773-1785.

Zhang, H., & Meadows, G. G. (2005) Chronic alcohol consumption in mice increases the proportion of peripheral memory T cells by homeostatic proliferation. *Journal of Leukocyte Biology*, 78(5), 1070-1080.

Zhang, C., & Cuervo, A. M. (2008). Restoration of chaperone-mediated autophagy in aging liver improves cellular maintenance and hepatic function. *Nature Medicine,* 14(9), 959-965.

Zhao, X. J., Dong, Q., Bindas, J., Piganelli, J. D., Magill, A., Reiser, J., et al. (2008). TRIF and IRF-3 binding to the TNF promoter results in macrophage TNF dysregulation and steatosis induced by chronic ethanol. *Journal of Immunology (Baltimore, Md.: 1950), 181*(5), 3049-3056.

7

Alcoholic Liver Disease and the Survival Response of the Hepatocyte Growth Factor

Luis E. Gómez-Quiroz, Deidry B. Cuevas-Bahena, Verónica Souza, Leticia Bucio and María Concepción Gutierrez Ruiz
Departamento de Ciencias de la Salud, Universidad Autónoma Metropolitana Iztapalapa, México, D.F., México

1. Introduction

Hepatocyte growth factor (HGF), also known as a scatter factor plays a major role in liver repair and regeneration during injury. HGF displays a complex network of signaling pathways that activate key functions for liver repair, survival and cellular redox control (Gomez-Quiroz, et al. 2008; Nakamura and Mizuno 2010) all these functions are initiated by the binding of HGF to its receptor c-Met which, after autophosphorylation, recruits a wide variety of signal transduction proteins.

After injury, liver initiates repair process which could be leaded by proliferation of the mature, and normally quiescent, hepatocytes or, when damage is extensive and mature hepatocytes are enable to proliferate, by the activation of progenitor cells population or oval cells (Riehle, et al. 2011)

It is well recognized that the repair process begins with the activation of Kupffer cells, the liver-resident macrophagues, which respond to damage secreting tumor necrosis factor alpha (TNF-α) and interleukin (IL-) 6, these cytokines induce the activation of signaling pathways in hepatocytes such as nuclear factor κB (NF-κB) and signal transducer and activator of transcription 3 (Stat3), respectively. In addition, hepatic stellate cells (HSC) and inflammatory cells initiate the production of HGF which together with TNF-α and IL-6 lead to a cooperative signal to overcome cell-cycle checkpoint controls and shift cells from G0 through G1, to S phase, leading to hepatocytes proliferation and repair.(Riehle et al. 2011)

2. HGF/c-Met and its function in liver repair

HGF gene is encoded on chromosome 7 band 7q21.1 and its product is a precursor glycopolypeptide of 697 amino acids which is proteolytic processed in the extracellular environment by the serine endoprotease urokinase-type plasminogen activator (uPA) (Naldini, et al. 1992) generating the mature HGF consisting in a heterodimeric disulphide-linked two polypeptide chains (α and β). The α-chain consists of 463 amino acids residues and four kringle domains. The β-chain consists of 234 amino acid residues. It is thought that *in vivo* HGF acts in a paracrine fashion, being produced by mesenchymal or stromal cells (Stoker, et al. 1987), and targeting epithelial cells nearby (Sonnenberg, et al. 1993).

Among the multiple biological function triggered by HGF is important underline: cell proliferation, apoptosis protection, morphogenesis, scattering, cell motility, invasion and metastasis (Hanna, et al. 2009). The signal transduction that drives all these effects starts by the ligand-induced dimerization and activation of the HGF receptor, the proto-oncogen c-Met (cellular-mesenchymal epithelial transition factor) (Ma, et al. 2003).

Human c-Met gene is located on chromosome 7 band 7q21-q31; the product is a 150-kDa polypeptide that, after glycosylation and proteolytic processing, generates the mature α-β heterodimer receptor composed of one extracellular 50-kDa α-chain linked by disulfide bonds to a transmembrane 140-kDa β-chain. The β-subunit encloses multiple sites of regulatory phosphorylation. Ligand binding to the receptor leads to autophosphorylation of the tyrosines 1230, 1234 and 1235 located within the activation loop of the tyrosine kinase domain and activates the intrinsic kinase activity of the receptor. (Ma et al. 2003).

HGF also induces tyrosine 1313 phosphorylation which is preferred by phosphoinositide 3-kinase (PI3K) binding, while in the multi-substrate signal transducer docking site, located in the C-terminus domain, phosphorylation of tyrosines 1349, and 1356 lead to the activation of adapter and effectors proteins such as Shc, Src, Gab1, Grb2, PI3K, SHP2, phospholipase C-γ (PLC-γ) among others (Bertotti and Comoglio 2003), these pathways have been widely characterized both *in vivo* and *in vitro*, and it has been well defined the difference between HGF and other growth factors with tissue repair activities such as epidermal growth factor (EGF), TNF-α, or IL-6. Under this context it has been reported that HGF promotes tubulogenesis by the activation of GAB1, SHP-2, and Stat3; survival and antiapoptosis by NF-κB, Stat3 and Erk1/2; and proliferation and growth by Grb2 and PI3K (Boccaccio, et al. 1998; Fan, et al. 2005; Maroun, et al. 1999; Maroun, et al. 2000; Trusolino, et al. 2010)

In addition of these phosphorylations, there are other regulatory sites within the β-subunit; in the juxtamembrane domain the phosphorylation of serine 956 and tyrosine 1093 have negative regulatory functions (Ma et al. 2003) which are involved in the receptor internalization after activation (Kermorgant and Parker 2005) and posterior degradation by ubiquitin-proteosome pathway (Jeffers, et al. 1997).

Functions elicited by HGF are particularly important for liver repair and regeneration after liver injury by alcohol, drugs, viral infections or partial hepatectomy. In fact, HGF was originally discovered as a potent mitogen of adult rat hepatocytes (Nakamura, 1984). HGF is produced in the liver by non-parenchymal cells, such as HSC, sinusoidal endothelial, Kupffer cells and immune cells; but also it can be produced by other distant organs in the body, including lungs, and kidneys where it displays repair process as well. (Grenier, et al. 2002; Nakamura and Mizuno 2010; Taieb, et al. 2002b).

In healthy humans circulating levels of HGF are always present, and can be affected by age, gender and pregnancy. It can be established a normal range from 0.26 to 0.39 ng/ml, however it is well known the increase in serum HGF after both, acute and chronic liver damage (Funakoshi and Nakamura 2003), and this increment depends on the kind of damage or disease. For example, in alcoholic liver cirrhosis the HGF levels reported is 0.78 ng/ml (Antoljak, et al. 2001), in patients with hepatocarcinoma the average level is 1.06 ± 1.45 ng/ml and in patients with fulminant hepatitis it could reach values of 16.40 ± 14.67 ng/ml (Funakoshi and Nakamura 2003). The increment shows a positive correlation with markers of liver failure such as serum bilirubin or gamma-glutamyl transpeptidase, and

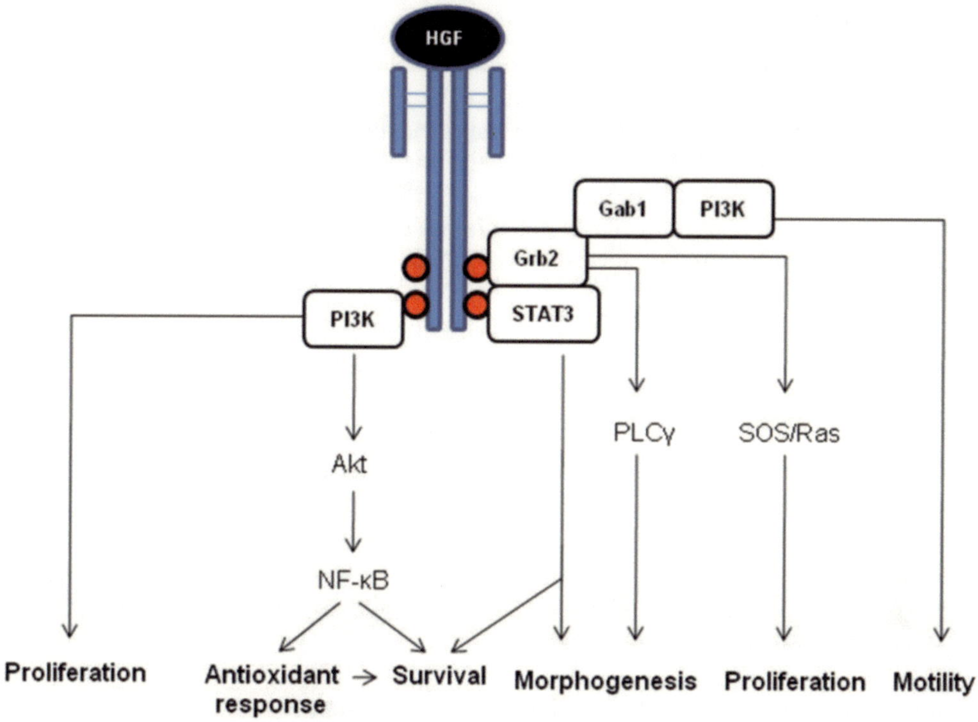

Fig. 1. Signaling pathways and effects elicited by HGF/c-Met. HGF, hepatocyte growth factor; Grb2, growth factor receptor-bound protein 2; Grb1 binding-associated binder1; PI3K, phosphoinositide-3-kinase; STAT3, signal transducer and activator of transcription 3; PLCγ, Phospholipase C gamma; SOS, son of sevenless, guanine nucleotide exchange factor; RAS, rat sarcoma, GTPase; Akt, Protein Kinase B; NF-κB, nuclear factor kappa B.

negative correlation with albumin content, suggesting that HGF levels can reflect the grade of illness and can be considered as a prognosis indicator.

The main evidence of the relevance of HGF on liver regeneration and repair came with the creation of the hepatocyte-specific c-Met signaling deletion mouse (MetKO) (Huh, et al. 2004). Loss of c-Met signaling appeared not to be detrimental to hepatocyte function under physiological conditions, but sublethal doses of Fas agonist (Jo2 antibody) induced a hypersensitization to damage generating massive liver apoptosis and necrosis, with no important effects in wild type mouse. Hepatocytes derived from MetKO mice exhibited sensitization to Jo2-induced apoptosis and impairment in motility and phagocytosis, activities which are required for a proper repair process (Gomez-Quiroz et al. 2008; Huh et al. 2004)

3. HGF and c-Met in alcoholic liver disease

Functions of HGF in ALD remains partially characterized. However it is clear that HGF and c-Met are involved in every stage of ALD, from inflammatory response to alcoholic steatohepatitis, fibrosis, cirrhosis and hepatocarcinoma (Cornella, et al. 2011; Tahara, et al. 1999; Taieb et al. 2002b).

3.1 Ethanol impairs HGF release from neutrophils

Ethanol-initiated damage lead to an inflammatory response characterized by neutrophilia and hepatic polymorphonuclear neutrophil (PMN) infiltration (Taieb et al. 2002b). We reported previously that acetaldehyde, the main metabolite of ethanol biotransformation, induces the production of IL-8, chemotactic factor for PMN, in HepG2 cells (Gomez-Quiroz, et al. 2003) and Taieb and coworkers (Taieb et al. 2002b) have shown that PMN are an important source of HGF specifically in patients with severe alcoholic hepatitis, finding that these patients presented higher levels of HGF (6.07 ± 0.738 ng/ml) in comparison with alcoholic hepatitis-free patients with cirrhosis (3.24 ± 0.438 ng/ml) and healthy controls (0.407 ± 0.027 ng/ml). Hepatic HGF levels correlated with the degree of hepatic PMN infiltration (P=0.0015, ρ=0.76). This study provides evidences that PMN cells are an important source of HGF, particularly in patients with large PMN infiltration, pointing out the PMN cells as coadjutants in liver repair, at least in acute processes.

Although PMN cells provide HGF to the injured liver, ethanol inhibits this effect. PMN cells treated with degranulation promoter agents (cytochalasin B and N-formyl-methionyl-leucyl-phenylalanine) induced the release of HGF, however the presence of different concentrations of ethanol significantly inhibited HGF degranulation in a concentration-dependent manner (Taieb, et al. 2002a), indicating that ethanol impairs HGF release from PMN cells obstructing liver repair process.

3.2 Free radicals, oxidative stress and ethanol metabolism

In terms of ethanol metabolism-induced oxidative stress, we can define two main levels of HGF-mediated protection. The first level is generating system regulation, particularly the microsomal ethanol oxidizing system (MEOS), and the second one is the control or neutralization of the free radicals formed as a consequence of ethanol metabolism.

A free radical is a molecule or atom that contains one or more unpaired electron, this characteristic makes them highly instable and reactive. In the cellular context, oxygen and nitrogen free radicals have a wide variety of actions ranging from modulation of gene expression to the induction of cell death.

Physiologically 1-2% of molecular oxygen is converted, by enzymatic and non-enzymatic mechanisms, to reactive oxygen species (ROS) which include hydrogen peroxide (H_2O_2), superoxide anion ($O_2^{\bullet-}$), singlet molecular oxygen ($^1O_2$), hydroxyl ($HO\bullet$), alkoxyl ($RO\bullet$), and Peroxyl ($ROO\bullet$) radicals (Cadenas 1989). In order to avoid the harmful effects of these molecules, cells enclose a battery of antioxidant defenses which include enzymatic and non-enzymatic components. Among the antioxidant enzymes superoxide dismutase (SOD), catalase, glutathione (GSH) peroxidase (GSHPx) and GSH reductase (GSHRd) sustain the major detoxifying activities. SOD1, 2 and 3 which are located in cytosol, mitochondria and plasma membrane respectively drive the transformation of $O_2^{\bullet-}$ in H_2O_2, although hydrogen peroxide is not a free radical, it is the precursor of the highest reactive and toxic specie among the ROS, the hydroxyl radical via either, Fenton reaction, which requires the presence of Fe^{3+} or Cu^{2+} for the process, or Haber-Weiss reaction. (Valko, et al. 2007)

To counteract this phenomenon H_2O_2 is transformed to H_2O by the action of catalase or GSHPx. GSHPx uses two molecules of GSH to reduce H_2O_2, generating the oxidized form of glutathione (GSSG) which can be regenerated to GSH by the action of GSHRd using NADPH as electron donor.

GSH is the naturally occurring major thiol. It is produced in the cytosol by the action of two enzymes, the γ-glutamyl cysteine ligase (also known as γ-glutamyl cysteine synthetase, γ-GCS) that catalyses the formation of the dipetide L-γ-glutamyl-L-cysteine, and by glutathione synthase which converts this dipeptide in GSH (L-γ-glutamyl-L-cysteinyl-Glycine).

The ability of GSH to deal with ROS is not restricted as a cofactor of GSHPx, because GSH has, by itself, the capacity to scavenge free radicals, as it happens with others non-enzymatic antioxidants such as vitamin C and E, and β-carotene .

Ethanol metabolism is mainly driven by both, alcohol dehydrogenase and MEOS which main member is cytochrome P450 (Cyp) 2E1, both enzymes generate acetaldehyde as primary metabolite, but only MEOS produces, in addition, ROS such as $O_2^{\bullet-}$, H_2O_2, and the highly toxic HO•, responsible of DNA, protein and lipid oxidation (Cadenas 1989). It has been reported that Cyp2E1 is induced by ethanol consumption principally in zone 3 hepatocytes. Biopsies from recently drinking subjects revealed an increment from 4- to 10-fold over normal values (Tsutsumi, et al. 1989).

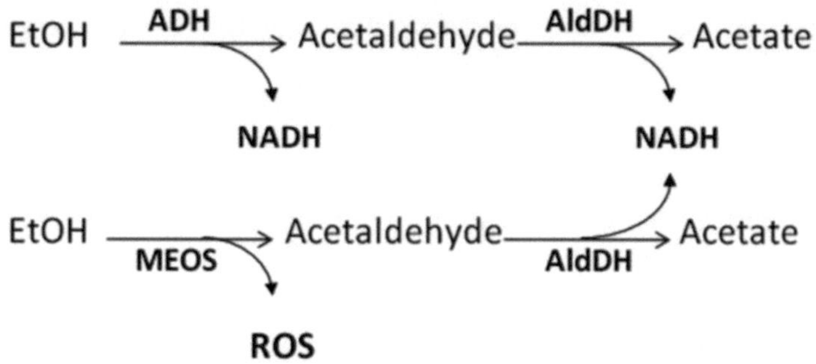

Fig. 2. Major alcohol metabolism processes. EtOH, ethanol; ADH, alcohol dehydrogenase; AldDH, aldeyde dehydrogenase; ROS, reactive oxygen species; MEOS, microsomal ethanol oxidizing system; NADH, reduced nicotine adenine dinucleotide.

Other Cyp isoforms have been implicated in ethanol metabolism, such as Cyp1A2 and Cyp3A4, thus the term MEOS characterizes the total microsomal ethanol oxidation, not only Cyp2E1 (Salmela, et al. 1998).

3.3 HGF regulates the ROS generating systems

Donato and coworkers reported in 1998 that HGF regulates the expression and activities of Cyp1A1/2, Cyp2A6, Cyp2E1 and, Cyp2B6 in human hepatocytes in primary culture (Donato, et al. 1998). Activities of Cyp1A2, Cyp3A4 and Cyp1A1/2 were significantly diminished at 72 h of HGF treatment (10 ng/ml). Particularly in five hepatocytes cultures from five different healthy donors, HGF treatment resulted in the reduction of Cyp2E1 activity ranging from 55 to 69% regarding not treated cultures. These effects were correlated with the decrease in the corresponding mRNA, suggesting that HGF transcriptionally and post-translationally downregulates some of the MEOS components. This regulation represents the first frontline of HGF-induced defense against the toxicity of ethanol.

In addition to the abrogation of MEOS components by HGF, it is reported that it can also downregulate another ROS generating systems such as NADPH oxidase (Gomez-Quiroz et al. 2008), which is involved in many liver diseases such as fibrosis(De Minicis, et al. 2010), hepatitis C virus infection (de Mochel, et al. 2010) and alcoholic liver disease where it is mainly activated in Kupffer cells leading to TNF-α production (Kono, et al. 2000).

3.4 HGF regulates the ROS produced by ethanol metabolism

The second HGF frontline against the oxidative effect of ethanol metabolism is leaded by the generation of antioxidants. It is well known that HGF/c-Met can regulate the activation of survival transcription factors such as NF-κB or Nrf2 (Gomez-Quiroz et al. 2008; Kaposi-Novak, et al. 2006; Valdes-Arzate, et al. 2009) which are responsible of the expression of a wide range of antioxidant, detoxifying and antiapoptotic proteins and it has been well documented elsewhere (Fan et al. 2005; Klaassen and Reisman 2010).

In vitro studies have revealed the prominent role of HGF in cellular survival against ethanol toxicity. One of the main problems to address the molecular mechanism of alcohol induced damage, at the cellular level, is that hepatocytes in primary culture loss the capacity to metabolize ethanol due to a downregulation in the MEOS and alcohol dehydrogenase. Cell lines expressing stable and constitutively Cyp2E1 and/or alcohol dehydrogenase have been established to sort the inconvenience in the absent of alcohol metabolism in normal hepatocytes in culture (Chen and Cederbaum 1998; Donohue, et al. 2006), particularly relevant is the cell line VL17A, which is a suitable *in vitro* model of ALD due to the expression of both Cyp2E1 and alcohol dehydrogenase (Donohue et al. 2006), which mimics much better conditions in normal hepatocytes than single gene transfected cells (Chen and Cederbaum 1998).

VL17A have been used to address the mechanism of HGF-induced protection in ALD (Valdez-Arzate 2009). HGF was capable to decrease ROS production, protein oxidation and lipid peroxidation damage due to ethanol metabolism, correlating with an increase in cell viability. Analysis of the mechanism involved in the HGF-induced protection against ethanol metabolism toxicity revealed that HGF induces the activation of NF-κB, with a concomitant expression of antioxidant enzymes such as catalase, SOD1, and γ-GCS, as well as an elevation in GSH synthesis as a consequence of the expression of γ-GCS. Inhibition of NF-κB, or the main upstream activators of this transcription factor (PI3K and Akt), significantly abrogated the protective role of HGF (Gomez-Quiroz et al. 2008; Valdes-Arzate et al. 2009)

HGF has demonstrated to increase the expression of catalse and GSHRd (Arends, et al. 2008). Catalase transforms H_2O_2 in H_2O, and GSHRd restores GSH from GSSG (Figure 2).

It has been widely characterized the relevance of GSH in ALD by Fernandez-Checa and coworkers (Fernandez-Checa, et al. 2002; Fernandez-Checa, et al. 1993; Fernandez-Checa, et al. 1996; Hirano, et al. 1992), and it is proposed as one of the key mechanism in the alcohol-induced hepatocellular damage, mainly by GSH depletion in mitochondria.

HGF has shown regulate strongly GSH homeostasis by inducing the expression of γ-GCS (Tsuboi 1999; Valdes-Arzate et al. 2009), and we are claiming that this is the main mechanism of protection against oxidative stress. In fact, c-Met KO mice are under oxidative stress due to the increment in the NADPH oxidase activity, and depletion in GSH. MetKO mice subjected to the carcinogenic agent N-nitrosodiethylamine were more susceptible to the development of tumors in the liver, presenting an increment in multiplicity, size and incidence. This effect was abrogated by the oral administration of N-acetyl cysteine (NAC) which is precursor of GSH synthesis (Takami, et al. 2007). These findings were correlated in *in vitro* studies, MetKO hepatocytes are more susceptible to Jo2-induced damage, effect that was abrogated by NAC treatment, which induced GSH reservoirs restoration (Gomez-Quiroz et al. 2008).

The main consequence in ROS generation is the induction of hepatocytes apoptosis. ROS can induce the activation of jun kinease signaling pathway leading to the activation of AP-1 transcription factor that promotes the expression of proapoptotic proteins such as FasL, TNF-α and Bak. ROS also targets mitochondria inducing membrane permeabilization and the release of proapoptotic proteins (cytochorme c, Smac/diablo, EndoG, among others(Serviddio, et al. 2010), which participate in the cell death process.

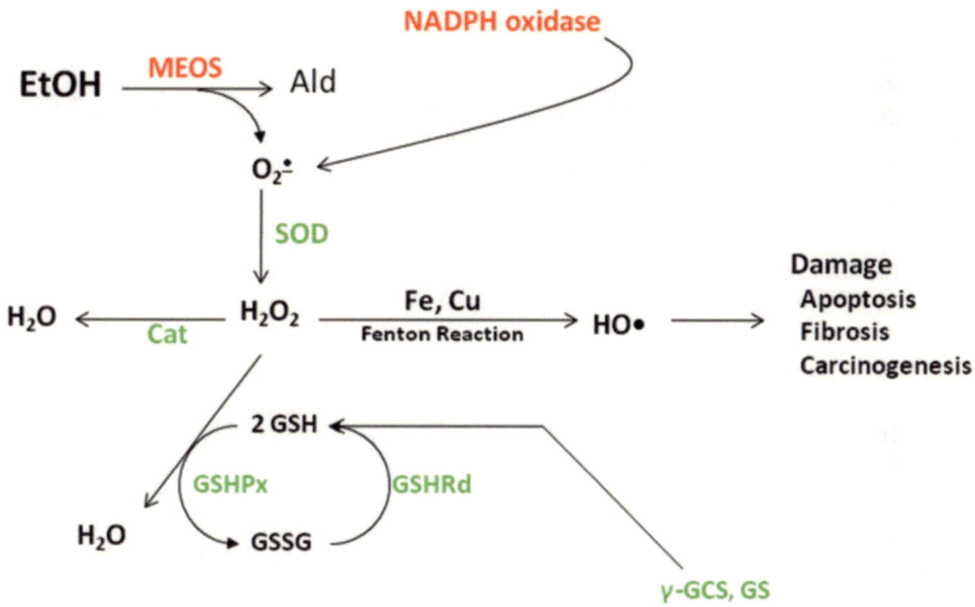

Fig. 3. Alcohol-mediated reactive oxygen species production and antioxidant response driven by HGF. Molecules downregulated (red) and upregulated (green) by HGF. EtOH, ethanol; MEOS, microsomal ethanol oxidizing system, Ald, Acetaldehyde; H_2O_2, hydrogen peroxide; $O_2^{\bullet-}$, superoxide anion; HO•,hydroxyl; SOD, Superoxide Dismutase; Cat, catalase; GSH Glutathione; GSHPX, Glutathione peroxidasa; Gluatathione –reductase; GSSG, Oxidized glutathione; γ-GCS, γ-glutamyl cysteine synthetase; GS, Glutathione Synthase.

It is well known the antiapoptotic effect of HGF, not only in hepatocytes, but in many cell types (Arends et al. 2008; Fan et al. 2005; Kitta, et al. 2001; Santangelo, et al. 2007). In addition to the control of ROS, HGF can induce the expression of antiapoptotic proteins by the activation of survival canonical pathways for example, Akt/NF-κB, Erk1/2 or Stat3, which induce Bcl2, Bcl-XL, and Mcl-1 expression (Gomez-Quiroz et al. 2008; Valdes-Arzate et al. 2009), but also HGF-induction of GSH supports its antiapoptotic function, based in the fact that NAC treatment significantly reduced the Jo2-induced apoptosis in hepatocytes, and pretreatment with BSO, an inhibitor of γ-GCS, abrogated the protective effect of both NAC and HGF(Gomez-Quiroz et al. 2008).

The evidence gathered here clearly shows the central role of HGF in the control of ethanol-induced oxidative stress and GSH homeostasis as key issues in the hepatoprotective mechanism in ALD (Figure 2).

3.5 Regulation of lipid homeostasis and recovery from alcohol-induced fatty liver

The mechanism of alcohol-induced fatty liver disease is complex and remains not fully characterized. The main mechanism proposed is that alcohol impacts at three levels.

The first level is the induction of oxidative stress, starting by MEOS, and continuing with mitochondria dysfunction due to a decrease in mitochondrial GSH reservoirs. The second level is the increase in TNF-α, which augments mitochondria failure, and ROS production and deregulates adiponectin, which promotes fatty acids oxidation. The third level is the activation of transcription factors involved in lipid biosynthesis and export.

Liver packages triglycerides into a very low density lipoproteins (VLDL), forming a complex with the apolipoprotein B 100 in a process facilitated by the microsomal triglyceride transfer protein (MTTP), which is downregulated in rats fed with an ethanol-containing liquid diet (Sugimoto, et al. 2002). The first and second levels converge in the generation of endoplasmic reticulum (ER) stress and in the increment in the activation of sterol regulatory element binding protein 1c (SREBP1c), which is in the third level. SREBP1c is a transcription factor that remains inactivated in ER, and after stimulus, migrates to the Golgi for further process and finally arrives to the nucleus where it promotes the expression of genes involved in fatty acids synthesis (Ferre and Foufelle 2010). Furthermore, the AMP-activated protein kinase (AMPK), a serine-threonine kinase, which stimulates both, fatty acid oxidation by the activation of the peroxisome proliferator-activated receptors alpha (PPARα) and glycolisis, and inhibits fatty acid synthesis due to the inactivation of acetyl-CoA carboxylase (ACC), leads to the decrease of malonyl-CoA, a precursor in fatty acid synthesis and inhibitor of the carnitine palmitoyl transferase 1, the rate-limiting enzyme in fatty acid oxidation (Dobrzyn, et al. 2004; Hardie and Pan 2002). AMPK also inhibits the activation of SREBP1c, presenting AMPK as a multimodal regulator of lipid metabolism in the liver. Animals fed with an alcohol-containing diet exhibit a decrease in the activity of AMPK resulting in the development of hepatic steatosis (Garcia-Villafranca, et al. 2008).

In addition, it has been proposed that the increase in $NADH/NAD^+$ ratio due to alcohol metabolism drives the inhibition of the tricarboxylic acids cycle and fatty acid oxidation, but also it can induce ER stress (figure 3) (Lieber 2004)

HGF involvement in lipid homeostasis has been experimentally demonstrated, Kaibori and collaborators reported that HGF is capable to induce lipid synthesis under liver regeneration (Kaibori, et al. 1998), and the genetic elimination of c-Met signaling in hepatocytes induced changes in the expression of many proteins related to lipid metabolism such as Acox1, ASS1, Crot, Cyp4a10, Cyp 4a14, Fasn, Lipc, among others (Kaposi-Novak et al. 2006).

One of the firsts studies focused to address the regulation of alcohol-induced fatty liver by HGF was reported in 1999 by Tahara and collaborators (Tahara et al. 1999), they observed that rats fed with an ethanol containing diet for 30 days developed hepatic steatosis. The administration of HGF for 7 days (37 days on the diet) reduced lipid deposition in liver tissue. The major mechanism observed was the increment on lipid secretion via VLDL by the induction of ApoB100 expression.

The second HGF effect related to steatosis control is the restoration of the mRNA levels and activity of MTTP. Injection of HGF on animals subjected to an alcoholic diet restored MTTP levels, this observation was corroborated in HepG2 cells which were exposed to HGF resulting an enhanced expression of both MTTP and ApoB100 (Sugimoto et al. 2002).

The induction of VLDL and MTTP by HGF seems not to be exclusive for alcohol-induced steatosis, due to Kosone and collaborators (Kosone, et al. 2007) found the same results in a model of fatty liver generated by a high-fat diet and confirmed in HepG2 cells the decrease in lipid content.

Another evidence of HGF-induced alcoholic steatosis protection comes from the effect of pioglitazone, this drug is used in the treatment of diabetes and non-alcoholic steatoshepatitis, but it has been postulated that it can be also used in the treatment of alcoholic steatohepatitis (Tomita, et al. 2004). Ethanol reduced the mRNA and protein levels of c-Met, and pioglitazone restored the c-Met expression decreasing the lipid content in liver tissue. Both HGF and pioglitazone showed downregulate the expression of key genes involved in lipid homeostasis such as SREBP 1c and stearoyl-CoA desaturase, improving the deleterious effects in the alcoholic fatty liver.

Finally, recently has been published that HGF can promote the activation of AMPK signaling pathway (Chanda, et al. 2009) inducing the suppression on lipid synthesis and gluconeogenesis.

3.6 Fibrosis

The main consequence in the chronic alcohol ingestion is liver fibrosis/cirrhosis which is characterized by the hyper-accumulation of connective tissue components, mainly collagen, and a disorganization of the normal hepatic structure of regenerative nodules. Many reports have clarified the preventive and therapeutic effects of HGF on liver fibrosis or cirrhosis (Inagaki, et al. 2008; Jones, et al. 2010; Matsuda, et al. 1995; Matsuda, et al. 1997; Ueki, et al. 1999; Xia, et al. 2006).

HGF treatment in animals challenged with different inducers of liver fibrosis suppressed the connective tissue components expression and hydroxyproline levels, preventing the onset of scar formation (Matsuda et al. 1997). The mechanism of HGF-induced anti-fibrotic protection is focused to antagonize the transforming growth factor beta (TGF-β) signaling pathway. TGF-β is the main profibrogenic factor, inducing the expression of collagen, fibronectin and hepatocytes apoptosis. The effect of HGF on TGF-β has been observed at different levels. In the model of fibrosis induced by the bile duct ligation, HGF showed suppress the expression of TGF-β and the conversion bile duct epithelial to mesenchymal transition (Xia et al. 2006). TGF-β suppression by HGF was also observed in the model of DEN-induced fibrosis (Ueki et al. 1999).

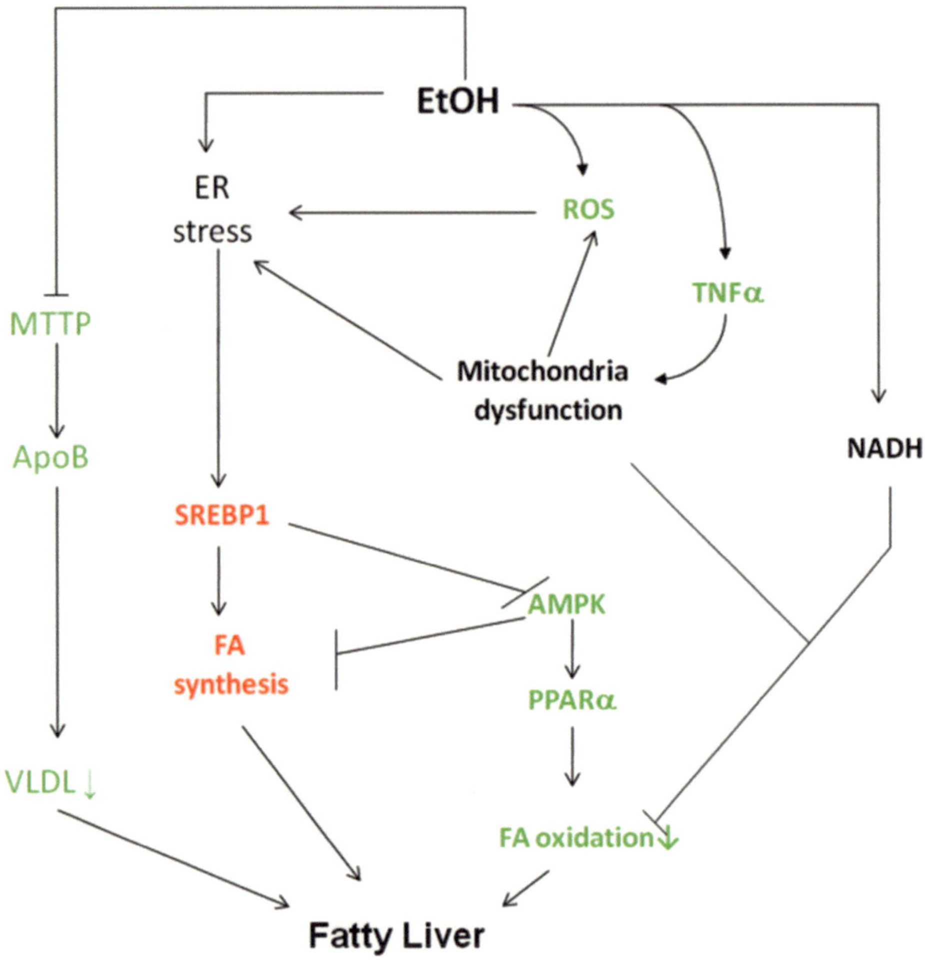

Fig. 4. Molecular mechanism of ethanol-mediated lipid deposition in the liver. Molecules or processes downregulated (red) and upregulated (green) by HGF. EtOH, ethanol; TNF-α, Tumor necrosis factor-alpha; ROS, reactive oxygen species; ER, Endoplasmic reticulum; NADH, Nicotine Adenine dinucleotide reduced; SREBP1c, sterol regulatory element binding protein 1c; AMPK, AMP-activated protein kinase; MTTP, microsomal triglyceride transfer protein; VLDL, very low density lipoproteins; PPAR-α; peroxisome proliferator-activated receptors alpha; FA, Fatty acid.

Another study showed that HGF decreased the expression of collagen 1A2 gene in a model of fibrosis induced by carbon tetrachloride by a mechanism dependent of the nuclear export of smad3 mediated by galectin-7 (Inagaki et al. 2008).

Recently an innovator system to study the anti-fibrotic and protective effect of HGF was developed (Jones et al. 2010). HGF was mixed with collagen and robotically printed onto standard glass slides to create arrays of 500 μm diameter spots, and then rat hepatocytes were seeded and challenged with 100 mM ethanol. Results showed that hepatocytes in the HGF-containing collagen spots presented less apoptosis comparing with those seeded in

HGF-free spots. To investigate impact on the fibrosis, a mix of hepatocytes and HSC were seeded and again challenged with alcohol. HSC were less activated (less fibrotic) in spots containing HGF compared to control. This *in vitro* study confirms the anti-fibrotic response of HGF

3.7 HGF, alcohol and cancer

Heavy long-term alcohol drinking (≥69.0 g alcohol/day in men, and ≥ 23.0 g alcohol/day in women) is a significant risk factor for the development of hepatocellular carcinoma (HCC) (Shimazu et al. 2011) . There is no efficient animal model to study the direct mechanism of alcohol-induced HCC, recently it has been reported that rats selectively bred for high alcohol preference with free access to water supplemented with 10% ethanol for 18 months developed hepatic neoplasia, ERK pathway activation, increased Cyp2E1 activity and oxidative stress (Yip-Schneider et al. 2011). As mentioned here, ethanol metabolism is the main harmful mechanism, due to ROS production; in addition ethanol increases the infiltration of inflammatory cells enhancing the oxidative damage, accelerating telomere shortening and favoring oncogenic mutation (Cornellá et al. 2011) in the carcinogenesis process.

The HGF functions, previously described inhere; strongly suggest the prominent role of this growth factor in the prevention of HCC. In fact, MetKO mice exhibited an accelerated DEN-induced hepatocarcinogenesis, demonstrating the protective and preventive roles of HGF in liver carcinogenesis (Takami et al. 2007), in this study, the accelerated tumor development was associated with increased rate of cell proliferation and prolonged activation of epidermal growth factor receptor (EGFR) signaling, MetKO mice also exhibited an elevated lipid peroxidation, decreased levels of GSH, and SOD expression increment, suggesting that oxidative stress could be a determinant factor for the acceleration of hepatocarcinogenesis. MetKO mice were more susceptible than WT mice to DEN-induced liver cancer increasing multiplicity, incidence and size of tumors. The negative effects of c-Met deletion were reversed by the chronic administration of NAC, blocking EGFR activation and reducing initiated hepatocarcinogenesis, confirming that c-Met deletion-induced oxidative stress is the main hallmark in the accelerated carcinogenesis and that c-Met integrity is required as a protective mechanism against chemical-induced carcinogenesis by the induction of cytoprotective enzymes such as antioxidant enzymes.

In contrast, a wide variety of human tumors exhibit sustained activation, overexpression or mutation of c-Met, including liver tumors. It is not hard to imagine that beneficial and protective roles of HGF in all stages of alcoholic liver disease are not longing in liver cancer. HGF-induced protection ends in the early stages of hepatocarcinogenesis. Once initiated the carcinogenic process, HGF and c-Met trigger signaling cascades resulting in proliferation, growth, survival, motogenesis and angiogenesis (Eder et al. 2009). Mouse and human cell lines that overexpress c-Met or/and HGF become tumorigenic and metastatic in athymic mice (Rong et al. 1994) and, in contrast, downregulation of c-Met or HGF expression decreases tumorigenic potential (Abounader et al., 2002), in fact, overexpression of c-Met or HFG are associated with poor prognosis and aggressive phenotype (Kaposi-Novak et al. 2006). In summary HGF/c-Met protects from carcinogenesis, but in established tumors induces the aggravation of the disease. Mutations in c-Met and HGF predispose to human cancer.

4. Conclusion

In conclusion HGF and c-Met are introduced as promissory therapeutic targets for the treatment of ALD, they can reverse or abrogate almost every stage of the disease, controlling the metabolism, the harmful molecules, the lipid homeostasis disturbing and the chronic effects of alcohol consumption. Although more research is needed to figure out the proper point of intervention in the signaling activated by HGF and c-Met, the experimental evidences gathered here support the promising success of HGF/c-Met.

5. Acknowledge

This work was partially funded by grants from the Consejo Nacional de Ciencia y Tecnología (CONACYT 61544 and 131707); by FUNDHEPA "Antonio Ariza Cañadilla" grant, and by the Universidad Autónoma Metropolitana-Iztapalapa.

6. References

Abounader R, Lal B, Luddy C, Koe G, Davidson B, Rosen EM & Laterra J. (2002) In vivo targeting of SF/HGF and c-met expression via U1snRNA/ribozymes inhibits glioma growth and angiogenesis and promotes apoptosis. FASEB J 16: 108-110.

Arends B, Slump E, Spee B, Rothuizen J & Penning LC (2008) Hepatocyte growth factor improves viability after H2O2-induced toxicity in bile duct epithelial cells. Comparative Biochemistry and Physiology C-Toxicology & Pharmacology 147 324-330.

Bertotti A & Comoglio PM 2003 Tyrosine kinase signal specificity: lessons from the HGF receptor. Trends Biochem Sci 28 527-533.

Boccaccio C, Ando M, Tamagnone L, Bardelli A, Michieli P, Battistini C & Comoglio PM (1998) Induction of epithelial tubules by growth factor HGF depends on the STAT pathway. Nature 391 285-288.

Cadenas E 1989 Biochemistry of oxygen toxicity. Annu Rev Biochem 58 79-110.

Cornella H, Alsinet C & Villanueva A (2011) Molecular pathogenesis of hepatocellular carcinoma. Alcohol Clin Exp Res 35 821-825.

Chanda D, Li T, Song KH, Kim YH, Sim J, Lee CH, Chiang JY & Choi HS (2009) Hepatocyte growth factor family negatively regulates hepatic gluconeogenesis via induction of orphan nuclear receptor small heterodimer partner in primary hepatocytes. J Biol Chem 284 28510-28521.

Chen Q & Cederbaum AI (1998) Cytotoxicity and apoptosis produced by cytochrome P450 2E1 in Hep G2 cells. Mol Pharmacol 53 638-648.

Cornella H, Alsinet C, Villanueva A. (2011) Molecular pathogenesis of hepatocellular carcinoma. Alcohol Clin Exp Res. 35 821-825

De Minicis S, Seki E, Paik YH, Osterreicher CH, Kodama Y, Kluwe J, Torozzi L, Miyai K, Benedetti A, Schwabe RF (2010) Role and cellular source of nicotinamide adenine dinucleotide phosphate oxidase in hepatic fibrosis. Hepatology 52 1420-1430.

de Mochel NS, Seronello S, Wang SH, Ito C, Zheng JX, Liang TJ, Lambeth JD & Choi J (2010) Hepatocyte NAD(P)H oxidases as an endogenous source of reactive oxygen species during hepatitis C virus infection. Hepatology 52 47-59.

Dobrzyn P, Dobrzyn A, Miyazaki M, Cohen P, Asilmaz E, Hardie DG, Friedman JM & Ntambi JM (2004) Stearoyl-CoA desaturase 1 deficiency increases fatty acid oxidation by activating AMP-activated protein kinase in liver. Proc Natl Acad Sci U S A 101 6409-6414.

Donato MT, Gomez-Lechon MJ, Jover R, Nakamura T & Castell JV (1998) Human hepatocyte growth factor down-regulates the expression of cytochrome P450 isozymes in human hepatocytes in primary culture. J Pharmacol Exp Ther 284 760-767.

Donohue TM, Osna NA & Clemens DL 2006 Recombinant Hep G2 cells that express alcohol dehydrogenase and cytochrome P450 2E1 as a model of ethanol-elicited cytotoxicity. Int J Biochem Cell Biol 38 92-101.

Eder PJ, Vande-Wounde GF, Boerner SA & LoRusso PM. (2009) Novel therapeutic Inhibitors of the c-Met Signaling pathways in Cancer. Clin Cancer Res 15:2207-2214.

Fan S, Gao M, Meng Q, Laterra JJ, Symons MH, Coniglio S, Pestell RG, Goldberg ID & Rosen EM (2005) Role of NF-kappaB signaling in hepatocyte growth factor/scatter factor-mediated cell protection. Oncogene 24 1749-1766.

Fernandez-Checa JC, Colell A & Garcia-Ruiz C (2002) S-Adenosyl-L-methionine and mitochondrial reduced glutathione depletion in alcoholic liver disease. Alcohol 27 179-183.

Fernandez-Checa JC, Hirano T, Tsukamoto H & Kaplowitz N (1993) Mitochondrial glutathione depletion in alcoholic liver disease. Alcohol 10 469-475.

Fernandez-Checa JC, Yi JR, Garcia Ruiz C, Ookhtens M & Kaplowitz N (1996) Plasma membrane and mitochondrial transport of hepatic reduced glutathione. Semin Liver Dis 16 147-158.

Ferre P & Foufelle F (2010) Hepatic steatosis: a role for de novo lipogenesis and the transcription factor SREBP-1c. Diabetes Obes Metab 12 Suppl 2 83-92.

Funakoshi H & Nakamura T 2003 Hepatocyte growth factor: from diagnosis to clinical applications. Clin Chim Acta 327 1-23.

Garcia-Villafranca J, Guillen A & Castro J (2008) Ethanol consumption impairs regulation of fatty acid metabolism by decreasing the activity of AMP-activated protein kinase in rat liver. Biochimie 90 460-466.

Gomez-Quiroz L, Bucio L, Souza V, Escobar C, Farfan B, Hernandez E, Konigsberg M, Vargas-Vorackova F, Kershenobich D & Gutierrez-Ruiz MC (2003) Interleukin 8 response and oxidative stress in HepG2 cells treated with ethanol, acetaldehyde or lipopolysaccharide. Hepatol Res 26 134-141.

Gomez-Quiroz LE, Factor VM, Kaposi-Novak P, Coulouarn C, Conner EA & Thorgeirsson SS (2008) Hepatocyte-specific c-Met deletion disrupts redox homeostasis and sensitizes to Fas-mediated apoptosis. J Biol Chem 283 14581-14589.

Grenier A, Chollet-Martin S, Crestani B, Delarche C, El Benna J, Boutten A, Andrieu V, Durand G, Gougerot-Pocidalo MA, Aubier M (2002) Presence of a mobilizable intracellular pool of hepatocyte growth factor in human polymorphonuclear neutrophils. Blood 99 2997-3004.

Hanna JA, Bordeaux J, Rimm DL & Agarwal S (2009) The function, proteolytic processing, and histopathology of Met in cancer. Adv Cancer Res 103 1-23.

Hardie DG & Pan DA (2002) Regulation of fatty acid synthesis and oxidation by the AMP-activated protein kinase. Biochem Soc Trans 30 1064-1070.

Hirano T, Kaplowitz N, Tsukamoto H, Kamimura S & Fernandez-Checa JC (1992) Hepatic mitochondrial glutathione depletion and progression of experimental alcoholic liver disease in rats. Hepatology 16 1423-1427.

Huh CG, Factor VM, Sanchez A, Uchida K, Conner EA & Thorgeirsson SS (2004) Hepatocyte growth factor/c-met signaling pathway is required for efficient liver regeneration and repair. Proc Natl Acad Sci U S A 101 4477-4482.

Inagaki Y, Higashi K, Kushida M, Hong YY, Nakao S, Higashiyama R, Moro T, Itoh J, Mikami T, Kimura T (2008) Hepatocyte growth factor suppresses profibrogenic signal transduction via nuclear export of Smad3 with galectin-7. Gastroenterology 134 1180-1190.

Jeffers M, Taylor GA, Weidner KM, Omura S & Vande Woude GF (1997) Degradation of the Met tyrosine kinase receptor by the ubiquitin-proteasome pathway. Mol Cell Biol 17 799-808.

Jones CN, Tuleuova N, Lee JY, Ramanculov E, Reddi AH, Zern MA & Revzin A (2010) Cultivating hepatocytes on printed arrays of HGF and BMP7 to characterize protective effects of these growth factors during in vitro alcohol injury. Biomaterials 31 5936-5944.

Kaibori M, Kwon AH, Oda M, Kamiyama Y, Kitamura N & Okumura T (1998) Hepatocyte growth factor stimulates synthesis of lipids and secretion of lipoproteins in rat hepatocytes. Hepatology 27 1354-1361.

Kaposi-Novak P, Lee JS, Gomez-Quiroz L, Coulouarn C, Factor VM & Thorgeirsson SS (2006) Met-regulated expression signature defines a subset of human hepatocellular carcinomas with poor prognosis and aggressive phenotype. J Clin Invest 116 1582-1595.

Kermorgant S & Parker PJ (2005) c-Met signalling: spatio-temporal decisions. Cell Cycle 4 352-355.

Kitta K, Day RM, Ikeda T & Suzuki YJ 2001 Hepatocyte growth factor protects cardiac myocytes against oxidative stress-induced apoptosis. Free Radic Biol Med 31 902-910.

Klaassen CD & Reisman SA (2010) Nrf2 the rescue: effects of the antioxidative/electrophilic response on the liver. Toxicol Appl Pharmacol 244 57-65.

Kono H, Rusyn I, Yin M, Gabele E, Yamashina S, Dikalova A, Kadiiska MB, Connor HD, Mason RP, Segal BH (2000) NADPH oxidase-derived free radicals are key oxidants in alcohol-induced liver disease. J Clin Invest 106 867-872.

Kosone T, Takagi H, Horiguchi N, Ariyama Y, Otsuka T, Sohara N, Kakizaki S, Sato K & Mori M (2007) HGF ameliorates a high-fat diet-induced fatty liver. Am J Physiol Gastrointest Liver Physiol 293 G204-210.

Lieber CS (2004) Alcoholic fatty liver: its pathogenesis and mechanism of progression to inflammation and fibrosis. Alcohol 34 9-19.

Ma PC, Maulik G, Christensen J & Salgia R (2003) c-Met: structure, functions and potential for therapeutic inhibition. Cancer Metastasis Rev 22 309-325.

Maroun CR, Holgado-Madruga M, Royal I, Naujokas MA, Fournier TM, Wong AJ & Park M (1999) The Gab1 PH domain is required for localization of Gab1 at sites of cell-cell contact and epithelial morphogenesis downstream from the met receptor tyrosine kinase. Mol Cell Biol 19 1784-1799.

Maroun CR, Naujokas MA, Holgado-Madruga M, Wong AJ & Park M (2000) The tyrosine phosphatase SHP-2 is required for sustained activation of extracellular signal-regulated kinase and epithelial morphogenesis downstream from the met receptor tyrosine kinase. Mol Cell Biol 20 8513-8525.

Matsuda Y, Matsumoto K, Ichida T & Nakamura T (1995) Hepatocyte growth factor suppresses the onset of liver cirrhosis and abrogates lethal hepatic dysfunction in rats. J Biochem 118 643-649.

Matsuda Y, Matsumoto K, Yamada A, Ichida T, Asakura H, Komoriya Y, Nishiyama E & Nakamura T (1997) Preventive and therapeutic effects in rats of hepatocyte growth factor infusion on liver fibrosis/cirrhosis. Hepatology 26 81-89.

Nakamura T & Mizuno S (2010) The discovery of hepatocyte growth factor (HGF) and its significance for cell biology, life sciences and clinical medicine. Proc Jpn Acad Ser B Phys Biol Sci 86 588-610.

Naldini L, Tamagnone L, Vigna E, Sachs M, Hartmann G, Birchmeier W, Daikuhara Y, Tsubouchi H, Blasi F & Comoglio PM (1992) Extracellular proteolytic cleavage by urokinase is required for activation of hepatocyte growth factor/scatter factor. EMBO J 11 4825-4833.

Riehle KJ, Dan YY, Campbell JS & Fausto N (2011) New concepts in liver regeneration. J Gastroenterol Hepatol 26 Suppl 1 203-212.

Rong, S., Segal, S., Anver, M., Resau, J. H. & Vande Woude, G. F. (1994) Invasiveness and metastasis of NIH 3T3 cells induced by Met-hepatocyte growth factor/scatter factor autocrine stimulation. *Proc. Natl Acad. Sci. USA* 91 4731–4735

Salmela KS, Kessova IG, Tsyrlov IB & Lieber CS (1998) Respective roles of human cytochrome P-4502E1, 1A2, and 3A4 in the hepatic microsomal ethanol oxidizing system. Alcohol Clin Exp Res 22 2125-2132.

Santangelo C, Matarrese P, Masella R, Di Carlo MC, Di Lillo A, Scazzocchio B, Vecci E, Malorni W, Perfetti R & Anastasi E 2007 Hepatocyte growth factor protects rat RINm5F cell line against free fatty acid-induced apoptosis by counteracting oxidative stress. J Mol Endocrinol 38 147-158.

Serviddio G, Bellanti F, Sastre J, Vendemiale G & Altomare E (2010) Targeting mitochondria: a new promising approach for the treatment of liver diseases. Curr Med Chem 17 2325-2337.

Shimazu T, Sasazuki S, Wakai K, Tamakoshi A, Tsuji I, Sugawara Y, Matsuo K, Nagata C, Mizoue T, Tanaka K, Inoue M, Tsugane S; Alcohol drinking and primary liver cancer: A pooled analysis of four Japanese cohort studies Int J Cancer. DOI: 10.1002/ijc.26255.

Sonnenberg E, Meyer D, Weidner KM & Birchmeier C (1993) Scatter factor/hepatocyte growth factor and its receptor, the c-met tyrosine kinase, can mediate a signal exchange between mesenchyme and epithelia during mouse development. J Cell Biol 123 223-235.

Stoker M, Gherardi E, Perryman M & Gray J (1987) Scatter factor is a fibroblast-derived modulator of epithelial cell mobility. Nature 327 239-242.

Sugimoto T, Yamashita S, Ishigami M, Sakai N, Hirano K, Tahara M, Matsumoto K, Nakamura T & Matsuzawa Y (2002) Decreased microsomal triglyceride transfer protein activity contributes to initiation of alcoholic liver steatosis in rats. J Hepatol 36 157-162.

Tahara M, Matsumoto K, Nukiwa T & Nakamura T (1999) Hepatocyte growth factor leads to recovery from alcohol-induced fatty liver in rats. J Clin Invest 103 313-320.

Taieb J, Delarche C, Ethuin F, Selloum S, Poynard T, Gougerot-Pocidalo MA & Chollet-Martin S (2002a) Ethanol-induced inhibition of cytokine release and protein degranulation in human neutrophils. J Leukoc Biol 72 1142-1147.

Taieb J, Delarche C, Paradis V, Mathurin P, Grenier A, Crestani B, Dehoux M, Thabut D, Gougerot-Pocidalo MA, Poynard T, et al. 2002b Polymorphonuclear neutrophils are a source of hepatocyte growth factor in patients with severe alcoholic hepatitis. J Hepatol 36 342-348.

Takami T, Kaposi-Novak P, Uchida K, Gomez-Quiroz LE, Conner EA, Factor VM & Thorgeirsson SS (2007) Loss of hepatocyte growth factor/c-Met signaling pathway accelerates early stages of N-nitrosodiethylamine induced hepatocarcinogenesis. Cancer Res 67 9844-9851.

Tomita K, Azuma T, Kitamura N, Nishida J, Tamiya G, Oka A, Inokuchi S, Nishimura T, Suematsu M & Ishii H (2004) Pioglitazone prevents alcohol-induced fatty liver in rats through up-regulation of c-Met. Gastroenterology 126 873-885.

Trusolino L, Bertotti A & Comoglio PM 2010 MET signalling: principles and functions in development, organ regeneration and cancer. Nat Rev Mol Cell Biol 11 834-848.

Tsuboi S (1999) Elevation of glutathione level in rat hepatocytes by hepatocyte growth factor via induction of gamma-glutamylcysteine synthetase. J Biochem 126 815-820.

Tsutsumi M, Lasker JM, Shimizu M, Rosman AS & Lieber CS (1989) The intralobular distribution of ethanol-inducible P450IIE1 in rat and human liver. Hepatology 10 437-446.

Ueki T, Kaneda Y, Tsutsui H, Nakanishi K, Sawa Y, Morishita R, Matsumoto K, Nakamura T, Takahashi H, & Okamoto E (1999) Hepatocyte growth factor gene therapy of liver cirrhosis in rats. Nat Med 5 226-230.

Valdes-Arzate A, Luna A, Bucio L, Licona C, Clemens DL, Souza V, Hernandez E, Kershenobich D, Gutierrez-Ruiz MC & Gomez-Quiroz LE (2009) Hepatocyte growth factor protects hepatocytes against oxidative injury induced by ethanol metabolism. Free Radic Biol Med 47 424-430.

Valko M, Leibfritz D, Moncol J, Cronin MT, Mazur M & Telser J (2007) Free radicals and antioxidants in normal physiological functions and human disease. Int J Biochem Cell Biol 39 44-84.

Xia JL, Dai C, Michalopoulos GK & Liu Y (2006) Hepatocyte growth factor attenuates liver fibrosis induced by bile duct ligation. Am J Pathol 168 1500-1512.

Yip-Scheider MT, Doyle CJ, McKillop IH, Wentz SC, Brandon-Warner E, Matos JM, Sandrasegaran K, Saxena R, Hennig ME, Wu H, Waters JA, Klein PJ, Froehlich JC,Max Schmidt C. (2011) Alcohol Induces Liver Neoplasia in a Novel Alcohol-Preferring Rat Model. Alcohol Clin Exp Res. DOI: 10.1111/j.1530-0277.2011.01568.x

8

Hepatic Myofibroblasts in Liver Fibrogenesis

Chiara Busletta, Erica Novo, Stefania Cannito,
Claudia Paternostro and Maurizio Parola
*Department of Experimental Medicine and Oncology,
Faculty of Medicine and Surgery, University of Torino
Italy*

1. Introduction

On a worldwide perspective chronic liver diseases (CLDs) are very common pathologic conditions which are characterized by reiteration of hepatocyte injury that is mainly induced by chronic infection by hepatitis B and C viruses (HBV and HCV), autoimmune injury and metabolic and/or toxic/drug - induced causes, with chronic alcohol consumption being predominant particularly in western countries. Chronic liver injury is reported to result in the chronic activation of both inflammatory and wound healing response that, in association with other major pathogenic mechanisms (oxidative stress, derangement of epithelial-mesenchymal interactions and possibly epithelial to mesenchymal transition, see later in section 3), can sustain persistent liver fibrogenesis (i.e., the process) and represent the prominent driving force for liver fibrosis (i.e., the result) (Parola and Robino, 2001; Friedman 2003; Bataller and Brenner, 2005; Friedman 2008b; Novo and Parola, 2008; Parola et al., 2008).

Literature data from the last two decades indicate that hepatic fibrogenesis in a CLD has to be envisaged as a dynamic and highly integrated molecular, tissue and cellular process that, irrespective of the aetiology, leads to the progressive accumulation of extracellular matrix (ECM) components in an attempt to limit hepatic injury. Persistent liver fibrogenesis is currently considered as the critical process responsible for the progression of any CLD to the end-points of liver cirrhosis and hepatic failure. According to current definition, cirrhosis should be regarded as an advanced stage of fibrosis, being characterized by the following major features: a) the formation of regenerative nodules of hepatic parenchyma surrounded and separated by fibrotic septa; b) the development of significant changes in organ vascular architecture, portal hypertension and related clinical complications (i.e., variceal bleeding, hepatic encephalopathy, ascites and hepatorenal syndrome) (Friedman, 2003, 2004; Pinzani and Rombouts, 2004; Bataller and Brenner, 2005; Friedman 2008b).

In any CLDs fibrotic progression can proceed through at least four distinct patterns of fibrosis that have close relationships with the underlying aetiology and are also related to the "topographic site" of tissue injury, the involvement of different populations of myofibroblasts (MFs) and the predominant pro-fibrogenic mechanism (Cassiman and Roskams, 2002; Pinzani and Rombouts, 2004; Parola et al., 2008; Parola and Pinzani, 2009).

1.1 Bridging fibrosis

This pattern of ECM deposition and fibrotic septa formation is typically described in the liver of patients carrying HBV- or HCV-related chronic hepatitis. As a result of portal-central bridging necrosis the pattern is characterized by the formation of a) portal-central fibrotic septa, that connect portal areas with the area of central vein, b) portal-portal fibrotic septa, that connect distinct portal areas, as well as of c) blind fibrotic septa in the parenchyma. As any pathologist may easily recall, to this pattern belong classic histopathological images of fibrotic septa leading to the obliteration of central veins and of early changes in vascular architecture and connections with the portal system, events that with the time favor the development of portal hypertension. The pattern of bridging fibrosis recognizes the chronic activation of wound healing as the major pathogenic mechanism driving fibrosis progression and, as detailed later in this chapter, fibrogenesis is predominantly sustained in these settings by hepatic populations of pro-fibrogenic MFs that originate mainly from hepatic stellate cells (HSCs) or, to a less extent, from either portal fibroblasts or from bone marrow - derived stem cells. Extensive literature data also suggest that oxidative stress and reactive oxygen species (ROS) offer an additional major contribution in sustaining liver fibrogenesis in this pattern of bridging fibrosis.

1.2 Perisinusoidal / Pericellular fibrosis

This specific pattern of fibrosis has been described in CLDs which follow either excess alcohol consumption (ASH or alcoholic steatohepatitis) or metabolic derangement and then progression from non-alcoholic fatty liver disease (NAFLD) to non-alcoholic steatohepatitis (NASH). In these clinical settings, which are increasingly common particularly in western countries, excess deposition of ECM components is first detected in the space of Disse leading to the peculiar "chicken-wire" pattern. MFs originating from the activation of hepatic stellate cells (HSC/MFs) are believed to represent the most relevant pro-fibrogenic cellular effectors in these conditions, with ROS and oxidative stress playing a predominant pro-fibrogenic and pathogenic role.

1.3 Biliary fibrosis

This is a pattern which in humans is typically detected in a number of conditions affecting the biliary tree (primary biliary cirrhosis, primary sclerosizing cholangitis, secondary biliary cirrhosis) that are characterized by a peculiar scenario involving concomitant proliferation of bile ductules and periductular MFs. In these clinical settings MFs mainly derive from periportal fibroblasts or, as recently suggested, by epithelial to mesenchymal transition (EMT) of cholangiocytes, an issue that at present is controversial and highly debated (see section 3.4). In any case, the biliary fibrosis scenario is dominated by the formation of portal-portal fibrotic septa that in human patients for long time do not significantly affect vascular connections with the portal system. Major pathogenic mechanisms sustaining this pattern of fibrosis have been identified either in alterations in the interactions between cholangiocytes and mesenchymal cells (with cholangiocyte transition into MF-like phenotype being still debated) or in alterations of redox equilibrium (i.e., oxidative stress).

1.4 Centrilobular fibrosis

Although this pattern is commonly included in the classification, centrilobular fibrosis is indeed unrelated to CLDs but, rather, is typically observed in those patients being affected by chronic heart failure: in these patients a significant alteration of venous outflow is realized that, with the time, leads to the formation of fibrotic septa developing among central vein areas (central-central septa) which, in turn, result in the unique scenario which is often described as of "reversed lobulation".

2. Hepatic myofibroblasts

Hepatic myofibroblasts (MFs) represent a heterogenous population of pro-fibrogenic cells, mostly positive for α-smooth muscle actin (α-SMA), that are mainly found in chronically injured livers (i.e., fibrotic and or cirrhotic) (Cassiman et al., 2002; Friedman, 2008a, 2008b; Parola et al., 2008; Parola and Pinzani, 2009) and, irrespective the specific aetiology of a CLD and of the prevalent pattern of fibrosis, sustain liver fibrogenesis in addition to injured hepatocytes, activated Kupffer cells and sinusoidal endothelial cells. Hepatic populations of MFs share a number of common properties which include high proliferative attitude, the ability to contract in response of vasoactive mediators, and the ability to actively participate to CLD progression by means of their multiple phenotypic responses. This includes excess deposition of ECM components and ECM altered remodelling as well as the synthesis and the release (paracrine/autocrine) of critical polypeptide mediators which sustain and perpetuate fibrogenesis, chronic inflammatory response and angiogenesis. Along these lines, hepatic MFs can be envisaged as a unique and crucial cellular crossroad where incoming paracrine and autocrine signals, including growth factors, inflammatory and angiogenic signals, chemokines, adipokines, as well as ROS, are integrated in order to "operate" phenotypic responses designed to sustain fibrogenesis and the progression of CLDs to the end-points of cirrhosis and hepatic failure.

As recently reviewed (Parola et al., 2008; Parola & Pinzani, 2009) progressive fibrogenesis is believed to be sustained by four main pro-fibrogenic mechanisms: a) chronic activation of the wound healing response, a mechanism that applies virtually to any CLDs and predominates in HBV or HCV chronic injury or autoimmune liver diseases; b) oxidative stress, with the generation of ROS and other oxidative stress - related reactive mediators, a mechanism that again applies to all CLDs but is predominant in either alcoholic liver disease (ALD) and NASH; c) derangement of epithelial-mesenchymal interactions, as detected in chronic cholangiopaties and, more generally, all the conditions of biliary fibrosis; d) EMT.

Some years ago it has been proposed a classification of the different hepatic populations of MFs which is based on the specific antigen profile and the tissue localization of these pro-fibrogenic cells in the context of a chronically injured liver (Cassiman et al., 2002). This classification recognizes at least three different kind of MFs.

2.1 Portal/septal MFs (PS/MFs)

These MFs are believed to originate mainly from portal fibroblasts (i.e., fibroblasts residing in the connective tissue of portal areas in normal conditions) through a process of activation/transdifferentiation. PS/MFs are typically detected in the expanded connective tissue around portal tracts (portal MFs) or in the inner part of fibrotic septa (septal MFs). Irrespective of their localization, they share a common and overlapping antigen repertoire that allows their recognition "in vivo". The antigen profile of human PS/MFs includes, in addition to α-SMA, expression of glial fibrillary acidic protein (GFAP), brain-derived nerve growth factor (BDNGF) and α-B-crystallin (ABCRYS).

2.2 Interface MFs (IF/MFs)

Interface MFs are α-SMA - positive cells detected at the edge between fibrotic septa and the surrounding parenchyma (i.e., where active fibrogenesis occurs). These cells can originate from activation/transdifferentiation of hepatic stellate cells, portal fibroblasts as well as from bone marrow - derived mesenchymal stem cells (Russo et al., 2006; Valfrè di Bonzo et al., 2008; Forbes & Parola, 2011) following their engraftment into chronically injured livers. Human IF/MFs express all the typical markers already mentioned (α-SMA, GFAP, BDNF, ABCRYS) as well as nerve growth factor (NGF), neural cell adhesion molecule (N-CAM) and neurotrophin-4 (NT-4).

2.3 Activated, MF-like, hepatic stellate cells (HSC/MFs)

HSC/MFs are α-SMA-positive cells found primarily in or around capillarised sinusoids of fibrotic/cirrhotic livers that by definition originate only through a process of activation/differentiation from hepatic stellate cells (HSC), a kind of cells which have their physiological location in the space of Disse and in normal conditions are believed to store vitamin A and retinoids, to contribute to the synthesis of the local ECM components as well as to act as liver specific pericytes. HSC/MFs are positively stained "in vivo" for α-SMA and can be recognized from other MFs for their positivity to a list of additional markers which includes neurotrophin-3 (NT-3), tyrosine kinase B or C (Trk-B, Trk-C), synaptophysin and p75, the low-affinity nerve growth factor receptor.

3. The multiple origin of hepatic myofibroblasts

A fascinating and still incompletely resolved issue is represented by the "in vivo" origin of hepatic MFs. According to current literature hepatic MFs mainly originate from hepatic stellate cells or from fibroblasts of portal areas through a process of activation and trans-differentiation. In addition, hepatic MFs have been reported to originate also from bone marrow - derived stem cells, including mesenchymal stem cells or circulating fibrocytes, able to engraft chronically injured liver (Forbes & Parola, 2011). It has also been proposed that myofibroblasts or pro-fibrogenic cells may originate from either hepatocytes or cholangiocytes through a process of EMT, an issue that is at present highly controversial and debated (see section 3.4). Although hepatic MFs may then originate from different sources the interested reader should note that these cells are likely to display the same pro-fibrogenic properties and phenotypic responses. Moreover, it has been proposed that HSC/MFs may play a critical role in the modulation of immune responses in CLDs and to strictly interact with either hepatic progenitor (stem) cells and/or with malignant cells of primary hepatocellular carcinomas or of metastatic cancers. In the following sections we will briefly summarize major information on the different intra- and extra-hepatic origin of MFs.

3.1 Hepatic stellate cells as a major intrahepatic source of MFs

Under physiological conditions HSC are perisinusoidal cells of still uncertain embryological origin which are responsible for at least four main functions: a) HSC are responsible for the synthesis of basal membrane like - ECM components of the subendothelial space of Disse where they are located; b) HSC are responsible for the storage and the metabolism of vitamin A and retinoids (HSC represent the main site of storage for these compounds in mammalians); c) HSC act as "liver specific pericytes" taking intimate contacts with liver sinusoidal endothelial cells (LSEC); d) HSC contribute significantly to hepatic development and regeneration following either acute liver injury of liver resection (Friedman 2008a).

HSC have been the first cell source of pro-fibrogenic MF-like cells to be identified and most of published studies performed on the pathogenic mechanisms of liver fibrosis deal with HSC/MFs. For these cells Scott Friedman's laboratory has proposed the two-step process of activation and trans-differentiation, i.e. the process that leads HSC to acquire the MF-like phenotype (Friedman, 2003, 2008a). HSC-MFs are currently believed to be involved in most of clinical conditions of CLDs, with a predominant involvement in the pattern of fibrosis progression defined as "perisinusoidal/pericellular fibrosis", recognising a metabolic or alcoholic aetiology. HSC contribute significantly also to the origin of IF/MFs and to the pattern of "bridging fibrosis" found in patients affected by chronic viral hepatitis (Friedman, 2008a,b; Parola et al., 2008).

Experimental and clinical studies dealing with HSC and HSC/MFs have been fundamental for our present knowledge concerning liver fibrogenesis and related molecular mechanisms by revealing that, under conditions of chronic liver injury, quiescent HSC located in the perisinusoidal space of Disse can undergo a peculiar process of activation. Human as well as rodent HSC undergo "in vitro"changes in morphology and operate phenotypical responses in their trans-differentiation from the original "storing or quiescent phenotype" to the one of activated MFs. The activated MF-like phenotype includes the following relevant pro-fibrogenic features (Friedman 2008a; 2008b; Pinzani and Marra, 2001; Pinzani and Rombouts, 2004; Bataller and Brenner, 2005; Parola et al., 2008): a) a high proliferative attitude in response to growth factors and other mediators; b) an increased ability to synthesize ECM components, mainly fibrillar collagens (i.e., collagen type I and type III), as well as of factors involved in ECM remodelling; c) the ability to migrate in response to chemoattractants; d) the property to produce and release growth factors (autocrine loops) and pro-inflammatory cytokines; e) the ability to contract in response to vasoactive compounds. All these changes and phenotypic responses are considered to be similar to those occurring "in vivo" and to represent a functional paradigm common to all pro-fibrogenic MFs, whatever the origin (Friedman 2008b; Parola et al., 2008; Parola and Pinzani 2009; Forbes & Parola, 2011).

3.2 Portal fibroblasts as an emerging additional intrahepatic source of MFs

Portal fibroblasts (PFs) in the normal liver are α-SMA positive cells characterized by a morphological phenotype and by an antigen repertoire which are close to those expressed by other fibroblasts. Moreover, PFs express the highly specific fibroblast marker TE7, that is not expressed by other potential cellular sources of MFs like HSC (Dranoff & Wells, 2010), as well as other rather specific markers including IL-6, fibulin 2, elastin and the ecto-ATPase nucleoside triphosphate diphosphohydrolase-2 (NTPD2). The origin of PFs is still uncertain and these cells may alternatively originate either from α-SMA positive cells of the ductal plate during human embryogenesis or, as recently proposed by a murine study, from a putative precursor in the early embryo development able to give also raise to HSCs (Asahina et al., 2009).

According to current literature PFs undergo myofibroblastic differentiation in the chronically injured liver and when cultured on plastic or glass. Portal myofibroblasts (P/MFs), like typical myofibroblasts, express large numbers of α-SMA-containing microfilament bundles arrayed in parallel to the long axis of the cell. At present no definitive evidence has been presented to establish whether P/MFs can proliferate and can be passaged in culture or whether they can revert to a non MF state either "in vitro" or "in vivo", as shown in the past for HSC and HSC/MFs.

Accumulating evidence suggest that PFs as well as P/MFs have a relevant role in liver fibrogenesis. In particular, evidence for the pro-fibrogenic role is unequivocal in experimental conditions of biliary fibrosis such as those from experimental models of cholestatic injury, namely the model of bile duct ligation (BDL) in rodents as recently reviewed (Dranoff and Wells, 2010). The first studies reported that PFs start to deposit matrix in portal areas following BDL before undergoing myofibroblastic differentiation; moreover, PFs proliferate very rapidly around bile ductular cells following BDL and desmin-negative MFs (not originating from HSC) appear early (i.e., within 48 hrs) after BDL adjacent to the proliferating ductules. More recent studies provide evidence suggesting that the pro-fibrogenic role of PFs and P/MFs in biliary fibrosis mostly relies on the fact that the injury to bile duct epithelial cells (BDEC) is a prerequisite for the differentiation of PFs into P/MFs. The elegant and now validated hypothesis is that, once damaged, BDEC start to express transforming growth factor β2 (TGFβ2) and release a number of growth factors and pro-inflammatory mediators, including platelet-derived growth factor -BB (PDGF-BB), interleukin-6 (IL-6) and monocyte chemotactic protein-1 (MCP-1 or CCL2), that can be responsible for differentiation of PFs (that express related receptors) towards the P/MF phenotype. This process closely resemble the process of HSC activation and even more relevant, emerging evidence indicate that the acquisition of the P/MF phenotype is apparently followed by a process of perpetuation in which P/MFs start to behave like HSC/MFs.

An emerging issue is that P/MFs may significantly contribute to CLD progression not only in biliary fibrosis but also in other clinical conditions characterised by bridging fibrosis irrespective of the aetiology. Indeed, as recently reviewed (Dranoff and Wells, 2010), the critical point is likely to be represented by the cross-talk between damaged and/or activated BDEC and PFs rather than the specific aetiology. Accordingly, several investigators have shown the existence of a direct correlation between the intensity of the so-called ductular reaction (a peculiar form of hyperplastic response of BDEC) and the severity of fibrosis in human liver disease of a variety of etiologies, including chronic HCV and NASH, as well as in animal models (Beaussier et al., 2007; Clouston et al., 2005; Fabris et al., 2007; Richardson et al., 2007). In particular, IL-6 and MCP-1 are emerging as important mediators of cell–cell communication between BDEC and PFs, with IL-6 being expressed specifically by BDEC and PFs expressing the IL-6 coreceptor glycoprotein 130 (gp130). It has been proposed the existence of a paracrine loop in which IL-6, by down-regulating NTPD2 on PFs (without altering PF myofibroblastic differentiation), can favor proliferation of BDEC that, in turn, provide stimuli like TGFβ2, PDGF and MCP-1 that sustain proliferation and MF-like differentiation of PFs.

As a final comment for the present section on the putative role of PFs and P/MFs in liver fibrogenesis, one should note that as proposed by Dranoff and Wells (2010) PFs and P/MFs may be as multifunctional as activated HSCs or HSC/MFs, then having a role in the liver progenitor cell niche and in hepatic progenitor cell expansion and differentiation (see paragraph 4 dedicated to the roles attributed to hepatic MFs for more details).

3.3 Bone marrow-derived cells as an extra-hepatic source of MFs

Clinical and experimental evidence indicates that under conditions of chronic liver injury, pro-fibrogenic MFs (mainly IF/MFs and, possibly, some P/MFs) may also originate from progressive recruitment of bone marrow-derived cells (Forbes et al., 2004; Kisseleva et al., 2006; Kallis et al., 2007; Henderson and Forbes, 2008; Friedman, 2008b; Parola et al. 2008; Forbes & Parola, 2011; Kisseleva & Brenner, 2011). This extrahepatic source of MFs is at present believed to offer a significant although modest contribution to liver fibrogenesis. Moreover, such a contribution, from a quantitative point of view, is likely to vary depending on both the aetiology and the progression rate of the specific form of CLD.

From an historical point of view, the first evidence for a bone marrow-derived origin of hepatic MFs was provided in 2004 (Forbes et al., 2004) in a study in which were analysed fibrotic liver obtained from two different kind of patients: a) from male patients (affected by CLDs of different aetiology) that had received liver transplants from female donors and subsequently developed CLD; b) from a female patient that received bone marrow transplant from a male donor and afterward developed HCV-related cirrhosis. By employing fluorescence in situ hybridization (FISH) for the Y chromosome together immune-histochemistry for MFs specific antigens, Authors showed unequivocally that a significant numbers of Y chromosome in fibrotic areas of were found in the nuclei of α-SMA positive cells having a MF phenotype. In the liver transplant cases, a percentage of α-SMA positive MFs ranging from 6.8% to 22.2% contained the Y chromosome whereas in the female recipient of a bone marrow transplant from a male donor, 12.4% of the MFs were positive for the Y chromosome. This first study was followed by other carefully designed experimental studies that confirmed the concept (i.e., MFs may originate from circulating cells derived from bone marrow recruited into chronically injured liver) and were instrumental to identify at least two distinct populations of bone marrow-derived MFs precursors, including circulating fibrocytes (Kisseleva et al., 2006) and mesenchymal stem cells (MSC; Russo et al., 2006; Valfrè di Bonzo et al., 2008).

In their study Kisseleva and coworkers performed experiments in which chimeric mice, transplanted with donor bone marrow from collagen alpha1(I)-green fluorescent protein (GFP)+ reporter mice, were subjected to the BDL model for biliary fibrosis. In response to injury, bone marrow-derived collagen-expressing GFP+ cells were detected in the liver tissues of chimeric mice and these bone marrow-derived cells, that were negative for α-SMA and desmin (then not originating from HSC/MFs), were found to co-express collagen-GFP+ and CD45+. This led Authors to suggest that these cells were representing a unique population of circulating fibrocytes that, in addition, increased numerically in bone marrow and spleen of chimeric mice in response to injury. These fibrocytes when cultured in the presence of TGF-β1 differentiated into α-SMA and desmin positive collagen-producing MFs, confirming then to be potentially able to contribute to liver fibrosis.

In the same year Russo and coworkers (Russo et al., 2006) employed female mice that were submitted to an experimental protocol consisting in: a) lethal irradiation, followed by b) transplant of either whole bone marrow or cell population enriched in MSC from mice male donors to be finally submitted to c) different protocols of fibrosis induction. BM-derived cells were tracked through FISH analysis for the Y chromosome FISH and results obtained indicated unequivocally that the bone marrow contributed significantly to hepatic stellate cell and MFs populations. Moreover, these bone marrow - derived MFs were able to actively synthesize collagen type 1 and originated largely from mesenchymal stem cells.

In a subsequent study (Valfrè di Bonzo et al., 2008), non-obese diabetic - severe combined immuno-deficient (NOD-SCID) mice were sub-lethally irradiated, transplanted with highly purified populations of ex-vivo expanded human MSC and then submitted to a protocol of chronic injury in order to induce fibrosis. When chimeric livers were then analyzed for expression of human transcripts and antigens it was found that a significant number of cells of human origin (identified by expression of HLA class I antigens) exhibited a myofibroblast-like morphology. Moreover, human MSC in their MF-like phenotype were found to respond by proliferation and or migration to PDGF-BB and MCP-1 which are known to be effective on HSC/MFs. This strongly suggests that the pattern of polypeptide mediators known to be generated in CLDs may have a role in the hepatic recruitment/engraftment of MSC.

Along these lines it seems correct to mention also a single study (Higashiyama et al., 2009), perhaps quite controversial (see Kallis and Forbes, 2009), that has questioned the real relevance of the phenomenon, suggesting that the contribution to liver fibrogenesis of MFs from bone marrow-derived cells recruited may be negligible.

3.4 Hepatocytes or cholangiocytes are an unlikely sources of MFs through EMT process

Epithelial to mesenchymal transition (EMT) must be envisaged as a fundamental biological process, paradigmatic of the concept of cell plasticity, that leads epithelial cells to lose their polarization and specialized junctional structures, to undergo cytoskeleton reorganization, and to acquire morphological and functional features of mesenchymal-like cells, including the ability to migrate and to produce and secrete components of the extracellular matrix (Cannito et al., 2010). Although EMT and the related opposite process of MET (mesenchymal to epithelial transition) have been originally described in embryonic development (i.e., where cell migration and tissue remodeling have a primary role in regulating morphogenesis in multicellular organisms), extensive literature data have recently provided evidence suggesting that the EMT process is a more general process that may have a significant role in several pathophysiological conditions, including cancer progression and organ fibrosis (Thiery and Sleeman, 2006; Acloque et al., 2009; Kalluri and Weinberg, 2009; Zeisberg and Neilson, 2009; Cannito et al., 2010).

Pertinent to this chapter, EMT has been proposed to have a pathogenic role in organ fibrosis and particularly in those conditions in which fibrosis may result from chronic and uncontrolled activation of wound-healing response, then in conditions where progressive fibrogenesis result in the progressive accumulation of ECM components, derangement of tissue and vascular architecture and eventually organ failure. The involvement of EMT in organ fibrosis was first claimed in experimental studies dedicated to the pathogenesis of kidney fibrosis (Iwano et al., 2002; Yang et al., 2002; Zeisberg and Kalluri, 2004) in which it was shown that a significant number of pro-fibrogenic kidney fibroblasts were positive for FSP1 (fibroblast specific protein 1), an antigen believed to be specific for fibroblast-like cells derived from local EMT. More recently, several studies (reviewed in Choi and Diehl, 2009; Cannito et al., 2010) have proposed that pro-fibrogenic cells may originate in CLDs through EMT involving either cholangiocytes (BDEC) or hepatocytes.

EMT of hepatocytes was suggested quite recently in an experimental study (Zeisberg et al., 2007) describing a progressive appearance in the injured livers of FSP-1 positive cells, although less than 10% of FSP-1+ cells were shown to co-express the typical and widely accepted MFs marker α-SMA. In such a study Authors also performed lineage-tracing experiments using *AlbCre*.R26Rstop*lacZ* double transgenic mice in order to investigate whether hepatocytes undergoing EMT may contribute significantly to fibrosis induced by chronic treatment with the hepatotoxin CCl_4. They reported that approx. 15% of hepatic cells were FSP-1 positive at the time of severe fibrosis and that approx. 5% of the hepatic cells were co-expressing either FSP-1 and albumin or FSP-1 and β-gal, then suggestive of EMT. Moreover, these authors also performed experiments showing that bone morphogenetic protein-7 (BMP-7), which is known to antagonize TGFβ1 signalling, significantly inhibited progression of liver fibrosis and almost abolished putative EMT-derived fibroblasts. Similar results, were described by another group that employed a transgenic mouse model of Smad7 over-expression in hepatocytes to counteract CCl_4 - induced fibrosis (Dooley et al; 2008). The latter study also reported preliminary morphological evidence for "in vivo" EMT in biopsies from chronic HBV patients in terms of positive hepatocyte nuclear staining for SNAI1 (a specific and EMT-related transcription factor).

Involvement of EMT of cholangiocytes or BDEC has been reported in either experimental and clinical conditions associated with a form of biliary fibrosis. The first report was published in 2006 (Xia et al., 2006) and provided evidence suggesting that BDEC undergoing the process of bile ductular reaction in the rat model of secondary biliary fibrosis due to bile duct ligation were co-expressing α-SMA and cytokeratin 19 (CK-19, a BDEC marker that also stain hepatic progenitor cells or HPCs). The same scenario was confirmed in the same model of BDL (rat and murine) by a series of elegant studies from the group of Anna Mae Diehl (reviewed in Choi and Diehl, 2009), the most relevant (Omenetti et al., 2008a, 2008b, and reference therein) being able to describe an apparently clear cause-effect relationships among EMT of BDEC, appearance of portal MFs and biliary fibrosis as well as the closely related major involvement of Hedgehog signalling pathway. Other studies from the same and other research groups described morphological evidence for EMT of BDEC also in liver biopsies from human patients affected by primary sclerosing cholangitis (PSC, Kirby et al., 2008), primary biliary cirrhosis (PBC, Jung et al., 2007; Robertson et al., 2007; Omenetti et al., 2008b) or biliary atresia (Diaz et al., 2008). Similar evidence has been reported EMT of BDEC in post-transplantation recurrence of PBC (Robertson et al., 2007) and the relevance of Hedgehog and TGFβ1-Smad2/3 signalling was reported also in human patients (Jung et al., 2007, 2008; Omenetti et al., 2008b; Robertson et al., 2007; Rygiel et al., 2008).

Following initial enthusiasm, however, a number of issues have very recently questioned whether EMT may be really involved in CLDs. A first cautionary issue is represented by actual re-evaluation of the specificity of FSP1 as a marker of EMT which comes from carefully performed experiments in kidney. Indeed, some studies have revealed that FSP1 is not at all a marker for fibroblasts but rather for leukocytes and other non-fibroblastic cell types (Le Hir et al., 2005; Lin et al., 2008). In addition, a recent elegant fate tracing study (using Cre/Lox techniques) has clearly shown that although genetically labelled primary proximal epithelial cells exposed in culture to TGFβ underwent apparent EMT becoming MF-like cells, no "in vivo" evidence was detected that epithelial cells may migrate outside of the tubular basement membrane and differentiate into interstitial MFs in a model of kidney fibrosis (Humphreys et al., 2010).

Whether liver fibrogenesis is concerned, the group of Brenner has very recently published three elegant experimental studies that are challenging the involvement of EMT of either hepatocytes or cholangiocytes (or BDEC) as a pathogenic mechanism in liver fibrogenesis. In a first study Authors employed triple transgenic mice expressing ROSA26 stop beta-galactosidase (beta-gal), albumin Cre, and collagen alpha1(I) green fluorescent protein (GFP), in order to have hepatocyte-derived cells permanently labeled by beta-gal and type I collagen-expressing cells labeled by GFP (Taura et al., 2010). These engineered hepatocytes underwent changes towards a fibroblast morphology if cultured in the presence of TGFβ1 but when authors isolated hepatic cells from the liver of triple transgenic mice after induction of fibrosis (carbon tetrachloride chronic model) they could not find cells expressing double-positivity for GFP and beta-gal. All beta-gal-positive cells exhibited the typical morphology of hepatocytes and did not expressed mesenchymal markers like α-SMA, FSP-1, desmin, or vimentin. On the other hand, GFP-positive areas in fibrotic livers were coincident with fibrotic septa but never overlapped with X-gal-positive areas and then Authors concluded that type I collagen-producing cells were not originating from hepatocytes.

A very similar conclusion was reached in a second study (Scholten et al., 2010) in which EMT was again investigated with Cre/LoxP system in order to map cell fate CK-19 positive BDEC in CK-19(YFP) or FSP-1(YFP) mice that were generated by crossing tamoxifen-inducible CK-19(CreERT) mice or FSP-1(Cre) mice with Rosa26(f/f-YFP) mice. MET of GFAP(+) HSCs was studied in GFAP(GFP) mice. Transgenic mice were then subjected to bile duct ligation or chronic carbon tetrachloride treatment. When the livers of fibrotic transgenic mice were analyzed specific immunostaining of CK-19(YFP) cholangiocytes showed no expression of EMT markers such as α-SMA, desmin, or FSP-1. Moreover, cells genetically labeled by FSP-1(YFP) expression did not coexpress neither the cholangiocyte marker CK-19 nor E-cadherin. These results led again Authors to conclude that EMT of BDEC were not contributing to liver fibrogenesis in murine models.

The third study by the group of Brenner was even more relevant because provided compelling evidence that FSP-1 (the putative marker of EMT-derived fibroblasts) in either human and experimental CLDs was not expressed by HSC or type I collagen-producing fibroblasts (Osterreicher et al. 2011). Moreover, FSP1-positive cells did not express classical myofibroblast markers, including α-SMA and desmin, and were not myofibroblast precursors in injured livers as evaluated by genetic lineage tracing experiments. According to what already described by studies on kidney fibrosis FSP1-positive cells expressed F4/80 and other markers of the myeloid-monocytic lineage and the overall characterization pointed out that FSP1 was expressed by a specific subset of inflammatory macrophages in liver injury, fibrosis, and cancer that differed from Kupffer cells for reduced expression of MMP-3 and TIMP-3.

Few months ago a study from the laboratory of Rebecca Wells provided what looks like as an unequivocal proof against EMT in the liver as a source of MFs (Chu et al. 2011). This study uses lineage tracing generated by crossing the alpha-fetoprotein (AFP) Cre mouse with the ROSA26YFP stop mouse in order to trace the fate of any cell ever expressing AFP. As expected, all the cholangiocytes and all the hepatocytes were genetically labeled, because they are derived from AFP-expressing precursor cells. Furthermore, AFP^+ progenitor cells were also irreversibly genetically marked. The critical result was that after inducing liver fibrosis using different models, none of the resulting myofibroblasts was found to originate from the genetically marked epithelial (AFP^+) cells.

As a final comment for this section, at present the real involvement of EMT as a pathogenic mechanism contributing to liver fibrogenesis in CLDs is then more than controversial, with accumulating evidence deposing against EMT from either hepatocytes or cholangiocytes. This has generated an intense debate that the interested reader may find recapitulated in three recently published editorials (Wells, 2010; Popov and Schuppan, 2010; Kisseleva & Brenner, 2011).

4. The role of hepatic myofibroblasts in liver fibrogenesis and chronic liver disease progression

In the previous section we outlined that hepatic MFs may originate from intra- and, to a less extent, extra-hepatic cellular sources; whether the origin of MFs from HSC or PFs is concerned (Friedman, 2008a; 2008b; Dranoff & Wells, 2010), this is likely to occur through a process of activation/transdifferentiation that is believed to involve common mediators, mechanisms and signalling pathways. Although this scenario may apply also to circulating bone marrow-derived cells recruited in the chronically injured liver, at present most of our knowledge derives from "in vivo" and "in vitro" studies performed on activated human or rodent HSC and then in the following sections we will mainly refer to the paradigm of HSC activation and transdifferentiation to HSC/MFs as well as to all those phenotypic responses which have been attributed to HSC/MFs.

As nicely outlined by Scott Friedman and coworkers, under condition of persisting chronic liver injury HSC activation is believed to progress in sequential stages of initiation and perpetuation (Friedman, 2008a; 2008b; Lee & Friedman, 2011). HSC initiation should be envisaged as an early response which is stimulated by several paracrine signals that lead quiescent HSC to acquire a transient and potentially reversible contractile and profibrogenic phenotype. This "transient" phenotype is typically characterized by the rapid induction of platelet-derived growth factor (PDGF)β receptor expression being then primed to respond to several additional growth factors and mediators that, in turn, will be crucial in eliciting major phenotypic responses operated by fully activated MF-like phenotype (i.e., perpetuation). These responses include proliferation, migration/chemotaxis, contractility, excess deposition and altered remodelling of ECM as well as the emerging role in modulating angiogenesis and the immune respose.

4.1 Proliferation and migration/chemotaxis of HSC/MFs

Cultured HSC/MFs proliferate in response to a number of mitogenic stimuli, including primarily PDGF, basic fibroblast growth factors (bFGF), angiotensin II (AT-II), vascular endothelial growth factor A (VEGF-A) and thrombin (Pinzani and Marra, 2001; Friedman, 2008b; Parola et al., 2008). The most powerful mitogenic stimulus is by far represented by PDGF, particularly by PDGF-BB homodimeric isoform which can be released in the scenario of a CLD by either activated Kupffer cells, sinusoidal endothelial cells, platelets or by activated MFs in a well established autocrine/paracrine loop. PDGF-BB mitogenic signalling pathways requires first interaction with PDGF β-receptor subunit (PDGFβR), which is a tyrosine kinase receptor, leading then to the activation of the classic downstream signalling involving Ras/ERK pathway, phosphatidyl-inositol 3-kinase (PI-3K), ERK5 and others (Pinzani and Marra, 2001; Friedman, 2008b). This pathway is also responsible for migratory response since PDGF-BB also represents the best characterized and most potent chemoattractant for HSC/MFs (Pinzani and Marra, 2001) as well as for MF-like cells from human MSC (Valfrè di Bonzo et al., 2008). Indeed, migration/chemotaxis of HSC/MFs and, more generally, of hepatic MFs represents a relevant pro-fibrogenic response that allow MFs to reach the site of injury and to align with both nascent and established fibrotic septa. Migration/chemotaxis of hepatic MFs is also elicited by MCP-1, AT-II, VEGF-A, Angiopoietin-1, C-X-C chemokine receptor type 3 (CXCR3) ligands and, interestingly, ROS (Novo et al., 2007; Friedman, 2008; Novo and Parola, 2008; Parola et al., 2008). Along these lines, a recently published study from our laboratory has established that all chemoattractant polypeptides activate, in both HSC/MFs or MFs derived from MSC, a common signalling involving phosphorylation of ERK1/2 and c-Jun-NH2 kinase 1/2 (JNK1/2) through a redox-dependent mechanism that requires a NADPH-oxidase - mediated increase in intracellular generation of ROS. Moreover, the same pro-migratory pathways can also be elicited by intracellular ROS in a polypeptide-independent manner (Novo et al., 2011).

4.2 ECM synthesis/remodelling by HSC/MFs and the concept of fibrosis reversion

Hepatic MFs are of course the main responsible for excess deposition of ECM components, particularly of fibrillar matrix (mainly collagen type I and III), which represent an undisputed hallmark of fibrotic and cirrhotic livers. Indeed, progressive fibrogenesis is typically characterized by the replacement of the low-density basement membrane of the subendothelial space of Disse with fibril-forming matrix, a scenario that negatively affect differentiated cell functions (mainly of hepatocytes). This scenario is believed to result primarily from a disequilibrium between excess deposition of fibrillar collagens as well as of other ECM components and a reduced/altered degradation and remodelling of fibrotic ECM. According to current literature HSC/MFs and likely all hepatic MFs have a predominant role in modulating both ECM deposition and remodelling.

Hepatic MFs synthesize ECM components primarily as a response to TGFβ1 which can be released in the scenario of a CLD by either activated inflammatory cells, mostly Kupffer cells or monocyte/macrophages recruited from circulation, as well as by HSC/MFs themselves in a paracrine and autocrine manner. TGFβ1 operates mainly through classic downstream signalling and then involving Smads-2 and -3. Connective tissue growth factor (CTGF) and cannabinoids have been also identified as potent profibrogenic signals for HSC/MFs

(Friedman, 2008b) and the list of putative pro-fibrogenic polypeptides also include vascular endothelial growth factor - A (VEGF-A) (Medina et al., 2004; Parola et al. 2008). To this list one should also add leptin, which is a key adipokine that has been implicated in fibrogenesis in relation to NAFLD development towards NASH (Marra & Bertolani, 2009; Lee & Friedman, 2011). In particular, leptin has been reported to promote HSC fibrogenesis and to enhance tissue inhibitor of metalloprotease type 1 (TIMP-1) expression (see later for the role of TIMP-1 over-expression). Leptin operates through its receptor (ObR) and leads to the stimulation of Janus kinase (Jak)-signal transduction and activates the Jak-signal transduction and activator of transcription (STAT) signalling pathway and, partially, through suppression of peroxisome proliferator-activated receptor-γ (PPARγ), the latter being an anti-fibrogenic nuclear receptor able to reverse HSC activation and to maintain HSC quiescence. The action of leptin is usually counteracted by the circulating levels of adiponectin and indeed adiponectin levels have been reported to decrease in liver fibrosis (Marra & Bertolani, 2009; Lee & Friedman, 2011).

Where ECM remodelling is concerned, according to current literature HSC/MFs mainly express metallo-proteinases (MMPs) able to degrade basement membrane (MMP-2, MMP-9, MMP3 or stromelysin) that are less efficient to degrade fibrillar matrix, with a low expression of MMP-1 (interstitial collagenase). HSC/MFs also overexpress tissue inhibitor of metalloproteinase type 1 (TIMP-1) that, in turn, can inhibit interstitial collagenases and act as anti-apoptotic factor for HSC/MFs. Deposition of fibrillar matrix and formation of fibrotic septa is also favoured by the fact that HSC/MFs and, likely, all hepatic MFs, develop resistance to induction of apoptosis (El-Sharkawy et al., 2005; Novo et al., 2006; Friedman, 2008b; Parola et al., 2008; Pinzani, 2009; Povero et al., 2010). Related to this concept are findings of the last decade suggesting that (Iredale, 2007; Parola et al., 2008; Pinzani, 2009; Povero et al., 2010) liver fibrosis and, possibly, initial stages of cirrhosis are potentially reversible in the presence of effective therapy and/or aetiology eradication. Experimental and clinical studies suggest that regression of histopathology develops as a result of increased apoptosis of HSC/MFs and MFs and is paralled by increased expression of interstitial collagenases by hepatic macrophages. However, it should be noted that based on the absence of any unequivocal clinical finding, most researchers still believe that advanced human cirrhosis (i.e., in the presence of a very significant derangement of vascular architecture) is unlikely to regress (Iredale, 2007; Henderson and Iredale, 2007; Parola et al., 2008; Pinzani, 2009; Povero et al., 2010).

4.3 HSCs as liver specific pericytes and the pro-angiogenic phenotype of HSC/MFs

Angiogenesis can be defined as dynamic, hypoxia-dependent and growth factor – mediated process leading to the formation of new vessels from pre-existing ones. Hepatic angiogenesis is considered as a key component of the wound healing response to liver fibrosis and is essential for liver regeneration but it plays a relevant role also in promoting hepatic carcinogenesis and then the angiogenic process is strictly regulated by several factors (Medina et al., 2004; Fernandez et al., 2009; Valfrè di Bonzo, 2010). In this scenario one should first consider that quiescent HSC have been proposed to act as liver specific pericytes and that under conditions of chronic liver injury HSC/MFs acquire features of smooth muscle cells and the ability to contract in response to vasoactive (Friedman 2008a, 2008b; Parola et al. 2008). HSC/MFs contractility is thought to contribute to both the genesis of increased portal resistance during early stages of fibrosis as well as, by contributing to angiogenesis, to the late and persistent increase in portal pressure found in the cirrhotic liver which is largely due to the distortion of hepatic angioarchitecture (i.e., a consequence of angiogenesis). HSC, in particular, are located in the perisinusoidal space of Disse and with their perisinusoidal processes can affect pericapillary resistance then contributing to modulate hepatic blood flow through contractility. HSC are sensitive to well known vasoactive mediators with contraction being elicited by Endothelin-1 (ET-1) whereas relaxation is induced by nitric oxide (NO) or carbon monoxide (CO).

Under conditions of chronic liver disease, vascular derangement and excess ECM deposition contribute to create an hypoxic milieu which is a major and physiological stimulus for angiogenesis. Along these lines, in recent years it has become clear that HSC may respond to hypoxia and contribute to angiogenesis, particularly when activated to the myofibroblast - like pro-fibrogenic phenotype. The interested reader may refer to recent more comprehensive reviews for more details (Medina et al., 2004; Fernandez et al., 2009; Valfrè di Bonzo et al., 2009). A number of critical concepts and findings correlating MFs, fibrogenesis and angiogenesis should be outlined.

First, angiogenesis and up-regulation of VEGF expression have been documented in experimental models of acute and chronic liver injury as well as in human fibrotic/cirrhotic liver, including chronic infection by HBV and HCV, and autoimmune diseases such as PBC and PSC. Moreover, in both experimental and clinical conditions angiogenesis and fibrogenesis develop in parallel and strict relationships between hypoxia, angiogenesis, VEGF expression and fibrogenesis have been outlined. Along these lines, VEGF expression is mostly limited to hepatocytes and to HSC/MFs and, possibly, other hepatic myofibroblasts. Other polypeptides have been involved in hepatic angiogenesis as a process associated with the fibrogenic progression process in CLDs, including, in particular, leptin and Hedgehog (Hh) ligands.

Where hepatic MFs are concerned, these cells have also been reported to play a significant pro-angiogenic role. As for recent literature data, HSC/MFs can be considered as a hypoxia - sensitive, cyto- and chemokine-modulated cellular crossroad between necro-inflammation, pathological angiogenesis and fibrogenesis (reviewed in Fernandez et al., 2009; Valfrè di Bonzo et al., 2009). This statement is justified by the fact that HSC and HSC/MFs react to conditions of hypoxia and leptin by up-regulating transcription and synthesis of VEGF, Angiopoietin 1, as well as of their related receptor VEGFR-2 and Tie2. Moreover, HSC/MFs respond to the action of VEGF and Angiopoietin 1 in terms of proliferation, increased deposition of ECM components and increased migration and chemotaxis (Novo et al., 2007) in a redox-dependent way involving activation of Ras/ERK and JNK1/2 signaling pathways (Novo et al., 2011).

According to this scenario, in both human and rat fibrotic/cirrhotic livers (Novo et al., 2007) α-SMA-positive MFs able to express concomitantly VEGF, Ang-1 or the related receptors VEGFR-2 and Tie-2, are found at the leading edge of tiny and incomplete developing septa, but not in larger bridging septa. This distribution is likely to reflect the existence of an early phase of CLD, occurring in developing septa, in which fibrogenesis and angiogenesis may be driven/modulated by HSC/MFs, and of a later phase occurring in larger and more mature fibrotic septa where the chronic wound healing is less active and fibrogenic transformation more established. In the late setting pro-angiogenic factors are expressed only by endothelial cells, a scenario that is likely to favour the stabilization of the newly formed vessels.

As a final comment, the reader should note that angiogenesis is at present debated as a potential therapeutic target in the treatment of CLDs since the bulk of available experimental data indicate that anti-angiogenic therapy is effective in preventing progressive fibrogenesis (reviewed in Fernandez et al., 2009; Valfrè di Bonzo et al., 2009). Interestingly, to block angiogenesis also results in a significant inhibition of the development of portal hypertension, porto-systemic collateral vessels and hyperdynamic splanchnic circulation.

4.4 HSC/MFs and their role in the modulation of inflammatory and immune response

Persisting inflammatory response in a CLD is considered as one of the major "driving forces" sustaining fibrogenesis. HSC/MF and, likely, all MFs behave like target cells for inflammatory cytokines and other pro-inflammatory signals, including: a) ROS and other oxidative stress - related mediators like 4-hydroxy-2,3-nonenal or HNE, generated as a consequence of hepatocyte injury and necrosis; b) apoptotic bodies (engulfing and activating); c) bacterial endotoxin or other endogenous activators of Toll Like Receptor 4 (TLR4) of innate immunity displayed by HSC/MFs. On the other hand, HSC/MFs have been unequivocally shown to represent the cell source (even in an autocrine manner) of a number of pro-inflammatory molecules, including TLR ligands, MCP-1 or CCL2 and other chemoattractants and chemokines (Pinzani & Marra, 2001; Bataller & Brenner, 2005; Friedman, 2008b).

As a matter of fact, HSC are both a source of chemokines as well as a cellular target for their action: HSC express several chemokine receptors including CXCR3, CCR5 and CCR7 and have been reported to express at least CCL2, CCL3,CCL5, CXCL1, CXCL8, CXCL9 and CXCL10 ligands (Sahin et al., 2010). Within this panel of chemokines, CCR5 interaction with its ligand (RANTES or CCL5) is induced by NF-kB signalling and can stimulate HSC proliferation and migration. Moreover (reviewed in Lee & Friedman, 2011) CCR1, CCR5 and CXCL4 deficient mice have been reported to be associated with reduced inflammation and fibrosis. On the other hand, CXCL9, through its receptor CXCR3 operates as an anti-fibrogenic mediators.

HSC do not only secrete inflammatory chemokines but, by also interacting with immune cells through expression of adhesion molecules (mainly intercellular- and vascular-cell adhesion molecule - 1, ICAM-1 and VCAM-1, respectively) can modulate hepatic immune response in addition to natural-killer (NK) cells, T-cells, dendritic cells and of course professional phagocytes (Kupffer cells and macrophages recruited from peripheral blood) a scenario that is likely to be relevant for fibrogenesis progression (reviewed in Friedman, 2008a; 2008b; Lee & Friedman, 2011). By expanding the concept previously introduced, HSC/MFs also express TLRs and then can respond to the presence of endotoxin (LPS). TLRs, which are pattern recognition receptors that sense pathogen-associated molecular patterns (PAMPs) to discriminate the products of microorganisms from the host, are expressed on Kupffer cells, endothelial cells, dendritic cells, biliary epithelial cells, HSC and hepatocytes in the liver. TLR signaling can induce potent innate immune responses in these cell types and this is relevant since the liver is constantly exposed to PAMPs, such as LPS and bacterial DNA through bacterial translocation from intestine, particularly in the settings of alcoholic liver disease (ALD). Recent evidence demonstrates the role of TLRs in the activation of hepatic immune cells and HSC during liver fibrosis. Activated human HSC/MFs express not only TLR4 but also CD14 and MD2, forming the LPS receptor; LPS then lead to activation of nuclear factor kB (NF-kB) and c-Jun amino-terminal kinase (JNK) isoforms resulting in the synthesis and release of chemokines and adhesion molecules. Moreover, crosstalk between TLR4 signaling and TGF-beta signaling in hepatic stellate cells has been reported, suggesting an additional pro-fibrogenic mechanism (Aoyama et al., 2010).

Concerning the immune modulatory action, a number of relevant issues should be outlined for HSC and MFs (the interested reader may refer to excellent comprehensive reviews (Unanue, 2007; Friedman, 2008a; 2008b; Lee & Friedman, 2011): a) HSC can act as professional antigen presenting cells (reviewed in Unanue, 2007), able to stimulate either lymphocyte proliferation or apoptosis; b) HSC can regulate leukocyte behaviour and are affected by specific lymphocyte populations, with CD8 lymphocytes being more pro-fibrogenic towards HSC/MFs than CD4 cells; c) HSC cells can induce locally immunotolerance throughout T cell suppression; d) natural killer (NK) cells seem able to selectively kill HSC/MFs, a scenario which is apparently stimulated by interferon and inhibited by ethanol.

4.5 HSC/MFs and their putative role in liver regeneration and cancer

At first the role of hepatic MFs in liver regeneration has been originally limited to the notion that these cells, particularly HSC/MFs, may contribute to sustain liver regeneration (for example following acute liver injury or partial hepatectomy) by producing growth factors for either mature hepatocytes or oval cells, bipotent progenitors of hepatocytes and cholangiocytes (Pinzani & Marra, 2001, Friedman 2008a, 2008b).

Recently, HSC/MFs have been reported to contribute to the so called "liver stem cell niche" and were shown to express the stem cell marker CD133 (Kordes et al., 2007). This has led Authors to propose that HSC and possibly HSC/MFs may then directly differentiate into stem or precursor cells. This is indeed a fascinating hypothesis in the scenario of liver regeneration that may even (see Friedman 2008b) offer a further possible explanation for the fact that fibrosis is a "near-absolute" requirement for the development of hepatocellular carcinoma (HCC). One should consider the following facts and hypothesis: a) neoplastic cells may be envisaged to derive either from hepatic progenitor cells (HPCs) or adult and DNA-damaged hepatocytes being sustained by paracrine or survival factors released by MFs or directly from HSC/MFs through a process of mesenchymal to epithelial transition into HPCs; the latter hypothesis is highly speculative, but supported by the notion that in HSC/MFs operate hedgehog and Wnt signalling, two pathways that have been implicated in stem cell differentiation and cancer. Another study went further in proposing an even more speculative and fascinating scenario (Yang et al., 2008) in which HSC may represent a type of oval cell thus being potentially able to generate hepatocytes to repopulate injured livers. In this elegant study, since quiescent HSC express glial fibrillary acidic protein (GFAP), mice in which GFAP promoter elements regulated Cre-recombinase were crossed with ROSA-loxP-stop-loxP-green fluorescent protein (GFP) mice to generate GFAP-

Cre/GFP double-transgenic mice. These mice were fed methionine choline-deficient, ethionine-supplemented diets to activate and expand HSC and oval cell populations. GFP-positive progeny of GFAP-expressing precursor cells were then characterized by immune-histochemistry. HSC, when activated by liver injury or culture, downregulated expression of GFAP but remained GFP(+); they became highly proliferative and began to co-express markers of mesenchymal and oval cells. These transitional cells apparently disappeared as GFP-expressing hepatocytes emerged, began to express albumin, and eventually repopulated large areas of the hepatic parenchyma. These findings led Authors to suggest that HSC are a peculiar type of precursor cell able to transit through a mesenchymal phase before to differentiate into hepatocytes during liver regeneration.

5. Major mechanisms sustaining liver fibrogenesis: a major focus on ROS and ethanol

According to current literature the mechanisms able to elicit and sustain liver fibrogenesis may be classified, from a general point of view, in three main groups including a) activation of chronic wound healing reaction, b) oxidative stress and c) altered modulation of epithelial-mesenchymal interactions.

The chronic activation of the wound-healing reaction is the most common and relevant mechanism in hepatic fibrogenesis which is characterized by the following key general features: a) the persistence of hepatocellular/cholangiocellular damage with variable degree of necrosis and apoptosis; b) a complex inflammatory infiltrate including mononuclear cells and cells of the immune system; c) the activation of different types of ECM-producing cells (HSC, portal myofibroblasts, etc.) with marked proliferative, synthetic and contractile features; d) marked changes in the quality and quantity of the hepatic ECM associated with very limited or absent possibilities of remodeling in the presence of a persistent attempt of hepatic regeneration (Pinzani & Rombouts, 2004; Parola et al., 2008).

In previous sections the attention has been already focussed on those main MF-related features that have outlined the role of several growth factors and cytokines involved in the chronic wound healing reaction and affecting the pro-fibrogenic potential of HSC/MF. For these reasons we will not further expand this issue and for more informations on pro-fibrogenic mechanisms related to chronic activation of wound healing the interested reader may refer to a number of comprehensive reviews generated within the last decade (Pinzani and Marra, 2001; Parola and Robino, 2001; Pinzani and Rombouts, 2004; Bataller and Brenner, 2005; El-Sharkawy et al., 2005; Friedman, 2003, 2008a, 2008b; Iredale, 2007; Lee & Friedman, 2011; Kallis et al., 2007; Parola et al., 2008). Moreover, since the topic of EMT has been already extensively discussed in the section dedicated to the origin of hepatic MFs the putative and controversial role of this process will be not further analyzed.

Whether the role of a derangement of epithelial - mesenchymal interactions is concerned, such a mechanism has been proposed as a major mechanism underlying fibrogenesis during the course of several cholangiopathies. Cholangiopathies are a group of progressive disorders representing a major cause of chronic cholestasis in adult and pediatric patients, and share a common scenario that involves coexistence of cholestasis, necrotic or apoptotic loss of cholangiocytes, cholangiocyte proliferation (i.e., ductular proliferation) as well as portal/periportal inflammation and fibrosis. All these conditions may be included in those leading to the pattern of biliary fibrosis and indeed it is well known that the ductular reaction can be considered as the most critical event: intense proliferation of these epithelial cells is associated with significant changes in the surrounding mesenchymal cells (first portal fibroblasts and then HSC with parenchyma invasion) and ECM. It has long been unclear whether the first event was represented by phenotypic changes in proliferating cholangiocytes or by changes in ECM leading to epithelial cell proliferation. However, an intense cross-talk between mesenchymal and epithelial (i.e.cholangiocytes) cells has been suggested to result in a release of cytokines and pro-inflammatory mediators possibly responsible for the overall mentioned scenario in cholangiopathies. As a matter of fact, cholangiocytes are now considered as active "actors" in pathological conditions by their ability to secrete chemokines like IL-6, tumour necrosis factor (TNF)α, IL-8 and MCP-1, as well as pro-fibrogenic factors (PDGF-BB, ET-1, CTGF, TGFβ2) : all these factors can be produced also by infiltrating immune, inflammatory or mesenchymal cells, and may affect in turn both epithelial cells and their intense cross-talk with mesenchymal cells sustaining the fibrogenic response (reviewed in Pinzani and Rombouts, 2004). The interested reader may refer for more details to a recent excellent review on the role of portal fibroblast and portal MFs and their interactions with activated/damaged cholangiocytes (Dranoff & Wells, 2010).

In this section we will then mostly focus our attention on the general role of oxidative stress and reactive oxygen species, with a specific reference to the case of ALD.

5.1 Oxidative stress and ROS in liver fibrogenesis: synopsis of general concepts and findings

Involvement of oxidative stress has been documented in all human major clinical conditions of CLDs as well as in most experimental models of liver fibrogenesis (Parola & Robino, 2001; Novo & Parola, 2008), but it is likely to represent the predominant pro-fibrogenic mechanism mainly in NAFLD/NASH and ASH (and then ALD). Oxidative stress in CLDs, resulting from increased generation of ROS and other reactive intermediates as well as by decreased efficiency of antioxidant defenses, does not represent simply a potentially toxic consequence of chronic liver injury but actively contributes to excessive tissue remodelling and fibrogenesis. In this section just a few major concepts, strictly limited to fibrogenesis, will be recalled and for more details, particularly on aetiology - dependent mechanisms leading to oxidative stress, the reader may refer to more extensive reviews (Parola and Robino, 2001; Bataller and Brenner, 2005; Novo & Parola, 2008; Bataller et al., 2011).

5.1.1 Oxidative stress and liver injury: redox-dependent injury is specific for hepatocytes

CLDs are characterized, whatever the aetiology, by persisting liver injury and hepatocyte loss and severe oxidative stress can be considered as a major cause for both necrotic and apoptotic cell death of parenchymal cells whether resulting from inflammatory flares (i.e., HCV or HBV infection) through increased ROS generation by leukocytes, ethanol consumption, hepatic iron overload, antioxidant status or other conditions. Some relevant concepts should be recalled (reviewed in Novo & Parola, 2008):

a. First, severe oxidative stress may lead to both hepatocyte necrosis and apoptosis, with necrosis mainly resulting from irreversible mitochondrial damage and/or inactivation of executioner caspases; moreover, both necrosis and apoptosis can be found on the same section, in association with the other events of the chronic scenario (inflammation, fibrogenesis, angiogenesis, etc.);

b. the level of ROS to which target cells are exposed may be critical in deciding whether these cells may survive or die, as described for the engagement of death receptors (DR) or TLR by respective ligands and the involvement of the critical kinase RIP (from Receptor Interacting Protein); along these lines, ROS-related sustained activation of JNK isoforms is a well characterized event leading to cell death in several conditions; moreover, in hepatocytes NF-kB inhibition sensitize cells to TNF-induced apoptosis by means of JNK sustained activation;
c. ROS-related mitochondrial damage is a typical example of two way-injury since mitochondria can represent not only a source of ROS (particularly when their integrity is deranged) but also a target for their action in relation to cell death; ROS are critical in mediating cell death of fatty hepatocytes due to excess of free fatty acids (FFAs) in the liver of NAFLD and NASH patients; this may happen in FFAs-related up-regulation of TNF, increased Fas ligand binding to Fas (CD-95) or induction of endoplasmic reticulum (ER)-stress and the so called "unfolded protein response" (UPR) ;
d. ER-stress, and then ROS, have been implicated also in hepatocyte apoptosis in chronic hepatitis C and ALD;
e. not all reactive species are dangerous for a target cells: for example, nitric oxide (NO) and related reactive nitrogen species (RNS) can theoretically promote or prevent apoptotic cell death by interfering with either mitochondrial-dependent or -independent signalling pathways.
f. although ROS and more generally oxidative stress can lead to hepatocyte death, human hepatic MFs have been reported to easily survive to ROS, HNE and other pro-oxidants (Novo et al., 2006) and that this relies on the MFs activation-related specific "survival attitude" involving up-regulation of Bcl2, over-activation of pro-survival pathways, including NF-kB-related ones, and down-regulation of Bax (Elsharkawy et al., 2005; Novo et al., 2006). Hepatic MFs can then survive to conditions of oxidative stress usually operating in CLDs that, rather (see later), are more likely to sustain their pro-inflammatory and pro-fibrogenic responses.

5.1.2 ROS and oxidative stress-related mediators affect inflammatory and pro-fibrogenic action of MFs

ROS and other reactive mediators such as 4-hydroxynonenal (HNE, a major aldehydic end-product of lipid peroxidation) can be generated outside MFs, here considered as potential "target" cells, being released either by activated inflammatory cells or injured hepatocytes. Indeed, oxidative stress, presumably by favouring mitochondrial permeability transition, is able to promote hepatocyte death (necrotic and/or apoptotic). In some of clinically relevant conditions generation of ROS within hepatocytes may represent a consequence of an altered metabolic state (like in NAFLD and NASH) or of ethanol metabolism (ALD, see next section), with ROS being then mainly generated by mitochondrial electron transport chain or through the involvement of selected cytochrome P450 isoforms like CYP2E1 (reviewed in Novo & Parola, 2008).

Mediators of oxidative stress, whatever the source, aetiology or metabolic condition, are involved in the up-regulation or modulation of the expression of pro-inflammatory cytokines and chemokines by different cells, (including inflammatory cells as well as HSC/MFs or, presumably, MF-like cells, mostly through activation of NF-kB (Elsharkawy et al., 2005; Novo et al., 2008). In addition, the following major concepts may be recalled: a) ROS are involved in the process of phagocytosis, possibly by leading to amplification of the stimulating signal that follows engagement of Fc receptors on the surface of phagocytic cells; b) ROS may have a role in apoptosis - related removal of leukocytes during inflammatory responses; c) HNE as well as other 4-hydroxy-2,3-alkenals (HAKs), have been reported to be able to stimulate leukocyte chemotaxis at very low concentrations; d) ROS and HNE elicit in vivo and in vitro up-regulation of the chemokine MCP-1, then sustaining recruitment/activation of monocytes/macrophages and Kupffer cells as well as chemotaxis of HSC/MFs.

On the other hand, oxidative stress - related mediators released by damaged or activated neighbouring cells can directly affect the behaviour of human HSC/MFs: ROS or the reactive aldehyde HNE have been reported to up regulate expression of critical genes related to fibrogenesis including procollagen type I, MCP-1 and TIMP-1, possibly through activation of a number of critical signal transduction pathways and transcription factors, including activation of JNK, activator protein-1 (AP-1) and, only for ROS, NF-kB (Parola and Robino, 2001; Novo & Parola, 2008). It has also been reported that ROS may positively modulate proliferation of rat HSC/MFs but here a discrepancy exist with data with human cells in which ROS and HNE, unable to stimulate cell growth at low pro-fibrogenic doses, may rather inhibit basal and PDGF - stimulated DNA synthesis or even induce cell death. On the other hand, low levels of extracellular superoxide anion, but not H_2O_2 or HNE, are able to stimulate migration of human HSC/MFs through activation of Ras/Erk and JNK1/2 signalling (reviewed in Novo & Parola, 2008; Novo et al., 2011).

In addition to "profibrogenic" extracellular release by neighbouring cells, ROS generation within human and rat HSC/MFs has been reported to occur in response to several known pro-fibrogenic mediators, including angiotensin II, PDGF and the adipokine leptin. ROS generation here depends on activation by the cited mediators of a non-phagocytic NADPH oxidase (NOX) that has been detected in either human or rat HSC/MFs. ROS generated within HSC/MFs are likely to act also as positive modulators or pro-fibrogenic signalling pathways, as shown by the fact that selective inhibition of NOX usually reduce the phenotypic response. Moreover, the potential relevance of ROS generation by NOX in fibrogenesis has been disclosed by a study in which mice lacking p47phox (i.e., a crucial subunit of NOX) were protected from development of experimental fibrosis (Bataller et al., 2003). Interestingly, intracellular and NADPH oxidase - related generation of ROS has been reported to follow "in vivo" and "in vitro" phagocytosis of apoptotic bodies from damaged hepatocytes by HSC/MFs, resulting in up-regulation of procollagen I expression (Zhan et al., 2006). More recently, as previously mentioned, our group has outlined that intracellular generation of ROS either linked to NADPH-oxidase activation following interactions of polypeptides with their receptors (PDGF, VEGF, MCP-1 and others) or in a ligand-independent manner, is a critical event in mediating migration of both HSC/MFs and bone marrow-derived MSC in their MF-like phenotype (Novo et al., 2011).

5.1.3 ROS, lipid peroxidation and immune response in human patients

Another relevant concept to mention is the fact that oxidative stress may contribute to CLDs progression also by affecting immune response. Experimental studies (alcohol fed rodents) and clinical data (patients affected by ALD, chronic HCV infection or NAFLD) indicate that oxidative stress is associated with the development of circulating IgG antibodies directed against epitopes derived from protein modified by lipid peroxidation products or against oxidized cardiolipin. Of relevance, titre of these antibodies correlate with disease severity and, as recently proposed for NAFLD patients, may serve as prognostic predictor of progression of NAFLD to advanced fibrosis (Albano et al., 2007 and reference therein). Along these lines, it should be also mentioned that a T cell mediated response towards lipid peroxidation derived antigens has been described in patients with advanced ALD (Stewart et al., 2004). Indeed, the body of evidence indicate that immune response triggered by oxidative stress may have a significant role in the progression of ALD, in the worstening of chronic hepatitis C by alcohol intake and, possibly, even in the progression of NAFLD.

5.2 Oxidative stress and ROS in alcoholic liver disease

As it is well known chronic ethanol consumption can lead to ALD, which encompasses a large spectrum of pathological liver changes, ranging from simple fatty liver with minimal injury to alcoholic steatohepatitis (ASH) and, in more advanced stages, fibrogenic progression to cirrhosis. Progression of ALD is now considered a multifactorial process involving nutritional, environmental and genetic factors, and ethanol consumption also represents one of the major host-related factors able to accelerate progression of fibrosis towards cirrhosis in chronic HCV patients and, possibly, in patients affected by CLDs with a different aetiology (Bataller & Brenner, 2005; Friedman, 2008b; Parola et al., 2008).

In the last two decades the role of ROS and oxidative stress in the pathogenesis of ethanol-induced liver injury has been extensively investigated (Arteel, 2003; Day & Cederbaum, 2006; Albano, 2008; Novo & Parola, 2008; Cubero et al., 2009) and here a number of relevant concepts may be recalled.

5.2.1 Major redox-related features in ALD

A first relevant issue is represented by the fact that both experimental and clinical data indicate unequivocally that oxidative stress and lipid peroxidation are involved, with antioxidants and free radical scavengers being able, at least in animal models, to afford prevention (reviewed in Novo & Parola, 2008; Cubero et al., 2009). Moreover, ALD progression is accompanied by a progressive decrease in hepatic antioxidant defenses, suggesting then that both increased generation of ROS and decreased ability to inactivate or metabolize ROS have a pathogenic role.

As a second point, one should note that ethanol-related ROS can be produced by the mitochondria respiratory chain, ethanol metabolizing (and ethanol-inducible) cytochrome P450 2E1 (CYP2E1) in hepatocytes, but not in HSCs, and NOXs of activated Kupffer cells or infiltrating neutrophils; moreover, NO produced by NO synthase of Kupffer cells and other reactive nitrogen species (RNS) has also been shown to contribute to ethanol-dependent hepatic injury (Arteel, 2003; Day & Cederbaum, 2006; Albano, 2008; Novo & Parola, 2008; Cubero et al., 2009). Indeed, in addition to the well known action of alcohol-dehydrogenase or ADH in metabolizing ethanol (when ethanol levels are low) CYP2E1 is an ethanol-inducible isoform mainly observed in hepatocytes that plays a role in oxidation in the presence of high ethanol circulating levels and in chronic alcohol consumption. CYP2E1 when metabolizing ethanol leads to the generation of acetaldehyde as well as of the ethanol-derived hydroxyethyl radical and major ROS including superoxide radical, hydrogen peroxide and hydroxyl-radical. Ethanol metabolism also leads to lipid peroxidation and related generation of reactive aldehydic end-products such as HNE and malonyldialdehyde (MDA).

Third, ethanol-induced oxidative stress is likely to contribute to liver steatosis found in alcoholics by causing an impairment in either mitochondrial lipid oxidation or lipoprotein secretions, the latter being related to enhanced degradation of ApoB100 and/or oxidative alteration of lipoprotein glycosilation in Golgi apparatus (Albano, 2008; Novo & Parola, 2008). Finally, CYP-2E1 generated ROS and formation of protein adducts by lipid peroxidation products may also affect proteasomal degradation, an event that has been proposed to lead to cytoplasmic aggregates of cytokeratins 8 and 18 and then the formation of Mallory's bodies (Bardag-Gorce et al., 2006).

5.2.2 Ethanol-mediated and redox-dependent effects on MFs related to paracrine release of ROS from surrounding cells, including HSC

When considering the role of redox-dependent events on the ALD-related fibrogenesis one may envisage a rather simplified scenario in which MFs represent the ideal target cells for ROS and other redox-related mediators released by the different hepatic cell populations operating in the complex microenvironment of ALD. Indeed, it is widely accepted that in early ALD (i.e., ASH) initiation of HSC activation is mainly due to paracrine stimulation by injured epithelial cells as well as inflammatory (macrophages plus neutrophils), endothelial as well as immune cells. Whether chronic ethanol consumption is concerned, a number of cell type - related issues (to be reconnected with previously mentioned concepts and findings) should be outlined (Albano, 2008; Novo & Parola, 2008; Cubero et al., 2009; Bataller et al., 2011):

a. Hepatocytes. Under conditions of chronic ethanol consumption hepatocyte contribution depend on the CYP2E1-dependent generation of ROS and on consequent generation of aldehydic end-products of lipid peroxidation (mainly HNE) as well as on the levels of acetaldehyde (ACA). ROS, ACA and HNE have been all connected with paracrine HSC activation. In addition to the already mentioned ability of ROS and HNE to increase collagen production it should be recalled that also ACA can up-regulate transcription of collagen type I (both COL1A1 and COL1A2) through a TGFβ-dependent mechanism. This is relevant since TGFβ is the most potent pro-fibrogenic cytokine being able not only to sustain HSC activation and excess synthesis of ECM components but also to suppress hepatocyte proliferation and even to induce their apoptosis. It has been also suggested that the ethanol-related altered ratio of $NAD^+/NADH$ and $NADP^+/NADPH$ may also favor an increased synthesis of angiotensin II which has been reported to be a powerful fibrogenic cytokine (Bataller & Brenner, 2005).
b. Kupffer cells (KC). Chronic ethanol consumption has been reported to impair gut permeability, an event potentially leading to overgrowth of Gram negative bacteria and subsequent translocation of endotoxin or lipopolysaccharide (LPS) from the intestinal lumen into portal circulation. LPS can trigger KC activation and indeed the influx of KC coincide with the appearance of HSC activation markers (α-SMA and

PDGF receptor-β or PDGFRβ). In addition to standard "macrophage-like" functions, one should consider that activation of KC leads to ROS generation through NOX, xanthine-oxidase, mitochondria or even CYP2E1 (detected in these cells), with ROS being then able to enhance HSC activation and collagen type I synthesis (Cubero et al., 2009). Along these lines, KC can also produce NO that has been described to counterbalance effect of ROS, then leading to decreased HSC proliferation, contractility and collagen type I synthesis; unfortunately, NO can also rapidly react with superoxide anion to generate peroxynitrite, a very powerful oxidizing intermediate whose effect on the synthesis of collagen type I and ECM components by HSC are at present unknown.

c. Liver sinusoidal endothelial cells (LSEC). Under conditions of chronic ethanol consumption major reactive intermediates like ACA and ROS can induce LSEC injury. Indeed, injured LSEC have been reported to react by up-regulating the expression of fibronectin isoforms and of a number of critical mediators able to target HSC or HSC/MFs including VEGF and leptin (Friedman 2003, 2008b; Marra & Bertolani, 2009). Injured LSEC may also convert latent TGFβ into the active form (Ikejima et al., 2002).
d. HSC/MFs. Once activated, HSC/MFs respond to stress conditions by secreting (paracrine/autocrine loops) inflammatory cytokines and chemokines such as mainly TNFα, TGFβ, IL-6, PDGF and CCL2 as well as other mediators like angiotensin II and the altered panel of MMPs and TIMPs described in section 4.2 . As mentioned before and pertinent to the condition of ALD, exposure to ROS, HNE and ACA HSC/MFs has been reported specifically to up-regulate synthesis of ECM components (reviewed in Novo & Parola, 2008; Cubero et al., 2009).

6. Conclusions and perspectives

The increasing knowledge on the pathogenesis of liver fibrogenesis (the process) leading to hepatic fibrosis (the result) has led to important changes in the clinical interpretation of the relevance of fibrogenic progression of any CLD. At present there is a need for an accurate and effective monitoring of the fibrotic progression of CLDs and for the effectiveness of the currently proposed treatments. Within the last five years more non-invasive/dynamic methods for the evaluation of liver fibrosis have been described that are beginning to be very useful, particularly if associated to the detection of critical non-invasive serum markers. This seems now mandatory in order to overcome the unavoidable limitations (lack of standardization, sampling error, inter-observer variability etc) of liver biopsy, although this invasive procedure is still regarded by most as the "gold standard" for assessing liver histology, disease activity and fibrosis progression. In addition, the identification of the genes involved in the progression of liver fibrosis would hopefully lead to the establishment of prognostic markers indicating a faster progression of fibrogenic CLDs and indeed several ongoing studies are addressing the relevance of gene expression and/or gene polymorphisms in defined subset of patients. However, in order to enable the rational development of therapeutic targets in CLDs we primarily need to continue to increase our knowledge on the complexity of the fibrogenic response, an issue that still remains a major objective of experimental and clinical studies designed to ascertain both the origin of fibrogenic cells (i.e., hepatic MFs) and, most important, of the mechanisms governing their "pathological behavior" in CLDs that results in the overall ability to sustain fibrotic progression of the disease towards the end-points of cirrhosis and related complications.

7. Acknowledgements

Authors gratefully acknowledge financial support received from the Ministero dell'Università e della Ricerca (MIUR, Rome - PRIN Project 2006067527, M.P.), Regione Piemonte (Torino, M.P. and E.N.), Fondazione CRT (Torino, M.P.) and Fondazione Bossolasco (Torino, C.P. and S.C.).

8. References

Acloque, H.; Adams, M.S.; Fishwick, K.; Bronner-Fraser, M. & Nieto M.A. (2009). Epithelial – mesenchymal transitions: the importance of changing cell state in development and disease. *J Clin Invest*, 119(6), pp.1438-1449. ISSN: 0021-9738.

Albano, E., Mottaran, E., Vidali, M., Reale, E., Saksena, S., Occhino, G., Burt, A.D. & Day, C.P. (2005). Immune response towards lipid peroxidation products as a predictor of progression of non-alcoholic fatty liver disease to advanced fibrosis. *Gut*, 54(7): pp.987-993. ISSN: 0017-5749.

Albano, E. (2008). Oxidative mechanisms in the pathogenesis of alcoholic liver disease. *Mol Aspects Med*, 29(1-2):pp.9-16. ISSN:0098-2997.

Aoyama, T., Paik, Y.H. & Seki, E. (2010). Toll-like receptor signalling and liver fibrosis. *Gastroenterol Res Pract*, Jul 25, available on line ahead of print. ISSN: 1687-6121.

Arteel, G.E. (2003). Oxidant and antioxidant in alcohol-induced liver disease. *Gastroenterology*, 124(3):778-790.ISSN: 0016-5085.

Asahina, K., Tsai, L.Y., Li, P., Ishii, M., Maxson, R.E., Sucov, H.M. & Tsukamoto, H. (2009). Mesenchymal origin of hepatic stellate cells, submesothelial cells, and perivascular mesenchymal cells during mouse liver development. *Hepatology*, 49 (3), pp.998-1011. ISSN: 0270-9139.

Bardag-Gorce, F., French, B.A., Nan, L., Song, H., Nguyen, S.K., Yong, H., Dede, J. & French, S.W. (2006). CYP2E1 induced by ethanol causes oxidative stress, proteasome inhibition and cytokeratin aggresome (Mallory body-like) formation. *Exp Mol Pathol*, 81(3):pp.191-201. ISSN: 0014-4800.

Bataller, R., Schwabe, R.F., Choi, Y.H., Yang, L., Paik, Y.H., Lindquist, J., Qian, T., Schoonhoven, R., Hagedorn, C.H., Leemasters, J.J. & Brenner, D.A. (2003). NADPH oxidase signal transduces angiotensin II in hepatic stellate cells and is critical in hepatic fibrosis. *J Clin Invest* 112(9): pp.1383-1394. ISSN: 0021-9738.

Bataller, R. & Brenner, D.A. (2005). Liver fibrosis. *J Clin Invest*, 115(2), pp.109-118. ISSN: 0021-9738.

Beaussier, M., Wendum, D., Schiffer, E., Dumont, S., Rey, C., Lienhart, A. & Housset, C. (2007). Prominent contribution of portal mesenchymal cells to liver fibrosis in ischemic and obstructive cholestatic injuries. *Lab Invest*, 87(3), pp.292-303. ISSN: 0023-6837.

Cannito, S., Novo, E., Valfrè di Bonzo, L., Busletta, C., Colombatto, S. & Parola, M. (2010). Epithelial-mesenchymal transition: from molecular mechanisms, redox regulation to implications in human health and disease. *Antioxid Redox Signal,* 12(12), pp.1383-1430. ISSN: 1523-0864.

Cassiman, D. & Roskams, T. (2002). Beauty is in the eye of the beholder: emerging concepts and pitfalls in hepatic stellate cell research. *J Hepatol,* 37(4), pp.527-535. ISSN: 0168-8278.

Choi, S.S. & Diehl, A.M. (2009). Epithelial-to-mesenchymal transitions in the liver. *Hepatology,* 50(6), pp.2007-2013. ISSN: 0270-9139.

Chu, A.S., Diaz, R., Hui, J.-J., Yanger, K., Zong,Y., Alpini, G., Stanger, B.Z. & Wells, R.G. (2011). Lineage tracing demonstrates no evidence of cholangiocyte epithelial-to-mesenchymal transition in murine models of hepatic fibrosis. *Hepatology,* 53(5), pp.1685-1695. ISSN: 0270-9139.

Clouston, A.D., Powell, E.E., Walsh, M.J., Richardson, M.M., Demetris, A.J., & Jonsson, J.R. (2005). Fibrosis correlates with a ductular reaction in hepatitis C: roles of impaired replication, progenitor cells and steatosis. *Hepatology,* 41(4), pp.809-818. ISSN: 0270-9139.

Cubero, F.J., Urtasun, R. & Nieto, N. (2009). Alcohol and liver fibrosis. *Sem Liver Disease,* 29(2), pp. 211-221. ISSN 0272-8087.

Dey, A. & Cederbaum, A.I. (2006). Alcohol and oxidative liver injury. *Hepatology,* 43(2 Suppl. 1): pp.S63-S74. ISSN: 0270-9139.

Díaz, R., Kim, J.W., Hui, J.J., Li, Z., Swain, G.P., Fong, K.S., Csiszar, K., Russo, P.A., Rand, E.B., Furth, E.E. & Wells R.G. (2008). Evidence for the epithelial to mesenchymal transition in biliary atresia fibrosis. *Hum Pathol,* 39(1), pp.102-115. ISSN: 0046-8177.

Dooley, S., Hamzavi, J., Ciuclan, L., Godoy, P., Ilkavets, I., Ehnert, S., Ueberham, E., Gebhardt, R., Kanzler, S., Geier, A., Breitkopf, K., Weng, H. & Mertens, P.R. (2008). Hepatocyte-specific Smad7 expression attenuates TGF-beta-mediated fibrogenesis and protects against liver damage. *Gastroenterology,* 135(2), pp.642-659. ISSN:0016-5085.

Dranoff, J.A. & Wells, R.G. (2010). Portal fibroblasts: underappreciated mediators of biliary fibrosis. *Hepatology,* 51(4), pp.1434-1444. ISSN:0270-9139.

Elsharkawy, A.M., Oakley, F. & Mann, D.A. (2005). The role and regulation of hepatic stellate cell apoptosis in reversal of liver fibrosis. *Apoptosis,* 10(5), pp.927-939. ISSN: 1360-8185.

Fabris, L., Cadamuro, M., Guido, M., Spirli, C., Fiorotto, R., Colledan, M., Torre, G., Alberti, D., Sonzogni, A., Okolicsanyi, L. & Strazzabosco, M. (2007). Analysis of liver repair mechanisms in Alagille syndrome and biliary atresia reveals a role for notch signaling. *Am J Pathol,* 171(2), pp.641-653. ISSN: 0002-9440.

Fernández, M., Semela, D., Bruix, J., Colle, I,. Pinzani, M. & Bosch, J. (2009). Angiogenesis in liver disease. *J Hepatol,* 50(3), pp.604-620. ISSN: 0168-8278.

Forbes, S.J., Russo, F.P., Rey, V., Burra, P., Rugge, M., Wright, N.A. & Alison, M.R. (2004). A significant proportion of myofibroblasts are of bone marrow origin in human liver fibrosis. *Gastroenterology,* 126 (4), pp.955-963. ISSN: 0016-5085.

Forbes, S.J. & Parola, M. (2011). Liver fibrogenic cells. *Best Practice & Research Clin Gastroenterol,* 25(2), pp.207-217. ISSN: 1521-6918.

Friedman, S.L. (2003). Liver fibrosis: from bench to bedside. *J Hepatol* 38, Suppl. 1, S38-S53. ISSN: 0168-8278.

Friedman, S.L. (2008a). Hepatic stellate cells: protean, multifunctional, and enigmatic cells of the liver. *Physiol Rev,* 88(1), pp.125-172. ISSN: 0031-9333.

Friedman, S.L. (2008b). Mechanisms of hepatic fibrogenesis. *Gastroenterology* 134(6), pp.1655-1669. ISSN: 0016-5085.

Henderson, N.C. & Iredale, J.P. (2007). Liver fibrosis: cellular mechanisms of progression and resolution. *Clinical Science,* 112 (5), pp.265-280. ISSN: 0143-5221.

Henderson, N.C. & Forbes, S.J. (2008). Hepatic fibrogenesis: from within and outwith. *Toxicology,* 254(3), pp.130-135. ISSN: 0300-483X.

Higashiyama, R., Moro, T., Nakao, S., Mikami, K., Fukumitsu, H., Ueda, Y., Ikeda, K., Adachi, E., Bou-Gharios, G., Okazaki, I. & Inagaki, Y. (2009). Negligible contribution of bone marrow-derived cells to collagen production during hepatic fibrogenesis in mice. *Gastroenterology,* 137(4), pp.1459-1466. ISSN: 0016-5085.

Humphreys, B.D., Lin, S.L., Kobayashi, A., Hudson, T.E., Nowlin B.T., Bonventre, J.V., Valerius, M.T., McMahon, A.P. & Duffield, J.S. (2010). Fate tracing reveals the pericyte and not epithelial origin of myofibroblasts in kidney fibrosis. *Am J Pathol,* 176(1), pp.85-97. ISSN: 0002-9440.

Ikejima, K., Takei, Y., Honda, H., Hirose, M., Yoshikawa, M., Zhang, Y.J., Lang, T., Fukuda, T., Yamashina, S., Kitamuram T. & Sato, N. (2002). Leptin receptor-mediated signaling regulates hepatic fibrogenesis and remodeling of extracellular matrix in the rat. *Gastroenterology* 122(5):1399-410. ISSN: 0016-5085.

Iredale, J.P. (2007). Models of liver fibrosis: exploring the dynamic nature of inflammation and repair in a solid organ. *J Clin Invest,* 117(3), pp.539-548. ISSN: 0021-9738.

Iwano , M., Plieth, D., Danoff, T.M., Xue, C., Okada, H. & Neilson E.G. (2002). Evidence that fibroblasts derive from epithelium during tissue fibrosis. *J Clin Invest,* 110(3), pp.341-350. ISSN: 0021-9738.

Jung, Y., Brown, K.D., Witek, R.P., Omenetti, A., Yang, L., Vandongen, M., Milton, R.J., Hines, I.N., Rippe, R.A., Spahr, L., Rubbia-Brandt, L. & Diehl, A.M. (2008). Accumulation of hedgehog-responsive progenitors parallels alcoholic liver disease severity in mice and humans. *Gastroenterology,* 134(5), pp.1532-1543. ISSN: 0016-5085.

Jung, Y., McCall, S.J., Li, Y.X. & Diehl, A.M. (2007). Bile ductules and stromal cells express hedgehog ligands and/or hedgehog target genes in primary biliary cirrhosis. *Hepatology,* 45(5): pp.1091-1096. ISSN: 0270-9139.

Kallis, Y.N., Alison, M.R. & Forbes S.J. (2007). Bone marrow stem cells and liver diseases. *Gut,* 56(5), pp.716-724. ISSN: 0017-5749.

Kallis, Y.N. & Forbes S.J. (2009). The bone marrow and liver fibrosis: friend or foe? *Gastroenterology,* 137(4), pp.1218-1221. ISSN: 0016-5085.

Kalluri, R. & Weinberg, R.A. (2009). The basics of epithelial – mesenchymal transition. *J Clin Invest,* 119(6), pp.1420-1428. ISSN: 0021-9738.

Kirby, J.A., Robertson, H., Marshall, H.L., Rygiel, K.A., Hudson, M., Jones, D.E., & Burt, A.D. (2008). Epithelial to mesenchymal transition in primary sclerosing cholangitis. *Liver Int*, 28(8), pp.1176-1177. ISSN: 1478-3223.

Kisseleva, T., Uchinami, H., Feirt, N., Quintana-Bustamante, O., Segovia, J.C., Schwabe, R.F. & Brenner, D.A. (2006). Bone marrow - derived fibrocytes partecipate in pathogenesis of liver fibrosis. *J Hepatol*, 45(3), 429-438. ISSN:0168-8278.

Kisseleva, T. & Brenner, D.A. (2011). Is it the end of the line for the EMT? *Hepatology* 53(5): pp.1433-1435. ISSN: 0270-9139.

Kordes, C., Sawitza, I., Muller-Marbach, A., Ale-Agha, N., Keitel, V., Klonowski-Stumpe, H. & Häussinger, D. (2007). CD133+ hepatic stellate cells are progenitor cells. *Biochem Biophys Res Commun*, 352(2), pp.410-417. ISSN: 0006-291X.

Lee, U.E. & Friedman, S.L. (2011). Mechanisms of liver fibrogenesis. *Best Practice & Research Clin Gastroenterol*, 25(2), pp.195-206. ISSN: 1521-6918.

Le Hir, M., Hegyi, I., Cueni-Loffing, D. & Kaissling, B. (2005). Characterization of renal interstitial fibroblast-specific protein 1 / S100A4-positive cells in healthy and inflamed rodent kidneys. *Histochem Cell Biol*, 123(4-5), pp.335-346. ISSN: 0948-6143.

Lin, S.L., Kisseleva, T., Brenner, D.A. & Duffield J.S. (2008). Pericyte and perivascular fibroblasts are the primary source of collagen-producing cells in obstructive fibrosis of the kidney. *Am J Pathol*, 173(6), pp.1617-1627. ISSN: 0002-9440.

Marra, F. & Bertolani, C. (2009). Adipokines in liver diseases. *Hepatology*, 50(3): pp.957-69. ISSN: 0270-9139.

Medina, J., Arroyo, A.G., Sanchez-Madrid, F. & Moreno-Otero, R. (2004). Angiogenesis in chronic inflammatory liver diseases. *Hepatology*, 39(5), pp.1185-1195. ISSN: 0270-9139.

Novo, E., Marra, F., Zamara, E., Valfrè di Bonzo, L., Monitillo, L., Cannito, S., Petrai, I., Mazzocca, A., Bonacchi, A., De Franco, R.S., Colombatto, S., Autelli, R., Pinzani, M. & Parola, M. (2006). Overexpression of Bcl-2 by activated human hepatic stellate cells: resistance to apoptosis as mechanism of progressive hepatic fibrogenesis. *Gut*, 55(8), pp.1174-1182. ISSN: 0017-5749.

Novo, E., Cannito, S., Zamara, E., Valfrè di Bonzo, L., Caligiuri, A., Cravanzola, C., Compagnone, A., Colombatto, S., Marra, F., Pinzani, M. & Parola, M. (2007). Proangiogenic cytokines as hypoxia - dependent factors stimulating migration of human hepatic stellate cells. *Am J Pathol*, 170(6), pp.1942-1953. ISSN: 0002-9440.

Novo, E., & Parola, M. (2008). Redox mechanisms in hepatic chronic wound healing and liver fibrogenesis. *Fibrogenesis & Tissue Repair*, 1(1), pp.5. ISSN: 1755-1536.

Novo, E., Busletta, C., Valfrè di Bonzo, L., Povero, D., Paternostro, C., Mareschi, K., Ferrero, I., David, E., Bertolani, C., Caligiuri, A., Cannito, S., Tamagno, E., Compagnone, A., Colombatto, S., Marra, F., Fagioli, F., Pinzani, M. & Parola, M. (2011). Intracellular reactive oxygen species are required for directional migration of resident and bone marrow-derived hepatic pro-fibrogenic cells. *J Hepatol*, 54(5): pp.964-974. ISSN:0168-8278.

Omenetti, A., Popov, Y., Jung, Y., Choi, S.S., Witek, R.P., Yang, L., Brown, K.D., Schuppan, D. & Diehl, A.M. (2008a). The hedgehog pathway regulates remodelling responses to biliary obstruction in rats. *Gut,* 57(9), pp.1275-82. ISSN: 0017-5749.

Omenetti, A., Porrello, A., Jung, Y., Yang, L., Popov, Y., Choi, S.S., Witek, R.P., Alpini, G., Venter, J., Vandongen, H.M., Syn, W.K., Baroni, G.S., Benedetti, A., Schuppan, D. & Diehl, A.M. (2008b). Hedgehog signaling regulates epithelial-mesenchymal transition during biliary fibrosis in rodents and humans. *J Clin Invest,* 118(10), pp.3331-3342. ISSN: 0021-9738.

Österreicher, C.H., Penz-Österreicher, M., Grivennikov, S.I., Guma, M., Koltsova, E.K., Datz, C., Sasik, R., Hardiman, G., Karin, M. & Brenner D.A. (2011). Fibroblast-specific protein 1 identifies an inflammatory subpopulation of macrophages in the liver. *Proc Natl Acad Sci USA,* 108(1): pp.308-313. ISSN: 0027-8424.

Parola, M. & Robino, G. (2001). Oxidative stress - related molecules and liver fibrosis. *J Hepatol,* 35(2), pp.297-306. ISSN: 0168-8278.

Parola, M. Marra, F. & Pinzani, M. (2008). Myofibroblast - like cells and liver fibrogenesis: emerging concepts in a rapidly moving scenario. *Mol Asp Med,* 29(1-2), pp.58-66. ISSN: 0098-2997.

Parola, M. & Pinzani, M. (2009). Hepatic wound repair. *Fibrogenesis & Tissue Repair,* 2(1), pp.4. ISSN: 1755-1536.

Pinzani, M. & Marra, F. (2001). Cytokine receptor and signalling in hepatic stellate cells. *Sem Liv Dis,* 21(3), pp.397-417. ISSN: 0272-8087.

Pinzani, M. & Rombouts, K. (2004). Liver fibrosis - from the bench to clinical targets. *Dig Liver Dis,* 36(4), pp.231-242. ISSN: 1590-8658.

Pinzani, M. (2009). Unravelling the spider web of hepatic stellate cell apoptosis. *Gastroenterology,* 136(7), pp.2061-2063. ISSN: 0016-5085.

Popov, Y. & Schuppan, D. (2010). Epithelial-to-Mesenchymal Transition in Liver Fibrosis: Dead or Alive? *Gastroenterology,* 139(3), pp.722-725. ISSN: 0016-5085.

Povero, D., Busletta, C., Novo, E., Valfrè di Bonzo, L., Cannito, S., Paternostro, C. & Parola, M. (2010). Liver fibrosis: a dynamic and potentially reversibile process. *Histology and Histopathology,* 25(8), pp.1075-1091. ISSN: 0213-3911.

Richardson, M.M., Jonsson, J.R., Powell, E.E., Brunt, E.M., Neuschwander-Tetri, B.A., Bhathal, P.S., Dixon, J.B., Weltman, M.D., Tilg, H., Moschen, A.R., Purdie, D.M., Demetris, A.J. & Clouston, A.D. (2007). Progressive fibrosis in nonalcoholic steatohepatitis: association with altered regeneration and a ductular reaction. *Gastroenterology,* 133(1), pp.80-90. ISSN: 0016-5085.

Robertson, H., Kirby, J.A., Yip, W.W., Jones, D.E. & Burt, A.D. (2007). Biliary epithelial-mesenchymal transition in posttransplantation recurrence of primary biliary cirrhosis. *Hepatology,* 45(4), pp.977-981. ISSN: 0270-9139.

Russo, F.P., Alison, M.R., Bigger, B.W., Amofah, E., Florou, A., Amin, F., Bou-Gharios, G., Jeffery, R., Iredale, J.P. & Forbes, S.J. (2006). The bone marrow functionally contributes to liver fibrosis. *Gastroenterology,* 130(6), pp.1807-1821. ISSN: 0016-5085.

Rygiel, K.A., Robertson, H., Marshall, H.L., Pekalski, M., Zhao, L., Booth, T.A., Jones, D.E., Burt, A.D. & Kirby, J.A. (2008). Epithelial-mesenchymal transition contributes to portal tract fibrogenesis during human chronic liver disease. *Lab Invest,* 88(2), pp.112-123. ISSN: 0023-6837.

Sahin, H., Trautwein, C. & Wasmuth, H.E. (2010). Functional roles of chemokines in liver disease models. *Nat Rev Gastroenterol Hepatol,* 7(12): pp.682-690. ISSN: 1759-5045.

Scholten, D., Osterreicher, C.H., Scholten, A., Iwaisako, K., Gu, G., Brenner, D.A. & Kisseleva, T. (2010). Genetic labeling does not detect epithelial-to-mesenchymal transition of cholangiocytes in liver fibrosis in mice. *Gastroenterology,* 139(3), pp.987-998. ISSN: 0016-5085.

Stewart, S.F., Vidali, M., Day, C.P., Albano, E. & Jones, D.E. (2004). Oxidative stress as a trigger for cellular immune response in patients with alcoholic liver disease. *Hepatology,* 39(1), pp.197-203. ISSN: 0270-9139.

Taura, K., Miura, K., Iwaisako, K., Osterreicher, C.H., Kodama, Y., Penz-Osterreicher, M. & Brenner, D.A. (2010). Hepatocytes do not undergo epithelial-mesenchymal transition in liver fibrosis in mice. *Hepatology,* 51(3), pp.1027-1036. ISSN: 0270-9139.

Thiery, J.P. & Sleeman, J.P. (2006). Complex networks orchestrate epithelial - mesenchymal transitions. *Nature Rev Mol Cell Biol,* 7(2), pp.131-142. ISSN: 1471-0072.

Unanue, E.R. (2007). Ito cells, stellate cells, myofibroblasts: new actors in antigen presentation. *Immunity,* 26(1), pp.9-10. ISSN: 1074-7613.

Valfrè di Bonzo, L., Ferrero, I., Cravanzola, C., Mareschi, K., Rustichelli, D., Novo, E., Sanavio, F., Cannito, S., Zamara, E., Bertero, M., Davit, A., Francica, S., Novelli, F., Colombatto, S., Fagioli, F. & Parola, M. (2008). Human mesenchymal stem cells as a two-edged sword in hepatic regenerative medicine: engraftment and hepatocyte differentiation versus profibrogenic potential. *Gut,* 57(2), pp.223-231. ISSN: 0017-5749.

Valfrè di Bonzo, L., Novo, E., Cannito, S., Busletta, C., Paternostro, C., Povero, D. & Parola, M. (2009). Angiogenesis and liver fibrogenesis. *Histology and Histopathology,* 24(10), pp.1323-1334. ISSN: 0213-3911.

Wells, R.G. (2010). The epithelial-to-mesenchymal transition in liver fibrosis: here today, gone tomorrow? *Hepatology,* 51(3), pp.737-740. ISSN: 0270-9139.

Xia, J.L., Dai, C., Michalopoulos, G.K. & Liu, Y. (2006). Hepatocyte growth factor attenuates liver fibrosis induced by bile duct ligation. *Am J Pathol,* 168(5), pp.1500-1512. ISSN: 0002-9440.

Yang, L., Shultz, R.W., Mars, W.M., Wegner, R.E., Li, Y., Dai, C., Nejak, K. & Liu, Y. (2002). Disruption of tissue-type plasminogen activator gene in mice reduces renal interstitial fibrosis in obstructive nephropathy. *J Clin Invest,* 110(10), pp.1525-1538. ISSN: 0021-9738.

Zeisberg, M. & Kalluri, R. (2004). The role of epithelial-to-mesenchymal transition in renal fibrosis. *J Mol Med,* 82(3), pp.175-181. ISSN:0946-2716.

Zeisberg, M., Yang, C., Martino, M., Duncan, M.B., Rieder, F., Tanjore, H. & Kalluri, R. (2007). Fibroblasts derive from hepatocytes in liver fibrosis via epithelial to mesenchymal transition. *J Biol Chem,* 282(32), pp.23337-23347. ISSN: 0021-9258

Zeisberg, M. & Neilson, E.G. (2009). Biomarkers for epithelial - mesenchymal transitions. *J Clin Invest,* 119(6), pp.1429-1437. ISSN: 0021-9738.

Zhan, S.S., Jiang, J.X., Wu, J., Halsted, C., Friedman, S.L., Zern, M.A. & Torok, N.J. (2006). Phagocytosis of apoptotic bodies by hepatic stellate cells induces NADPH oxidase and is associated with liver fibrosis in vivo. *Hepatology,* 43(3), pp.435-445. ISSN:0270-9139.

9

Up-to-Date Insight About Membrane Remodeling as a Mechanism of Action for Ethanol-Induced Liver Toxicity

Odile Sergent, Fatiha Djoudi-Aliche and Dominique Lagadic-Gossmann
EA 4427 SeRAIC/IRSET, Université de Rennes 1, IFR 140, UFR des Sciences Pharmaceutiques et Biologiques, 2, av Pr Léon Bernard, 35043 Rennes cédex, France

1. Introduction

Hepatocellular death is a key mechanism in alcoholic liver diseases. Although ethanol has been described for many years as capable of increasing membrane fluidity, it is only recently that this fluidizing effect has been reported to be involved in ethanol-induced liver toxicity. In addition, in the last decade, a better understanding of plasma membrane has led to suggest that this membrane is not a random association of lipids, but is rather heterogeneous, with various microstructures enriched in specific components depending on their affinity. Special attention has been paid on lipid rafts that are cholesterol- and sphingolipid- rich microstructures, conferring them higher rigidity compared to other plasma membrane microdomains. As lipid rafts can also activate or suppress cell signaling pathways, lipid raft discovery provides new arguments for several researchers to revisit the fluidizing effect of ethanol by studying the possible ethanol-induced physical and biochemical alteration of lipid rafts. Thus, in this chapter, we have considered to review the capacity of ethanol to induce a membrane remodeling, depicted as an increase in membrane fluidity and alterations of physical and biochemical properties of lipid rafts, and its relationship with ethanol liver toxicity.

2. Membrane fluidity

The Singer-Nicolson fluid mosaic model indicates that membranes consist of a phospholipid bilayer, where lipids, in a fluid phase, act as solvent for proteins (Singer & Nicolson, 1972). In this chapter, membrane fluidity means the relative freedom of motion for membrane components, especially phospholipids, and represents the combination of various types of mobility (Figure 1). Membrane fluidity is principally determined by the acyl chain swinging movement and phospholipid rotation. Thus, short chains and double bonds in acyl chains of phospholipids create spaces in the bilayer and promote membrane fluidization. At the opposite, the rigid steroid nucleus of cholesterol, lying next to the first 9 or 10 carbon atoms of the phospholipid acyl chains, prevents the swinging movement of the acyl chains thereby stiffening membranes. For the evaluation of this membrane parameter, most studies have used either electron paramagnetic resonance (EPR) with spin-labeled fatty acids, or polarization of fluorescence with hydrophobic fluorescence polarization probes. An increased membrane fluidity for EPR is usually assessed by a decrease of order parameter (S), and for fluorescence, by a decrease of polarization (P), anisotropy (A) or microviscosity (η).

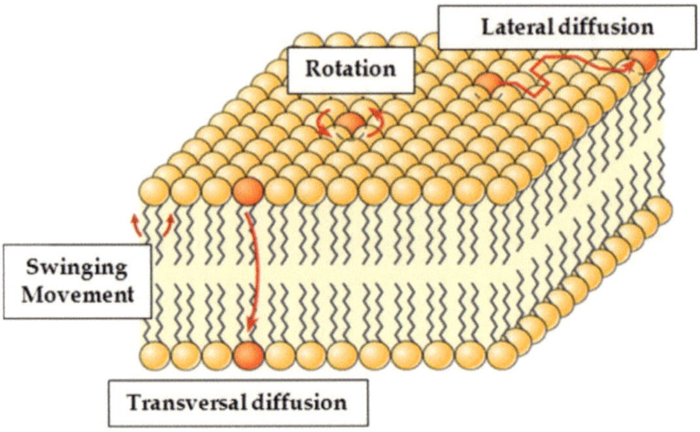

Fig. 1. Different types of mobility of phospholipids.

Any alteration of the optimal range for membrane fluidity has influence on many biological functions such as membrane enzyme and receptor activities, or transmembrane transport processes (Ho et al, 1994; Schachter, 1984; Stubbs et al, 1988). Furthermore, more recently, it was also shown its fundamental role in cell signalling responses to xenobiotic stress (polycyclic aromatic hydrocarbons, cisplatin or ethanol), leading to cell death such as apoptosis (Rebillard et al, 2007; Sergent et al, 2005; Tekpli et al, 2011).

2.1 Plasma liver membranes

Since the end of the seventies, many papers have provided strong evidence that ethanol very rapidly induces a fluidization of membranes as reported by several reviews (Goldstein, 1987; Rottenberg, 1992; Wood & Schroeder, 1988).

2.1.1 Tissue type-dependent effect of ethanol

Using electron paramagnetic resonance, Chin and Goldstein (1977a) were the first to demonstrate the ability of ethanol used at low concentrations (from 20 mM - 40 mM) to increase *in vitro* membrane fluidity of erythrocyte and synaptosomal plasma membranes. In addition, they showed that continuous exposure of mice to ethanol provided in the diet for a short period (8 days) (Chin & Goldstein, 1977b) or by inhalation (3 days) (Lyon & Goldstein, 1983) respectively restored a membrane fluidity near controls or even rigidified membranes in the inner hydrophobic regions, testifying an adaptation. Thus, in alcoholic patients, erythrocytes exhibited a decrease in membrane fluidity (Beaugé et al, 1985; Parmahamsa et al, 2004). However, the effect of ethanol on plasma membranes is different for the liver. Indeed, they become more fluid, mainly in the inner hydrophobic regions, for chronically ethanol-intoxicated rats (Schüller et al, 1984; Yamada & Lieber, 1984) and an increase in fluidity was also observed in plasma membranes isolated from Reuber H35 rat hepatoma cells (Polokoff et al, 1985) or WRL-68 human hepatic cells (Gutierrez-Ruiz et al, 1995) following a long term treatment with ethanol (3 or 4 weeks). Such an effect could contribute to the special sensitivity of liver to ethanol toxicity. At the opposite, other organelles in the liver did not exhibit any membrane fluidification after ethanol intoxication of rats (Table 1). It should be noted that, when primary hepatocytes isolated from chronically ethanol-treated rats were cultured before the evaluation of plasma membrane fluidity by fluorescence polarization, an increased ordering was observed (Benedetti et al, 1991).

Organelles	Methods	Type of Lipid Bilayer Environnement	Membrane Fluidity (compared to controls)	References
Mitochondria	Electron Paramagnetic Resonance	Polar region	=	Waring et al, 1981
	Fluorescence Polarization	Polar region	⇩	Castro et al, 1991
	Fluorescence Polarization	Polar region	⇩	Colell et al, 1997
Microsomes	Electron Paramagnetic Resonance	Polar region	⇩	Ponnappa et al, 1982
	Electron Paramagnetic Resonance	Apolar core region	=	Taraschi et al, 1985
	Electron Paramagnetic Resonance	Apolar core region	=	Aloia et al, 1985
Plasma membranes	Fluorescence Polarization	Apolar core region	⇧	Schüller et al, 1984
	Fluorescence Polarization	Apolar core region	⇧	Yamada and Lieber, 1984

Table 1. Effect of chronic ethanol intoxication on membrane fluidity of various organelles in the liver. (In all experiments, rats were fed a diet containing 36 % of total calories as ethanol for 30 to 40 days.)

Whatever exposure modes (ingestion, inhalation or intraperitoneal injections) (Chin & Golstein, 1977b; Lyon & Golstein, 1983; Johnson et al, 1979), erythrocyte and synaptosomal plasma membranes isolated from ethanol-treated mice did not exhibit an increase in membrane fluidity after a further *in vitro* ethanol addition in contrast to membranes isolated from untreated mice. Such an *in vitro* resistance was also observed in erythrocyte membranes from alcoholic patients (Beaugé et al, 1985). Even though liver plasma membranes remained more fluid after chronic rat intoxication (Schüller et al, 1984; Yamada & Lieber, 1984) or after long term ethanol treatment of cultured hepatocytes (Gutierrez-Ruiz et al, 1995; Polokoff et al, 1985), these isolated membranes also exhibited an *in vitro* resistance to the disordering effect of a further direct addition of ethanol. Finally, most of the papers quoted in table 1 indicated such a process for microsomes or mitochondria. This phenomenom could be related to several changes in membrane lipid composition (Johnson et al, 1979) *ie* an increase in cholesterol within brain and liver cell membranes in rats (Chin et al, 1978) and in monkeys (Cunningham et al, 1983), an increased ratio of saturated to polyunsaturated fatty acids (Johnson et al, 1979), or reduced concentrations of sialic acid and galactose in the membrane surface of human erythrocytes (Beaugé et al, 1985).

2.1.2 Molecular mechanisms whereby ethanol could increase membrane fluidity

These mechanisms, summarized in figure 2, can occur simultaneously. The first described mechanism was in brain membranes and concerns physical properties of ethanol which allow it to directly interact with the lipid bilayer, thus triggering a direct membrane disorder (Goldstein, 1984; Gurtovenko & Anwar, 2009; Marquês et al, 2011; Rottenberg, 1992). This theory was particularly developed in the field of drug tolerance and physical dependence, but, in the liver, other mechanisms were also described. First, it was proposed that the fluidizing effect of chronic ethanol treatment could be related to changes in membrane lipid composition as acyl chain saturation and cholesterol are well-described to affect membrane fluidity. Thus, Yamada et al (1984) related the increase in membrane fluidity of liver plasma membranes after chronic ethanol feeding to a decrease in cholesterol plasma membrane content by an unknown mechanism. In hepatoma cells chronically exposed to ethanol for 3 weeks, the increase in membrane fluidity of plasma membranes was linked to the elevation of the ratio phosphatidylcholine/sphingomyelin (Polokoff et al, 1985). However, the main distinction of liver is that most of the ethanol metabolism occurs in this organ. Thus, ethanol metabolism appeared to play a key role since blocking ethanol metabolism by methylpyrazole inhibited changes in membrane fluidity both in acute intoxicated primary rat hepatocytes (Sergent et al, 2005), and in chronically treated hepatoma cells (Polokoff et al, 1985). Logically, as ethanol metabolism was involved, our team was interested in looking at the involvement of oxidative stress following an acute ethanol intoxication of primary rat hepatocytes. Using antioxidant such as thiourea (reactive oxygen species (ROS) scavenger) or vitamin E (lipid peroxidation inhibitor), we showed that oxidative stress played a role in the fluidizing effect of ethanol (Sergent et al, 2005). This new mechanism explained how ethanol could very rapidly (30 minutes) increase membrane fluidity since ROS production could be detected as soon as 15 minutes. Several molecular mechanisms can be proposed to explain the influence of oxidative stress on membrane fluidity. First, lipid peroxidation by-products could increase membrane fluidity either by interacting with membrane proteins (Buko et al, 1996; Subramaniam et al, 1997), or more directly by their own rearrangement (Jain et al, 1994; Gabbita et al, 1998). ROS, by oxidizing tubulin could also disrupt microtubule cytoskeleton, thereby increasing membrane fluidity (Yoon et al, 1998; Remy-Kristensen et al, 2000). In our model of primary rat hepatocytes, paclitaxel (a microtubule stabilizer) prevented from the fluidizing effect of ethanol (unpublished data).

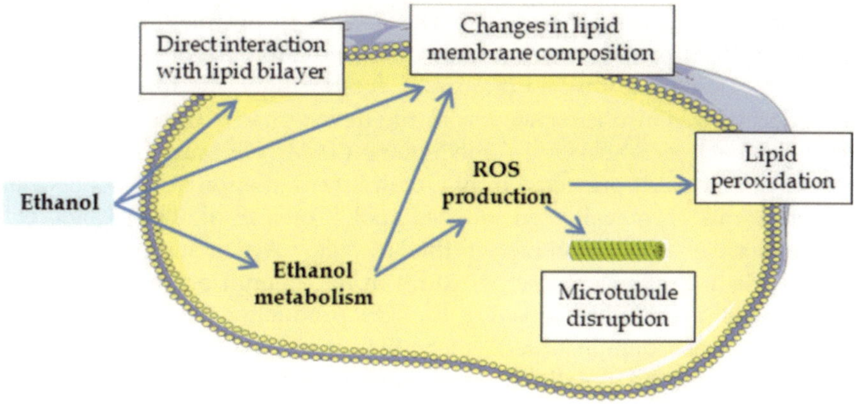

(ROS : reactive oxygen species).

Fig. 2. Possible molecular mechanisms for ethanol to increase membrane fluidity.

2.2 Liver mitochondria membranes

As shown above, a great body of evidence indicated that, in inner membranes of mitochondria, ethanol intoxication induced a decrease rather than an increase in fluidity. This was demonstrated for chronically intoxicated rats but also with HepG2 human hepatocytes treated with acetaldehyde, a product of ethanol metabolism (Lluis et al, 2003), providing a further proof of the involvement of ethanol metabolism in membrane fluidity changes. In addition, this decrease was related to an elevation of cholesterol content in mitochondria which concerns both outer and inner membranes. Finally, the acetaldehyde stimulation of cholesterol incorporation into mitochondria membranes was attributed to endothelium reticulum stress.

2.3 Membrane pharmacology of ethanol liver toxicity by manipulation of membrane fluidity

Since the eighties, many studies suggested the influence of ethanol fluidizing effect on membrane protein activities (McCall et al, 1989; Mills et al, 1985; Rubin & Rottenberg, 1982). Only recently, researchers became interested in determining the role of membrane fluidity changes in ethanol-induced hepatocellular death. Thus, manipulation of plasma membrane fluidity by exposing primary rat hepatocytes to membrane stabilizing agents (ursodeoxycholic acid (UDCA) or ganglioside GM1 (GM1)) led to the inhibition of ethanol-induced cell death, while fluidizing compounds (tween 20 or A_2C) enhanced it (Sergent et al, 2005). In order to explain how plasma membrane fluidity could affect cell death, oxidative stress was also studied. At the opposite of fluidizing compounds, membrane stabilizing agents were shown to protect from ethanol-induced lipid peroxidation, ROS production and the elevation of another prooxidant factor, namely low-molecular-weight iron. Low-molecular-weight iron consists of iron species that can trigger oxidative stress by catalyzing the formation of a highly reactive free radical, the hydroxyl radical. It should be noted that UDCA and GM1 displayed a protection towards ethanol-induced ROS production only when ROS were evaluated after 1 or 5 hours of incubation with ethanol. At 15 minutes, no protection was afforded by membrane stabilizing agents, unlike the inhibitor of ethanol metabolism, 4-methyl-pyrazole. This led us to postulate a sequence of events whereby the early ROS formation was mainly due to ethanol metabolism and the late phase to the increase in membrane fluidity (Figure 3). Interestingly, the increased mitochondrial membrane ordering was also associated with the development of oxidative stress. Indeed, stabilizing agents such as S-adenosyl-L methionine (SAME) or taurine conjugate of UDCA (tauroursodeoxycholic acid) protected from glutathione depletion in mitochondria obtained from the liver of rats chronically fed with ethanol (Colell et al, 1997; Colell et al, 2001). Reduced glutathione, the main non protein thiol in cells, plays an important role to detoxify hydrogen peroxide and other organic peroxides in mitochondria. Glutathione depletion in mitochondria made them more sensitive to ROS production and subsequent oxidative stress. Thus, it was demonstrated that the increased mitochondrial membrane microviscosity impaired the glutathione transporter which normally allows the glutathione transport from cytosol to mitochondrial matrix (Coll, 2003; Lluis et al, 2003) (Figure 3).

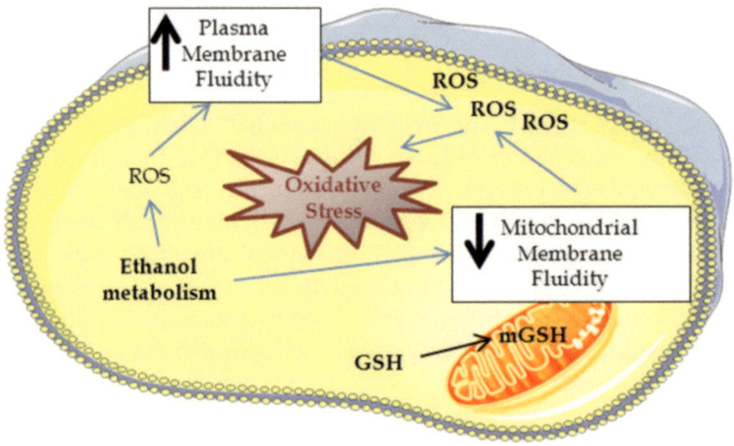

(GSH : reduced glutathione; ROS : reactive oxygen species).

Fig. 3. Relationship between membrane fluidity and ethanol-induced oxidative stress.

Cholesterol involvement in this process should be pointed out. Indeed, as mitochondrial membrane enrichment in cholesterol was responsible for the decreased mitochondrial membrane fluidity, lovastatin, an inhibitor of hydroxymethylglutaryl coenzyme A involved in cholesterol synthesis, was able to protect hepatocytes from acetaldehyde sensitization to tumor necrosis factor (TNF)α (Lluis et al, 2003). Similarly to membrane stabilizing agents, membrane fluidizer (A_2C) restored the initial glutathione transport rate and mitochondrial content (Coll et al, 2003; Lluis et al, 2003). However, the use of membrane fluidizers should be done with caution since, from our results about the involvement of plasma membrane fluidization in ethanol-induced cell death, it appears that they can be injurious for hepatocytes. At the opposite, UDCA and its conjugates seem to be good candidates for a potential therapeutic use, because, due to their membrane stabilizing properties (Güldütuna et al, 1993), they restore the normality in membrane fluidity for every type of membranes. Thus, in case of ethanol intoxication, they were able to prevent both the increase of plasma membrane fluidity, as we observed in primary rat hepatocytes (Sergent, 2005), and the decrease in mitochondria membranes of hepatocytes from ethanol-fed rats (Colell et al,

2001). In addition, UDCA was also shown to protect rats from the increase in liver plasma membrane fluidity due to chronic ethanol intake and hence from liver lipid peroxidation and necrosis (Oliva et al, 1998). However, although UDCA is a therapeutically relevant bile acid, already used for preventing human primary biliary cirrhosis (Poupon et al, 2003; Corpechot et al, 2011), it did not exhibit any beneficial effect on a 6-month survival of patients with severe alcohol-induced cirrhosis, but possibly because of inappropriate dosage (Pelletier et al, 2003).

3. Lipid rafts

Because of the well-described effect of ethanol on plasma membrane fluidity, it is not surprising that some researchers about alcoholic liver diseases were interested in the possible involvement of lipid rafts in ethanol toxicity. Indeed, plasma membrane is not constituted by a random lipid distribution but rather by a selective lateral lipid segregation due to self-associative properties of sphingolipid and cholesterol, leading to the concept of "lipid rafts" (Simons & Toomre, 2000; Lingwood & Simons, 2010). Thus, lipid rafts are detergent-resistant, sphingolipid- and cholesterol-rich microdomains of the plasma membrane, which form highly ordered spatial nanoscale assemblies separated from other membrane regions composed of more unsaturated and loosely packed fatty acids (Figure 4).

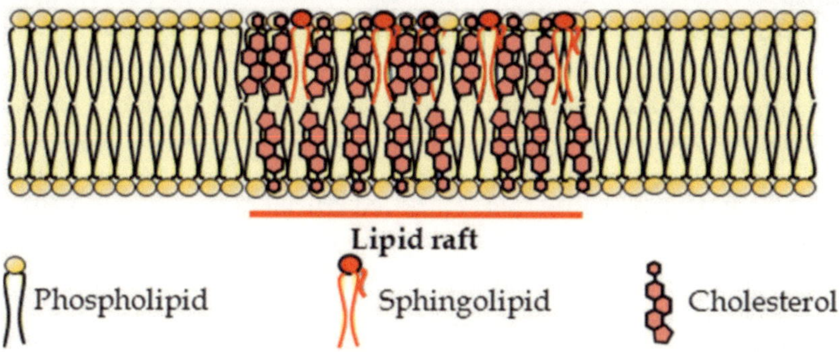

Fig. 4. Schematic representation of a lipid raft (without proteins).

Lipid rafts as nanoscale assemblies are dynamics and after cell stimulation, can coalesced to larger levels to form raft platforms (Harder & Engelhardt, 2004). Concerning proteins, lipid rafts are notably enriched in glycosylphosphatidylinositol (GPI) proteins, receptors such as cell death receptors and Toll-like receptors (TLR), and signaling proteins like mitogen-activating protein kinases, protein kinases C etc. Some proteins are raft residents, whereas others are recruited after cell stimulation with receptor-specific ligands. In addition, based on their mobility, lipid rafts, through their aggregation, can form platforms that assembly many proteins on a same place leading to the formation of a receptor cluster, which can then activate or suppress signaling pathways (Pike, 2003; Schmitz & Orso, 2002). One might suppose that ethanol, through its capacity to increase liver plasma membrane fluidity, can disturb these microdomains and hence, various cell signaling pathways. Consequently, in the last past decade, new investigations were undertaken to possibly link lipid rafts to ethanol toxicity. Researches were conducted in two directions: the main one concerned perturbation of innate immunity *via* TLR4 signaling and the other one, hepatocyte cell death *via* the activation of phospholipase C (PLC) signaling.

3.1 Lipid rafts in the TLR4 signaling dysfunction by ethanol

Several components of innate immunity contribute to the pathogenesis of alcoholic liver disease (Gao et al, 2011). Here, we will mainly focus on lipopolysaccharide (LPS)/TLR4 signaling pathways because of the necessary translocation of TLR4 receptor into lipid rafts for its activation.

3.1.1 Involvement of LPS/TLR4 signaling pathway in alcoholic liver disease

Strong evidence suggest that the immune cells of the liver (phagocytic cells such as neutrophils or resident Küpffer cells, and lymphocytes such as natural killer [NK] cells or T cells) play a crucial role in alcoholic liver disease including steatosis, hepatitis and fibrosis (Suh & Jeong, 2011). Thus, Küpffer cells are main actors in the immune response against endotoxin/lipopolysaccharide (LPS) *via* Toll-Like Receptor type 4 (TLR4) signaling pathway leading to the production of pro-inflammatory mediators such as cytokines (TNF-α, interleukin [IL]-1, IL-6), chemokines (monocyte chemotactic protein-1 [MCP-1]), ROS and profibrogenic factors (transforming growth factor [TGF]-β, platelet-derived growth factor [PDGF]), which subsequently activate hepatic stellate cells for the production of extracellular matrix (Jeong & Gao, 2008) (Gao et al, 2011) (Figure 5). Indeed, it is well established that ethanol intake, by increasing gut permeabilization, allows the uptake of LPS in portal circulation (Parlesak et al, 2000) promoting liver ethanol toxicity (Nanji et al, 1994). In addition, in the liver, TLR4 is also expressed on recruited macrophages, hepatocytes, sinusoidal endothelial cells and hepatic stellate cells (Seki & Brenner, 2008). Consequently, *via* TLR4 signalling, these last cells can also contribute to liver inflammation by releasing proinflammatory cytokines and chemokines. Finally, TLR4 signalling in hepatic stellate cells can also participate to the development of alcoholic fibrosis by enhancing TGF-β signalling (Seki et al, 2007). Therefore, TLR4 receptor appeared crucial in the development of alcoholic liver disease (Gao et al, 2011).

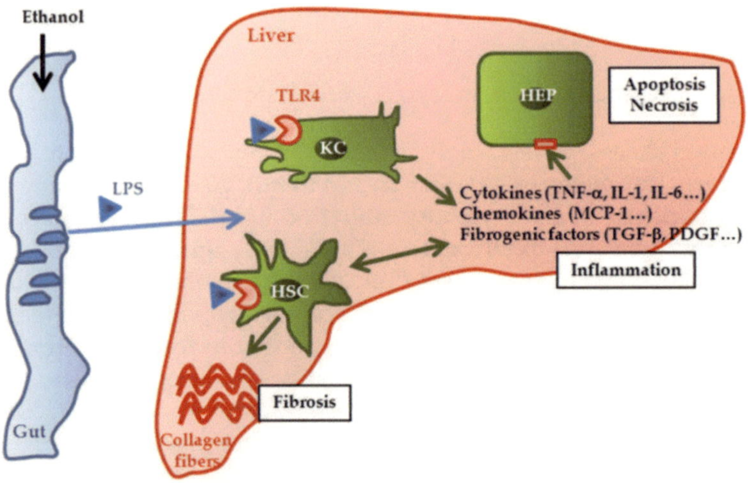

(HEP : hepatocytes; HSC: hepatic stellate cells; KC : Küpffer cells; IL : interleukin; LPS : lipopolysaccharide; MCP-1 : monocyte chemotactic protein-1 ; PDGF : platelet-derived growth factor; TGF: tumor growth factor; TLR4 : Toll-like receptor 4; TNF : tumor necrosis factor)

Fig. 5. Contribution of TLR4 receptor to the pathogenesis of alcoholic liver disease.

3.1.2 Effects of ethanol on the recruitment of TLR4 into lipid rafts

LPS does not bind TLR4 receptor directly, but is rather first bound to cell surface co-receptors, the cluster of differentiation 14 (CD14) and the myeloid differentiation protein 2 (MD-2), without cytoplasmic domains (Fitzgerald, 2004). However, TLR4 is the integrator of cell signalling since it has intracellular signaling domains. Close interactions between these membrane receptors are made possible by their recruitment and assembly within lipid rafts (Schmitz & Orso, 2002; Triantafilou et al, 2002). Thus, CD14 is a glycosyl phosphatidylinositol-linked protein which therefore constitutively resides in lipid rafts, while TLR4 needs translocation into rafts for the complex formation (Dolganiuc et al, 2006). Two features of the ethanol effect on TLR4 and other receptor signaling could be distinguished depending on ethanol concentration. 1) At high concentration (≥ 50 mM), ethanol prevented from LPS-induced redistribution pattern of the co-receptor CD14 within lipid rafts, and from the translocation of TLR4 receptor into rafts (Table 2). This alteration could partly explain why ethanol consumption is recognized as a risk factor for concomitant bacterial or viral infections (Nelson and Kolls, 2002; Szabo, 1999). Dai et al (2005) and Dolganiuc et al (2006) suggested that ethanol, at the concentration of 50 or 86 mM, may disrupt lipid rafts because similar effects were obtained with lipid raft disrupters. However, a protein raft marker, flotillin did not exhibit any alteration and no clear evidence of lipid raft disruption was given, since the cholesterol decrease was detected in culture media instead of lipid rafts. They also attributed changes in partitioning cellular membrane in raft and nonraft structures to the increase in bulk membrane fluidity (Dolganiuc et al, 2006) without checking this influence by the use of membrane stabilizing agents or measuring the increase in membrane fluidity directly in lipid rafts. Their hypothesis would be that ethanol by this way could disrupt lipid protein interactions (Szabo et al, 2007). Only at very high concentrations (200 mM), a lipid raft disruption was really observed in RAW 264.7 macrophages (Fernandez-Lizarbe et al, 2008). However, at 50 mM, in primary rat cortical astrocytes, a partial disruption of lipid raft could be detected suggesting that ethanol at this concentration induced both effects : i) disruption leading to the inhibition of lipid raft - induced cell signalling, and ii) promotion of TLR4 recruitment in lipid rafts (see below)) (Blanco et al, 2008). More recently, it was also demonstrated an ethanol inhibition of lipid raft-mediated T-Cell Receptor (TCR) signalling in human CD4+ T cells and in Jurkat T cells, but no alteration of lipid raft markers was observed suggesting that ethanol had no direct effect on lipid rafts (Ghare et al, 2011). Interestingly, the authors proposed a post-translational modification of proteins to explain the inhibition of protein translocation into lipid rafts. These mechanisms could also be explored for the other models. 2) At lower concentration (≤ 50 mM), mimicking LPS effects both in macrophages and astrocytes, ethanol induced the recruitment of TLR4 into lipid rafts, thus allowing the activation of TLR4 dependent cell signalling (Table 2). A similar process was also observed for IL-1R1 (IL1 receptor 1) (Blanco et al, 2008). Thus, ethanol triggered cytokine and other inflammatory mediator secretion *via* lipid raft-dependent signalling pathway. According to Blanco et al (2008), low ethanol concentrations (10 - 50 mM) may facilitate protein-protein and protein-lipid interactions within the membrane microdomains to promote receptor recruitment into the lipid rafts. Even if this effect has not yet been directly described in the liver, lipid rafts might participate to the mechanisms involved in the enhancement by chronic ethanol treatment of liver inflammation associated with the activation of IL-1R1 receptor in rat liver and hepatocytes (Valles et al, 2003), or TLR4 in immune cells (Szabo & Bala, 2010).

Ethanol Concen tration	Cell Type	Ethanol effects on		References
		lipid raft biochemical properties	receptor signalling and inflammation	
86 mM	RAW macrophage like cell line	- Alteration of the redistribution pattern of CD14 in lipid rafts after LPS stimulation	- Decrease in LPS-induced TNFα production - Similar effect with nystatin, a lipid raft disrupter	Dai et al, 2005
50 mM	Chinese hamster ovary cell line (CHO) Primary human monocytes	- Alteration of the redistribution pattern of CD14 in lipid rafts after LPS stimulation - Decrease in LPS-induced TLR4 translocation into lipid rafts -Increase in residual TLR4 in the nonraft fractions - No changes in flotillin, a protein raft marker	- Decrease in LPS-induced TNFα production and NF-kB activation - Similar effects with methyl-β-cyclodextrin, a lipid raft disrupter	Dolganiuc et al, 2006
10 mM 50 mM 200 mM	RAW macrophage like cell line Primary mice peritoneal macrophages	-10 mM : CD14 and TLR4 translocation into lipid rafts -50 mM: CD14 translocation into lipid rafts, but at a lesser extent for TLR4 -10 and 50 mM : translocation of proteins associated with TLR4 response into lipid rafts -200 mM : No translocation of TLR4 into lipid rats and disruption of lipid rafts	- Direct production of TNFα (10 mM : by 2.4 fold; 50 mM: by 1.8 fold; 100 mM : no effect)	Fernandez-Lizarbe et al, 2007

Table 2. (Continued)

Ethanol Concen tration	Cell Type	Ethanol effects on		References
		lipid raft biochemical properties	receptor signalling and inflammation mediators	
10 mM 50 mM	Primary rat cortical astrocytes	- 10 mM: translocation of IL-1R1 and TLR4 into lipid rafts; recruitment of activated signalling proteins into rafts (P-IRAK and P-ERK) - 50 mM : idem, but at a lesser extent, with a slight disruption	- Expression of IL-1R1 and TLR4 receptors in cell lysates was abolished by lipid raft disrupters (saponin, or methyl-β-cyclodextrin) - Internalization of IL-1R1 receptor in caveosomes	Blanco et al, 2008
25 mM 75 mM	Primary human CD4+ T cells Jurkat T cell line	- Inhibition of PHA or anti-CD23/CD28 antibodies induced Lck, LAT or PLCγ recruitment into lipid rafts - No changes in lipid raft protein marker (flotillin)	Decrease in IL2 expression and down-regulation of TCR signaling	Ghare et al, 2011

(ERK : extracellular regulated kinase; IL : interleukin; IRAK : interleukin-1 receptor associated kinase; LAT : linker for activation of T cells; lck : lymphocyte-specific protein tyrosine kinase; LPS : lipopolysaccharide; NF-kB : nuclear factor kappa B; PHA : phytohaemagglutinin; PLC: phospholipase C; TCR : T cell receptor; TNF : tumor necrosis factor).

Table 2. Effects of acute ethanol exposure on lipid raft-mediated receptor activation. (In these studies, rafts were isolated by their *in vitro* property to resist to solubilization in non-ionic detergents at low temperature and to float and concentrate in low-density sucrose (Brown & Rose, 1992), leading to raft and non-raft fractions.)

3.2 Lipid rafts in ethanol-induced hepatocyte damage

Another approach was to consider the role of lipid rafts in ethanol-induced oxidative stress. The occurrence of oxidative stress in alcoholic liver disease and its relationship with ethanol liver damage have been extensively documented (Albano, 2008; Cederbaum et al, 2009; De Minicis & Brenner, 2008; Wu & Cederbaum, 2009), but less is known about the possible role of lipid rafts. Thus, it was shown by our team that lipid raft disrupters were able to protect from ethanol-induced ROS production and lipid peroxidation in primary rat hepatocytes (Nourissat et al, 2008). In addition, we have showed for the first time that oxidative changes within lipid rafts are a prerequisite for the oxidative stress to develop in rat hepatocytes.

Thus, ethanol metabolism, by producing a rapid and mild oxidative stress, was able to induce oxidative damage within lipid rafts leading to their clustering following protein crosslinkages (Figure 6).

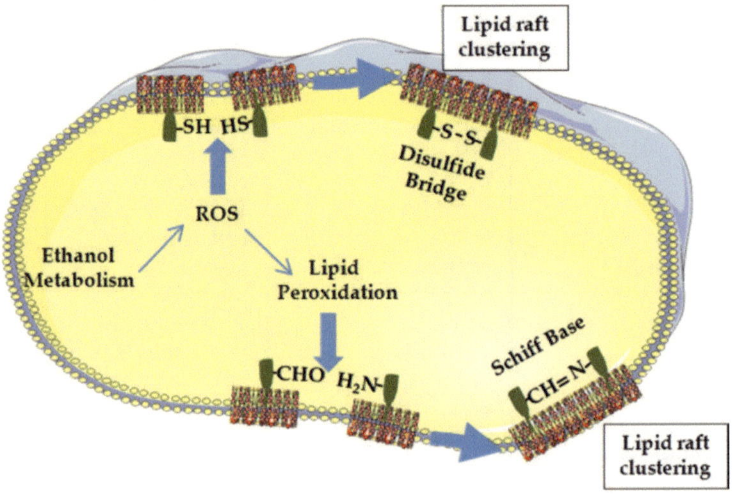

(CHO : carbonyl group; ROS : reactive oxygen species; SH : thiol group)

Fig. 6. Ethanol-induced lipid raft clustering *via* oxidative stress and protein crosslinkage.

Protein crosslinkages were obtained by the formation of disulfide bridges from two intermolecular thiol (SH) groups from several rafts, and by the formation of adducts with malondialdehyde, a well-known product of lipid peroxidation in ethanol treated-rat hepatocytes (Nourissat et al, 2008). This aldehyde like 4-hydroxynonenal can react with nucleophile residues in proteins to form carbonyl groups which then may form Schiff base with a lysine of another protein. Such a protein can be included in another raft leading to raft clustering (Figure 6). Interestingly, according to experiments performed on the translocation of TLR4 (see above) which proposed a role for membrane fluidity without fully demonstrating it, we expressly proved the involvement of the fluidizing effect in the ethanol-induced lipid raft clustering by the use of membrane stabilizer or fluidizers. In addition, ethanol was shown to be able to fluidize lipid rafts, but at a lesser extent compared to bulk membranes. These results also confirmed our previous results which showed the pivotal role of the increased membrane fluidity in ethanol-induced cell death of rat hepatocytes (Sergent et al, 2005), thereby emphasizing on the contribution of membrane remodeling in ethanol liver toxicity. Finally, lipid raft clustering also participated to the activation of phospholipase C-γ-dependent signaling pathway. Indeed, this clustering induced translocation of phospholipase C-γ into rafts, which induced elevation of low-molecular-weight-iron, a potent prooxidant factor, and hence, lipid peroxidation. To summarize, ethanol metabolism, by producing a mild oxidative stress can rapidly affect both membrane fluidity and lipid rafts, thus promoting lipid raft aggregation (Figure 7). Then, this lipid raft clustering, by activating phospholipase C-γ dependent signaling pathway, may in turn trigger amplification of oxidative stress and cell death (Figure 7).

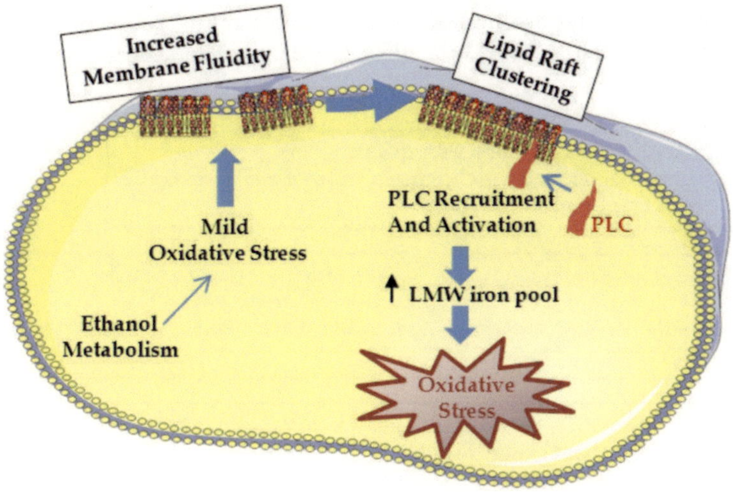

(LMW iron: low molecular weight iron; PLC: phospholipase C)

Fig. 7. Amplification of oxidative stress *via* lipid raft clustering during acute ethanol intoxication of rat hepatocytes.

In this context, new therapeutic approach, called membrane lipid therapy (Escriba et al, 2006), could be a very effective strategy to protect hepatocytes from membrane-dependent oxidative damage in alcoholic liver damage, especially as an increasing body of evidence indicated that some dietary compounds such as plant flavonoids (Tarahosky et al, 2008) or fatty fish long-chain polyunsaturated n-3 fatty acids (n-3 PUFAs) (Wassal & Stillwell, 2009) might modify physical and chemical properties of lipid rafts. Thus, n-3 PUFAs have been extensively described as efficient modifiers of lipid and protein composition of lipid rafts in many cell types such as T lymphocytes (Fan et al, 2004; Stulnig, 2001), Caco-2 cells (Duraisamy et al, 2007), retinal vascular endothelial cells (Chen et al, 2007) and macrophages (Wong et al, 2009). In this context, the nutritional significance of lipid rafts has been recently pointed out (Yaqoob and Shaikh, 2010).

4. Conclusion

Taken altogether, these studies show that physical alterations of membranes (changes in membrane fluidity and microstructures) can be considered as an additional mechanism involved in ethanol liver toxicity. It is only in the last past decade that membrane remodeling appeared to be linked to ethanol liver toxicity (Figure 8). Therefore, further studies are needed in order to determine the role of lipid rafts in chronic ethanol intoxication, to further explore the downstream cell signaling after lipid raft clustering such as pathways involved in the elevation of low-molecular weight iron cell content, or to understand whether receptor recruitment in lipid raft might participate to alcoholic liver disease. In addition, other investigation should shed light on the possible beneficial effect of the modulation of membrane fluidity and lipid raft. Thus, statins that are already currently used in patients suffering from hypercholesterolemia, have demonstrated their efficiency to protect hepatocytes from acetaldehyde sentization to TNF (Lluis et al, 2003), and might also be proposed to disrupt lipid rafts. Finally, nutritional compounds such as plant flavonoids or fatty fish long-chain polyunsaturated n-3 fatty acids might represent a new therapeutic approach for patients with alcoholic liver disease based upon modulation of the membrane structures.

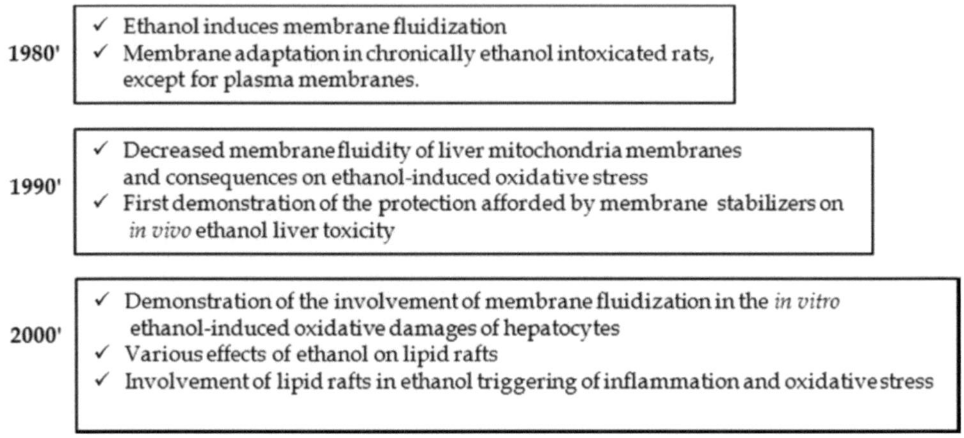

Fig. 8. Evolution of the "membrane remodelling" concept for alcoholic liver diseases.

5. Acknowledgement

The authors gratefully acknowledge IREB (Institut de Recherches Scientifiques sur les Boissons, Paris, France) for its financial support. They also wish to thank "Région Bretagne", which provided a grant for Fatiha Djoudi. The authors are also very grateful to Martine Chevanne for her skilfull technical assistance.

6. References

Albano, E. (2008). Oxidative mechanisms in the pathogenesis of alcoholic liver disease. *Molecular Aspects of Medicine*, Vol.29, No.1-2, (February-April 2008), pp.9-16, ISSN 0098-2997.

Aloia, R.C.; Paxton, J.; Daviau, J.S.; Van Gelb, O.; Mekusch, W.; Truppe; W.; Meyer, J.A. & Brauer, F.S. (1985). Effect of chronic alcohol consumption on rat brain microsome lipid composition membrane fluidity and Na+-K+-ATPase activity. *Life Sciences*, Vol.36, No. 10, (March 1985), pp.1003-1017, ISSN 0024-3205.

Beaugé, F.; Stibler, H & Borg S. (1985). Abnormal fluidity and surface carbohydrate content of the erythrocyte membrane in alcoholic patients. *Alcoholism: Clinical and Experimental Research*, Vol.9, No.4, (July-August 1985), pp.322-326, ISSN 0145-6008.

Benedetti, A.; Tangorra, A.; Baroni, G.S.; Ferretti, G.; Marucci, L.; Jezequel, A.M. & Orlandi, F. (1994). Plasma membrane order parameter in periportal and perivenular hepatocytes isolated from ethanol-treated rats. *American Journal of Physiology*, Vol.266, No.2Pt1, (February 1994), pp.G282-G291, ISSN 0193-1857.

Blanco, A.M.; Perez-Arago, A.; Fernandez-Lizarbe, S. & Guerri, C. (2008). Ethanol mimics ligand-mediated activation and endocytosis of IL-1RI/TLR4 receptors via lipid rafts caveolae in astroglial cells. *Journal of Neurochemistry*, Vol.106, No.2, (July 2008), pp.625-639, ISSN 0022-3042.

Brown, D.A. & Rose, J.K. (1992). Sorting of GPI-anchored proteins to glycol-lipid enriched membrane subdomains during transport to the apical cell surface. *Cell*, Vol.68, No.3, (February 1992), pp.533-544, ISSN 0092-8674.

Buko, V.; Artsukevich, A.; Zavodnik, I.; Maltsev, A.; Suhko, L.; Zimmermann, T. & Dianzani, M.U. (1996). Interactions of malondialdehyde and 4-hydroxynonenal with rat liver plasma membranes and their effect on binding of prostaglandin E2 by specific receptors. *Free Radical Research*, Vol.25, No. 5, (November 1996), pp.415-420, ISSN 1071-5762.

Castro, J.; Cortés, J.P. & Guzman, M. (1991). Properties of the mitochondrial membrane and carnitine palmitoyltransferase in the periportal and the perivenous zone of the liver. Effects of chronic ethanol feeding. *Biochemical Pharmacology*, Vol.41, No.12, (Jun 1991), pp.1987-1995, ISSN 0006-2952.

Cederbaum, A.I.; Lu, Y. & Wu, D. (2009). Role of oxidative stress in alcohol-induced liver injury. *Archives in Toxicology*, Vol.83, No.6, (June 2009), pp.519-548, ISSN 0340-5761.

Chen, W.; Jump, D.B.; Esselman, W.J. & Busik, J.V. (2007). Inhibition of cytokine signaling in human retinal endothelial cells through modification of caveolae/lipid rafts by docosahexaenoic acid. *Investigative Ophtalmology and Visual Science*, Vol.48, No.1, (January 2007), pp.18-26, ISSN 0146-0404.

Chin, J.H. & Goldstein, D.B. (1977a). Effects of low concentrations of ethanol on the fluidity of spin-labeled erythrocyte and brain membranes. *Molecular Pharmacology*, Vol.13, No.3, (May 1977), pp.435-441, ISSN 0026-895x.

Chin, J.H. & Goldstein, D.B. (1977b). Drug tolerance in biomembranes. *Science*, Vol.196, No. 4290, (May 1977), pp.684-685, ISSN 0036-8075.

Chin, J.H.; Parson, L.M. & Goldstein D.B. (1978). Increased cholesterol content of erythrocyte and brain membranes in ethanol-tolerant mice. *Biochimica et Biophysica Acta*, Vol.513, No.3, (September 1978), pp.358-363, ISSN 0270-9139.

Coll, O.; Colell, A.; Garcia-Ruiz, C.; Kaplowitz, N. & Fernandez-Checa, J.C. (2003). Sensitivity of the 2-oxoglutarate carrier to alcohol intake contributes to mitochondrial glutathione depletion. *Hepatology*, Vol. 38, No.3, (September 2003), pp.692-702, ISSN 0270-9139.

Colell, A.; Garcia-Ruiz, C.; Morales, A.; Ballestta, A.; Ookhtens, M.; Rodés, J.; Kaplowitz, N. & Fernandez-Checa, J.C. (1997). Transport of reduced glutathione in hepatic mitochondria and mitoplasts from ethanol-treated rats: Effect of membrane physical properties and S-adenosyl-L-Methionine. *Hepatology*, Vol.26, No.3, (September 1997), pp.699-708, ISSN 0270-9139.

Colell, A.; Coll.O.; Garcia-Ruiz, C.; Paris, R.;Tiribelli, C.; Kaplowitz, N.; Fernandez-Checa, J.C. Tauroursodeoxycholic acid protects hepatocytes from ethanol-fed rats against tumor necrosis factor-induced cell death by replenishing mitochondrial glutathione. *Hepatology*, Vol.34, No.5, (November 2001), pp.964-971, ISSN 0270-9139.

Corpechot, C.; Chazouillères, O. & Poupon, R. (2011). Early primary biliary cirrhosis : biochemical response to treatment and prediction of long-term outcome. *Journal of Hepatology*, (2011), in press, ISSN 0168-8278.

Cunningham, C.C.; Bottenus, R.E.; Spach, P.I & Rudel, L.L. (1983) Ethanol-induced changes in liver microsomes and mitochondria from the monkey, Macaca fascicularis. *Alcoholism : Clinical and Experimental Research*, Vol. 7, No. 4, (September 1983), pp.424-430, ISSN 0145-6008.

Dai, Q.; Zhang, J. & Pruett, S.B. (2005). Ethanol alters cellular activation and CD14 partitioning in lipid rafts. *Biochemical and Biophysical Research Communications*, Vol.332, No.1, (June 2005), pp. 37-42, ISSN 0006-291x.

De Minicis, S. & Brenner, D.A. (2008). Oxidative stress in alcholoc liver disease : role of NADPH oxidase complex. *Journal of Gastroenterology and Hepatology*, Vol.23, Suppl.1, (2008), pp.S98-S103, ISSN 0815-9319.

Dolganiuc, A.; Bakis, G.; Kodys, K.; Mandrekar, P. & Szabo, G. (2006). Acute ethanol treatment modulates toll-like receptor-4 association with lipid rafts. *Alcoholism : Clinical and Experimental Research*, Vol.30, No.1, (January 2006), pp.76-85, ISSN 0145-6008.

Duraisamy, Y.; Lambert, D.; O'Neill, C.A. & Padfield, P.J. (2007). Differential incorporation of docosahexaenoic acid into distinct cholesterol-rich membrane raft domains. *Biochemical and Biophysical Research Communications*, Vol.360, No.4, (September2007), pp.885-890, ISSN 0006-291x.

Escriba, P.V. (2006). Membrane-lipid therapy : a new approach in molecular medicine. *Trends in Molecular Medecine*, Vol.12, No.1, (January 2006), pp.34-43, ISSN 1471-4914.

Fan, Y.-Y.; Ly, L.H.; Barhoumi, R.; McMurray, D.N.; Chapkin, R.S. (2004). Dietary docosahexaenoic acid suppresses T cell protein kinase C theta lipid raft recruitment and IL-2 production. *Journal of Immunology*, Vol. 173, No.10, (November 2004), pp.6151-6160, ISSN 0022-1767.

Fernandez-Lizarbe, S.; Pascual, M.; Gascon, M.S.; Blanco, A. & Guerri, C. (2008). Lipid rafts regulate ethanol-induced activation of TLR4 signaling in murine macrophages. *Molecular Immunology*, Vol.45, No.7, (April 2008), pp.2007-2016, ISSN 0161-5890.

Fitzgerald, K.A.; Rowe, R.C. & Golenbock, D.T. (2004). Endotoxin recognition and signal transduction by the TLR4/MD2-complex. *Microbes and Infection,* Vol.6, No.15, (December 2004), pp.1361-1367, ISSN 1286-4579.

Gabbita, S.P.; Subramaniam, R.; Allouch, F.; Carney, J.M. & Butterfield, D.A. (1998). Effects of mitochondrial respiratory stimulation on membrane lipids and proteins : an electron paramagnetic resonance investigation. *Biochimica et Biophysica Acta,* Vol.1372, No.2, (July 1998), pp.163-173, ISSN 0006-3002.

Gao, B.; Deki, E.; Benner, D.A.; Frideman, S.; Cohen, J.I.; Nagy; L.; Szabo, G. & Zakhari, S. (2011). Innate immunity in alcoholic liver disease. *American Journal of Physiology,* Vol. 300, No.4, (April 2011), pp.G516-G525, ISSN 0193-1857.

Ghare, S.; Patil, M.; Hote, P.; Suttles, J.; McClain, C.; Barve, S. & Joshi-Barve, S. (2011). Ethanol inhibits lipid raft-mediated TCR signaling and IL-2 expression: potential mechanism of alcohol-induced immune suppression. *Alcoholism : Clinical and Experimental Research*, Vol.35, No.8, (August 2011), pp.1-10, ISSN 0145-6008.

Goldstein, D.B (1984). The effects of drugs on membrane fluidity. *Annual Review of Pharmacology and Toxicology*, Vol.24, (1984), pp.43-64, ISSN 0362-1642.

Goldstein, D.B. (1987). Ethanol-induced adaptation in biological membranes. *Annals of the New York Academy of Sciences*, Vol.492, (April 1987), pp.103-111, ISSN 0077-8923.

Güldütuna, S.; Zimmer, G., Imhof, M.; Bhatti; S.; You, T. & Leuschner, U. (1993). Molecular aspects of membrane stabilization by ursodeoxycholate. *Gastroenterology*, Vol.104, No.6, (June 1993), pp. 1736-1744, ISSN 0016-5085.

Gurtovenko, A.A. & Anwar, J. (2009). Interaction of ethanol with biological membranes : the formation of non-bilayer structures within the membrane interior and their significance. *The Journal of Physical Chemistry B*, Vol.113, No. 7, (February 2009), pp.1983-1992, ISSN 1520-6106.

Guttiérez-Ruiz, M.C.; Gomez, J.L.; Souza, V. & Bucio, L. (1995). Chronic and acute ethanol treatment modifies fluidity and composition in plasma membranes of a human hepatic cell line (WRL-68). *Cell Biology and Toxicology*, Vol.11, No.2, (April 1995), pp.69-78, ISSN 0742-2091.

Harder, T. & Engelhardt, K.R. (2004). Membrane microdomains in lymphocytes - from lipid rafts to protein scaffolds. *Traffic*, Vol.5, No.4, (April 2004), pp.265-275, ISSN 1600-0854.

Ho, C.; Williams, B.W.; Kelly, M.B. & Stubbs, C.D. (1994) Chronic ethanol intoxication induces adaptative changes in the membrane protein/lipid interface. *Biochimica et Biophysica Acta*, Vol.1189, No.7, (January 1994), pp.135-142, ISSN 0006-3002.

Jain, S.; Thomas, M.; Kumar, P. & Laloraya, M. (1994). Appearance of homogeneous smectic multilamellar microenvironments in biomembranes undergoing superoxide-initiated lipid peroxidation : lipid-dienyl radical acccumulation and fluidity management in lipid bilayers. *Biochemistry and Molecular Biology International*, Vol.33, No.5, (August 1994), pp.853-862, ISSN 1039-9712.

Jeong, W.I & Gao, B. (2008). Innate immunity and alcoholic liver fibrosis. *Journal of Gastroenterology and Hepatology*, Vol.23, No. Suppl.1, (2008), pp.S112-S118, ISSN 0815-9319.

Johnson, D.A.; Lee, N.M.; Cooke R. & Loh, H.H. (1979). Ethanol-induced fluidization of brain lipid bilayers : required presence of cholesterol in membranes for the expression of tolerance. *Molecular Pharmacology*, Vol. 15, No., (1979), pp.739-746, ISSN 0026-895x.

Lingwood, D. & Simons, K. (2010). Lipid rafts as a membrane-organizing principle. *Science*, Vol. 237, No., (January 2010), pp.46-50, ISSN 0036-8075.

Lluis, J.M.; Colell, A.; Garcia-Ruiz, C.; Kaplowitz, N. & Fernandez-Checa, J.C. (2003). Acetaldehyde impairs mitochondrial glutathione transport in HepG2 cells through endoplasmic reticulum stress. *Gastroenterology*, Vol.124, No.3, (March 2003), pp.708-724, ISSN 0016-5085.

Lyon, R.C. & Goldstein D.B. (1983). Changes in synaptic membrane order associated with chronic ethanol treatment in mice. *Molecular Pharmacology*, Vol.23, No.1, (January 1983), pp.86-91, ISSN 0026-895x.

Marquês, J.T.; Viana, A.S. & De Almeida, R.F. (2011) Ethanol effects on binary and ternary supported lipid bilayers with gel/fluid domains and lipid rafts. *Biochimica and Biophysica Acta*, Vol.1808, No.1, (January 2011), pp.405-414, ISSN 00036-3002.

McCall, D.; Henderson, G.I.; Gray, P. & Schenker, S. Ethanol effects on active Na+ and K+ transport in cultured fetal rat hepatocytes. *Biochemical Pharmacology*, Vol.38, No.16, (August 1989), pp.2593-2600, ISSN

Mills, P.R.; Meier, P.J.; Boyer, J.L. & Gordon, E.R. The effect of ethanol and calcium on fluid state of plasma membranes of rat hepatocytes. *Alcohol*, Vol.2, No.1, (January-February 1985), pp.153-156, ISSN 0006-2952.

Nanji, A.A.; Khettry, U. & Sadrzadeh, S.M. (1994). Lactobacillus feeding reduces endotoxemia and severity of experimental alcoholic liver disease. *Proceedings of the Society for Biology and Medicine*, Vol.205; No.3, (March 1994), pp.243-247, ISSN 0037-9727.

Nelson, S. & Kolls, J.K. (2002). Alcohol, host defence and society. *Nature reviews. Immunology*, Vol.2, No.3, (March 2002), pp.205-209, ISSN 1471-1733.

Nourissat, P.; Travert, M.; Chevanne M.; Tekpli, X.; Rebillard, A.; Le Moigne-Müller, G.; Rissel, M.; Cillard, J.; Dimanche-Boitrel, M.-T.; Lagadic-Gossmann, D. & Sergent, O. (2008). Ethanol induces oxidative stress in primary rat hepatocytes through the early involvement of lipid raft clustering. *Hepatology*, Vol.47, No.1, (January 2008), pp.59-70, ISSN 0270-9139.

Oliva, L.; Beaugé, F.; Choquart, A.M.; Guitaoui, M. & Montet, J.C. (1998). Ursodeoxycholate alleviates alcoholic fatty liver damage in rats. *Alcoholism : Clinical and Experimental Research*, Vol.22, No.7, (October1998), pp.1538-1543, ISSN 0145-6008.

Parlesak, A.; Schäfer, C.; Schütz, T. Bode, J.C. & BodeC. (2000). Increased intestinal permeability to macromolecules and endotoxemia in patients with chronic alcohol abuse in different stages of alcohol-induced liver disease. *Journal of Hepatology*, Vol.32, No.5, (May 2000), pp.742-747, ISSN 0168-8278.

Parmahamsa, M.; Reddy, K.R. & Varadacharyulu, N. (2004). Changes in composition and properties of erythrocyte membrane in chronic alcoholics. *Alcohol & Alcoholism*, Vol.39, No.2, (March-April 2004), pp.110-112, ISSN 0735-0414.

Pelletier, G.; Roulot, D.; Davion, T.; Masliah, C.; Causse, X.; Oberti, F.; Raabe, J.J.; Van Lemmens, C.; Labadie, H. & Serfaty, L. A randomized controlled trial of ursodeoxycholic acid in patients with alcohol-induced cirrhosis and jaundice. *Hepatology*, Vol.37, No.4, (April 2003), pp.887-892, ISSN 0270-9139.

Pike,L.J. (2003). Lipid rafts : bringing order to chaos. *Journal of Lipid Research*, Vol.44, No.4, (April 2003), pp.655-667, ISSN 0022-2275.

Polokoff, M.A.; Simon, T.J.; Harris A.; Simon, F.R & Iwahashi. (1985). Chronic ethanol increases liver plasma membrane fluidity. *Biochemistry*, Vol.24, No.13, (June 1985), pp.3114-3120, ISSN 0006-2960.

Ponnappa, B.C.; Waring, A.J.; Hoeck, J.B.; Rottenberg, H. & Rubin, E. (1982). Chronic ethanol ingestion increases calcium uptake and resistance to molecular disordering by ethanol in liver microsomes. *The Journal of Biological Chemistry*, Vol.257, No.17, (September 1982), pp.10141-10146, ISSN 0021-9258.

Poupon, R.E.; Lindor, K.D.; Pares, A.; Chazouilleres, O.; Poupon, R. & Heathcote, E.J. (2003). Combined analysis of the effect of treatment with ursodeoxycholic acid on histologic progression in primary biliary cirrhosis. *Journal of Hepatology*, Vol. 39, No.1, (July 2003), pp.12-16, ISSN 0168-8278.

Rebillard, A.; Tekpli, X.; Meurette, O.; Sergent, O.; LeMoigne-Muller, G.; Vernhet, L.; Gorria, M.; Chevanne, M.; Christmann, M.; Kaina, B.; Counillon, L.; Gulbins, E.; Lagadic-Gossmann, D. & Dimanche-Boitrel, M.-T. (2007). Cisplatin-induced apoptosis involves membrane fluidification via inhibition of NHE1 in human colon cancer cells. *Cancer Research*, Vol.67, No.16, (August 2007), pp.7865-7874, ISSN 0008-5472.

Remy-Kristensen, A.; Duportail, G.; Coupin, G. & Kuhry, J.G. (2000). The influence of microtubule integrity on plasma membrane fluidity in L929 cells. *Molecular Membrane Biology*, Vol.17, No.2, (April-June 2000), pp.95-100, ISSN 0968-7688.

Rottenberg, H. (1992). Liver cell membrane adaptation to chronic alcohol consumption, In : *Drug and Alcohol Abuse Reviews, Vol.2 : Liver Pathology and Alcohol*, R.R. Watson (Ed.), 91-115, The humana Press, ISBN 978-0-89603-206-4, Totowa, New Jersey, USA.

Rubin, E. & Rottenberg, H. (1982). Ethanol-induced injury and adaptation in biological membranes. *Federation Proceedings*, Vol.41, No.8, (June 1982), pp. 2465-2471, ISSN 0014-9446.

Schachter D. Fluidity and function of hepatocyte plasma membranes. (1984). *Hepatology*, Vol. 4, No.1, (January-February 1984), pp.140-151, ISSN 0270-9139.

Schmitz, G. & Orso, E. (2002). CD14 signaling in lipid rafts : new ligands and co-receptors, *Current Opinion in Lipidology*, Vol.13, No.5, (October 2002), pp.513-521, ISSN 0957-9672.

Schüller, A.; Moscat, J.; Diez, E.; Fernandez-Checa, C.; Gavilanes F.G. & Muncio, A.M. (1984). The fluidity of plasma membranes from ethanol-treated rat liver. *Molecular and Cellular Biochemistry*, Vol.64, No.1, (September 1984), pp.89-95, ISSN 0300-8177.

Seki, E; De Minicis, S.; Osterreicher, C.H.; Kluwe, J.; Osawa, Y.; Brenner D.A. & Schwabe, R.F. (2007).TLR4 enhance TGF-beta signaling and hepatic fibrosis. *Nature Medicine*, Vol.13, No.11, (November 2007), pp.1324-1332, ISSN 1078-8956.

Seki, E. & Brenner, D.A. (2008). Toll-like receptors and adaptator molecules in liver disease: update. *Hepatology*, Vol.48, No.1, (July 2008), pp.322-335, ISSN 0270-9139.

Sergent, O.; Pereira, M.; Belhomme, C.; Chevane, M.; Huc, L. & Lagadic-Gosmman, D. (2005). Role for membrane fluidity in ethanol-induced oxidative stress in primary rat hepatocytes. *The Journal of Pharmacolgy and Experimental Therapeutics*, Vol. 313, No.1, (April 2005), pp.104-111, ISSN 0022-3665.

Simons, K. & Toomre, D. Lipid rafts and signal transduction. *Nature Reviews. Molecular Cell Biology*, Vol.1, No.1, (October 2000), pp.31-39, ISSN 1471-0072.

Singer, S.J. & Nicolson, G.L. (1972). The fluid mosaic model of the structure of cell membranes. *Science*, Vol.175, No.23, (February 1972), pp.720-731, ISSN 0036-8075.

Stubbs, C.D.; Williams, D.B.; Pryor, C.L. & Rubin, E. (1988) Ethanol-induced modifications to membrane lipid structure : effect on phospholipase A_2 membrane interactions. *Archives of Biochemistry and Biophysics*, Vol. 262, No.2, (May 1988), pp.560-573, ISSN 0003-9861.

Stulnig, T.M.; Huber, J.; Leitinger, N.; Imre, E.-M., Angelisova, P.; Nowotny, P. & Waldhausl W. (2001). Polyunsaturated eicosapentaenoic acid displaces proteins from membrane rafts by altering raft lipid composition. *Journal of Biological Chemistry*, Vol.276, No., pp.37335-37340.

Suh, Y.-G. & Jeong, W.-I. (2011). Hepatic stellate cells and innate immunity in alcoholic liver disease. *World Journal of Gastroenterology*, Vol.17, No.20, (May 2011), pp.2543-2551, ISSN 1007-9327.

Subramaniam, R.; Roediger, F.; Jordan, B.; Mattson, M.P.; Keller, J.N.; Waeg, G. & Butterfield, D.A. (1997). The lipid peroxidation product, 4-hydroxy-2-trans-nonenal, alters the conformation of cortical synaptosomal membrane proteins. *Journal of Neurochemistry*, Vol.69, No.3, (September1997), pp.1161-1169, ISSN 0022-3042.

Szabo, G. (1999). Consequences of alcohol consumption on host defense. *Alcohol and Alcoholism*, Vol.34, No.6, (November-December 1999), pp.830-841, ISSN 0735-0414.

Szabo, G.; Dolganiuc A.; Dai, Q. & Pruett, S.B. (2007). TLR4, ethanol and lipid rafts : a new mechanism of ethanol action with implications for other receptor-mediated effects. *Journal of Immunology*, Vol.178, No.3, (February 2007), pp.1243-1249, ISSN 0022-1767.

Szabo, G. & Bala, S. (2010). Alcoholic liver disease and the gut-liver axis. *World Journal of Gastroenterology*, Vol.16, No.11, (March 2010), pp.1321-1329, ISSN 1007-9327.

Tarahosky, Y.S.; Muzafarov, E.N. & Kim, Y.A. (2008). Rafts making and rafts braking : how plant flavonoids may control membrane heterogeneity. *Molecular and Cellular Biochemistry*, Vol.314, No.1-2, (July 2008),pp.65-71, ISSN 0300-8177.

Taraschi, T.F.; Wu, A. & Rubin, E. (1985). Phospholipid spin probes measure the effects of ethanol on the molecular order of liver microsomes. *Biochemistry*, Vol.24, No., (1985), pp.7096-7101, ISSN 0021-2960.

Tekpli, X.; Holme, J.A.; Sergent, O. & Lagadic-Gossmann, D. (2011). Importance of plasma membrane dynamics in chemical-induced carcinogenesis. *Recent Patents on Anti-Cancer Drug Discovery*, Vol.6, (2011), in press, ISSN 1574-8928.

Triantafilou, M.; Miyake, K.; Golenbock, D.T. & Triantafilou, K. (2002). Mediators of innate immune recognition of bacteria concentrate in lipid rafts and facilitate lipopolysaccharide-induced cell activation. *Journal of Cell Science*, Vol.115, No.Pt12, (June 2002), pp. 2603-2611, ISSN 0021-9533.

Valles, S.L.; Blanco, A.M.; Azorin, I.; Guasch, R.; Pascual, M.; Gomez-Lechon, M.J.; Renau-Piqueras, J. & Guerri, C. (2003). Chronic ethanol consumprion enhances interleukin-1 mediated signal transduction in rat liver and in cultured hepatocytes. *Alcohol: Clinical and Experimental Research*, Vol.27, No.12, (December 2003), pp.1979-1986, ISSN 0145-6008.

Waring, A.J.; Rottenberg, H.; Ohnishi, T. & Rubin, E. (1981). Membranes and phospholipids of liver mitochondria from chronic alcoholic rats are resistant to membrane disordering by ethanol. *Proceedings of the National Academy of Sciences of the United States of America*, Vol.78, No.4, (April 1981), pp.2582-2586, ISSN 0027-8424.

Wassal, S.R. & Stillwell, W. (2009). Polyunsaturated fatty-acid-cholesterol interactions : domain formation in membranes. *Biochimica et Biophysica Acta*, Vol. 1788, No.1, (January 2009), pp.24-32, ISSN 0006-3002.

Wong, S.W.; Kwon, M.-J.; Choi, A.M.K.; Kim, H.-P.; Nakahira, K. & Hwang, D.H. (2009). Fatty acids modulate toll-like receptor 4 activation through regulation of receptor dimerization and recruitment into lipid rafts in a reactive oxygen species-dependent manner. *Journal of Biological Chemistry*, Vol. 284, No.40, (October 2009), pp.27384-27392, ISSN 0021-9258.

Wood, W.G. & Schroeder, F. (1988). Membrane effects of ethanol : bulk lipid versus lipid domains. *Life Science*, Vol.43, No.6, (1988), pp.467-475, ISSN 0024-3205.

Wu, D. & Cederbaum, A.I. (2009). Oxidative stress and alcoholic liver disease. *Seminars in Liver Disease*, Vol.29, No.2, (May 2009), pp.141-154, ISSN 0272-8087.

Yamada, S. & Lieber C.S. (1984). Decrease in microviscosity and cholesterol content of rat liver plasma membranes after chronic ethanol feeding. *The Journal of Clinical Investigation*, Vol.74, No.6, (December 1984), pp.2285-2289, ISSN 0021-9738.

Yaqoob, P. & Shaikh, S.R. (2010). The nutritional and clinical significance of lipid rafts. *Current Opinion in Clinical Nutrition and Metabolic Care*, Vol.13, No.2, (March 2010), pp.156-166, ISSN 1363-1950.

Yoon, Y.; Török, N; Krueger, E; Oswald, B & McNiven M.A. (1998). Ethanol-induced alterations of the microtubule cytoskeleton in hepatocytes. *The American Journal of Physiology*, Vol.274, No.4Pt1, (April 1988), pp.G757-G766, ISSN 0002-9513.

10

Crucial Role of ADAMTS13 Related to Endotoxemia and Subsequent Cytokinemia in the Progression of Alcoholic Hepatitis

Masahito Uemura[1*], Yoshihiro Fujimura[2], Tomomi Matsuyama[1], Masanori Matsumoto[2], Hiroaki Takaya[1], Chie Morioka[1] and Hiroshi Fukui[1]

[1]*Third Department of Internal Medicine, and*
[2]*Department of Blood Transfusion Medicine, Nara Medical University, Kashihara, Nara*
Japan

1. Introduction

Excessive alcohol consumption causes a variety of liver diseases including alcoholic steatosis, alcoholic hepatitis (AH), liver fibrosis, cirrhosis and hepatocellular carcinoma (Mandayam et al. 2004). Alcoholic steatosis is, generally, a benign lesion if the patient abstains from alcohol intake, whereas AH observed in the approximately 20% of heavy drinkers is much more serious and requires treatment with the development of hepatocellular necrosis and inflammation (Menon et al., 2001). The severe form of AH, severe alcoholic hepatitis (SAH), is characterized by multiorgan failure with manifestations of acute hepatic failure and is associated with high morbidity and mortality (Haber et al., 2003; Ishii et al., 1993; Maddrey et al., 1978; Mookerjee et al., 2003; Sougioultzis, 2005). Alcohol-induced liver injury (ALD) occurs through the multiple steps involving a range from innate immune cells to the liver parenchymal cells, and out of many factors contributing to the pathogenesis of ALD gut-derived endotoxin plays a central role in the induction of steatosis, inflammation, and fibrosis in the liver (Bode & Bode, 2005; Fukui et al., 1991; Mandrekar & Szabo, 2009; McClain et al, 2005; Nolan, 2010; Vidali et al., 2008). AH is a multifactorial process involving gut-derived endotoxin-induced Kupffer cell activation via hepatic reticuloendothelial dysfunction and increased intestinal permeability, and subsequent cytokine stimulation. Additional factors include ethanol metabolism to toxic products, oxidative stress, acetaldehyde adducts, nutritional impairment and impaired hepatic regeneration (Haber et al., 2003; Ishii et al., 1993, Mookerjee et al., 2003; Nath & Szabo, 2009; Nolan, 2010; Sakaguchi et al., 2011; Sougioultzis et al., 2005; Tsukamoto et al., 2009; Wu & Cederbaum, 2009). In SAH pathogenesis, endotoxemia may trigger enhanced pro-inflammatory cytokine production, potentially causing a systemic inflammatory response syndrome together with microcirculatory disturbances, systemic haemodynamic derangements, and subsequent multiorgan failure (Fukui, 2005; Haber et al., 2003; Ishii et al., 1993; Mookerjee et al., 2003; Sougioultzis et al., 2005).

---

* Corresponding Author

ADAMTS13 (a disintegrin-like and metalloproteinase with thrombospondin type-1 motifs 13) is a metalloproteinase that specifically cleaves multimeric von Willebrand factor (VWF) between Tyr1605 and Met1606 residues in the A2 domain (Moake 2002; Fujimura et al., 2002). In the absence of ADAMTS13 activity (ADAMTS13:AC), unusually large VWF multimers (UL-VWFMs) are released from vascular endothelial cells (ECs) and improperly cleaved, causing them to accumulate and to induce the formation of platelet thrombi in the microvasculature under conditions of high shear stress. Currently, a severe deficiency in ADAMTS13:AC, which results either from genetic mutations in the *ADAMTS13* gene (Upshaw-Schulman syndrome, USS) (Fujimura et al., 2002; Kokame et al., 2002; Levy et al., 2001, Moake, 2002) or acquired autoantibodies against ADAMTS13 (Furlan et al., 1998; Tsai & Lian, 1998), is thought to be a specific feature of thrombotic thrombocytopenic purpura (TTP) (Amorosi & Ultmann, 1966; Moschcowitz, 1924).

In 2000, we demonstrated that a decreased plasma ADAMTS13:AC in patients with cirrhotic biliary atresia can be fully restored after liver transplantation, indicating that the liver is the main organ producing ADAMTS13 (Matsumoto et al., 2000). One year later, northern blot analysis showed that the 4.6-kilobase ADAMTS13 mRNA was highly expressed in the liver (Levy et al., 2001; Soejima, et al., 2001; Zheng et al., 2001), and subsequently both *in situ* hybridization and immunohistochemistry clearly indicated that ADAMTS13 is produced exclusively in hepatic stellate cells (HSCs) (Uemura et al., 2005a). Platelets (Suzuki et al., 2004), vascular ECs (Turner et al., 2006), and kidney podocytes (Manea et al., 2007) also have been implicated as ADAMTS13-producing cells, but the amount produced by these cell types in the liver appears to be far less than that produced by HSCs.

Mannucci et al. (Mannucci et al., 2001) originally reported a reduction of the ADAMTS13:AC in advanced liver cirrhosis (LC). Since HSCs were shown to be the major producing cells of ADAMTS13 in the liver (Uemura et al., 2005a), much attention has been paid to the potential role of ADAMTS13 in the pathophysiology of liver diseases associated with sinusoidal and/or systemic microcirculatory disturbances (Feys et al., 2007; Ishikawa et al., 2010; Ko et al., 2006; Kobayashi et al., 2009; Lisman et al., 2006; Matsuyama et al., 2007; Matsumoto et al., 2007; Okano et al., 2010; Park et al., 2002; Pereboom et al., 2009; Uemura et al., 2005b; Uemura et al., 2008a; Uemura et al., 2008b; Uemura et al., 2010; Yagita et al., 2005). ADAMTS13:AC is significantly decreased in patients with hepatic veno-occlusive disease (VOD) (Matsumoto et al., 2007; Park et al., 2002), AH (Ishikawa et al.,2010; Matsuyama et al., 2007; Uemura et al., 2005b, Uemura et al., 2008b), LC (Feys et al., 2007; Uemura et al., 2008a), and patients undergoing living-donor related liver transplantation (Ko et al., 2006; Kobayashi et al.,2009; Pereboom et al., 2009) and partial hepatectomy (Okano et al.,2010). Furthermore, hepatitis C virus (HCV)-related LC patient with ADAMTS13 inhibitor (ADAMTS13:INH) typically develops TTP (Yagita et al., 2005).

In this review, we will address interesting findings from our previous studies showing that plasma ADAMTS13:AC and its related parameters are potentially involved in the severity of liver disturbances and the development of multiorgan failure in patients with AH (Ishikawa et al., 2010; Matsuyama et al., 2007; Uemura et al., 2005b; Uemura et al., 2008b). We will focus on the importance of ADAMTS13 determination for a better understanding of pathophysiology and/or for possible therapeutic approaches of ADAMTS13 supplementation in this disease.

2. Alcohol-related thrombocytopenia and effects of alcohol on hemostasis

Alcohol-related thrombocytopenia is independent of nutritional state or the presence of liver functional abnormalities, anemia, or leucopenia (Lindenbaum & Hargrove, 1968; Paintal et al., 1975; Post & Desforges, 1968a, 1968b; Rubin & Rand, 1994). Both quantitative and qualitative platelet abnormalities appear during alcohol consumption (Cowan, 1980). A decrease in circulating platelets was first reported in 3 alcoholics who responded to folic acid administration (Sullivan & Herbert, 1964). Subsequently, alcohol has been shown to exert a direct toxic effect on blood platelets in 5 chronic alcoholics with ten episodes of thrombocytopenia (Lindenbaum & Hargrove, 1968) and in 8 patients with acute alcoholism (Post & Desforges, 1968a), who showed no evidence of liver cirrhosis, splenomegaly, folate deficiency, or massive hemorrhage, indicating the presence of alcohol-related thrombocytopenia. Additionally, thrombocytopenia was observed in alcoholics on intravenous injection of ethanol (Post & Desforges, 1968b). The platelet counts in patients with alcohol-related thrombocytopenia return to normal quickly (2-3 days) after ingestion of ethanol is discontinued. Thereafter, the number of platelets increases, and maximum counts occur 5-21 days after cessation of alcohol (Cowan & Hines, 1971), when rebound thrombocytosis after alcohol abuse in some patients may contribute to thromboembolic disease (Haselager & Vreeken, 1977). Potential mechanisms for alcohol-related thrombocytopenia may involve a suppressive effect of alcohol on megakaryocyte maturation and platelet release (Sullivan & Herbert, 1964), reduced platelet survival time (Cowan, 1980), alterations of platelet structure (Cowan, 1980), and abnormalities of platelet metabolism involving adenosine nucleotides and eicosanoids (Cowan, 1980). The spectrum of platelet function defects in alcoholics is complex. In actively drinking alcoholic patients admitted to the hospital for detoxification, platelet aggregation in platelet-rich plasma is considerably reduced in response to agonists (Haut & Cowan, 1974; Neiman et al., 1989; Rubin & Rand, 1994), whereas platelet aggregation is greater in chronic alcoholics compared to normal healthy controls both on admission and 1 week after hospitalization (Arai et al., 1986). It is necessary to clarify the role of platelet function not only in platelet aggregation *in vitro*, but also in platelet-endothelial interactions under shear stress during alcohol-related thrombocytopenia (Siegel-Axel & Gawaz, 2007).

Alternatively, recent epidemiologic studies have consistently shown that regular light-to-moderate alcohol intake protects against ischemic stroke including coronary heart disease and peripheral arterial disease (Camargo et al., 1997; Lippi et al., 2010; Mukamal et al., 2001; Rimm et al., 1996). Such beneficial effects may be attributable to a number of factors including the inhibition of platelet aggregation and adhesion, the decrease in plasma levels of VWF, fibrinogen, and coagulation factor VII, or the increase in nitric oxide bioavailability and high-density lipoprotein cholesterol (Lippi et al., 2010; Rubin R, 1999). In contrast, soft blood clots are often observed in cadaveric blood in cases of sudden death after excess alcohol consumption, which enhances the procoagulant status via VWF release, and IL-6-related interaction with lipopolysaccharide (LPS) (Kasuda et al., 2009). Additionally, both chronic alcoholism and acute alcohol intoxication have increasingly been recognized as risk factors for circulatory disorders, including thrombotic complications and hemorrhage (Hillbom & Kaste, 1982; Hillbom & Kaste, 1983, Numminen et al., 2000). Patients with chronic alcoholism show a higher incidence of pulmonary infarction, cerebral infarction, and venous thrombosis in their extremities after abstinence (Haselager & Vreeken, 1977; Hillbom et al., 1985; Walbran et al., 1981), probably due to alterations of haemostatic and fibrinolytic parameters that may be largely influenced by drinking pattern, nutritional balance, and genetic background (Arai et al., 1986; Enomoto et al., 1991; Lippi et al., 2010; Mukamal et al., 2001).

3. Hepatic microcirculation and microcirculatory disturbances in ALD

Hepatic microcirculation comprises a unique system of capillaries, called sinusoids, which are lined by three different cell types: sinusoidal endothelial cells (SECs), HSCs, and Kupffer cells (Kmieć, 2001). The SECs modulate microcirculation between hepatocytes and the sinusoidal space through the sinusoidal endothelial fenestration. The SECs have tremendous endocytic capacity, including for VWF and the extracellular matrix, and secrete many vasoactive substances (Kmieć, 2001). The HSCs are located in the space of Disse adjacent to the SECs, and regulates sinusoidal blood flow by contraction or relaxation induced by vasoactive substances (Rockey, 2001). Kupffer cells are intrasinusoidally-located tissue macrophages, and secrete potent inflammatory mediators during the early phase of liver inflammation (Kmieć, 2001). Intimate cell-to-cell interaction has been found between these sinusoidal cells and hepatocytes (Kmieć, 2001, Rockey, 2001).

Vascular ESs play a pivotal role in hemostasis and thrombosis (Fujimura et al., 2002; Moake, 2002). VWF is a marker of endothelial cell activation (damage), and plays an essential role in hemostasis (Fujimura et al., 2002; Moake, 2002). In the normal state, VWF immunostaining is usually positive in large vessels, but negative in the SECs (Hattori et al., 1991). On the occurrence of liver injury accompanied by a necroinflammatory process, the SECs become positive for VWF, presumably in association with the capillarization of hepatic sinusoids (Schaffner & Popper, 1963). Subsequently, platelets adhere to subendothelial tissue mediated by UL-VWFM. ADAMTS13 then cleaves UL-VWFM into smaller VWF multimers. This interaction of ADAMTS13 and UL-VWFM is the initial step in hemostasis (Fujimura, et al., 2002; Moake, 2002).

Hepatic microcirculatory disturbances are considered to play an important pathogenic role in ALD. These disturbances include narrowing of the sinusoidal space due to ballooned hepatocytes and perisinusoidal fibrosis (French et al., 1984), imbalances between endothelin and nitric oxide (Oshita et al., 1993), and contraction of HSCs (Itatsu et al., 1988). After liver injury, fibrogenesis within the Disse's space and a decrease in the number of sinusoidal endothelial fenestrations together with narrowing of their diameter may lead to neocapillarization of the endothelium (Horn et al., 1987; Mak & Lieber, 1984). Sinusoidal lining cells and the scar-parenchyma interface are stained by anti-VWF antibodies, even at the early stages of ALD (Urashima et al., 1993), indicating capillarization of the SECs. Interestingly, in SAH patients, mild to severe hepatic veno-occlusive disease (VOD) was frequently observed (Goodman & Ishak, 1982; Kishi et al., 2000), and the degree of ascites became more severe as VOD progressed (Kishi et al., 2000), suggesting that the hepatic circulatory disturbance involves not only the sinusoidal microcirculation but also the hepatic terminal veins.

In patients with LC and fulminant hepatitis, VWF plasma levels are remarkably high (Albornoz et al., 1999; Ferro et al., 1996; Langley et al., 1985). In LC, immunostaining for VWF antigen (VWF:Ag) shows positive cells predominantly at the scar-parenchyma interface, within the septum, and in the sinusoidal lining cells (Knittel, et al., 1995), and many fibrin thrombi are demonstrated in the hepatic sinusoid in patients with fulminant hepatitis (Rake et al., 1971), and in rats with dimethylnitrosamine (DMN) induced acute hepatic failure (Fujiwara et al., 1988). Portal or hepatic vein thrombosis is often observed in advanced LC (Amitrano et al., 2004; Wanless et al., 1995), and microthrombi formation is seen in one or multiple organs in one-half of autopsied cirrhotic patients (Oka & Tanaka, 1979). Such a hypercoagulable state in liver diseases may be involved in hepatic parenchymal destruction, the acceleration of liver fibrosis and disease progression (Northup et al., 2008; Pluta et al., 2010).

A deficiency of anticoagulant proteins (antithrombin, protein C and protein S) and the high levels of several procoagulant factors (Factor VIII and VWF) may contribute to hypercoagulability in advanced liver diseases (Northup et al., 2008). Locally, the SEC dysfunction could lead to the development of a hypercoagulable state at the hepatic sinusoids corresponding to the site of liver injury, even in the presence of a systemic hypocoagulable state (Northup et al., 2008). Considering that ADAMTS13 is synthesized in HSCs and its substrate, UL-VWFM, is produced in transformed SECs during liver injury, decreased plasma ADAMTS13:AC may involve not only sinusoidal microcirculatory disturbances, but also subsequent progression of liver diseases, finally leading to multiorgan failure. Based on these findings, it is of particular interest to evaluate the activity of plasma ADAMTS13:AC in patients with liver diseases including AH and SAH.

4. Cleavage of UL-VWFM byADAMTS13

Although the mechanism by which TTP develops in the absence of ADAMTS13:AC has not been fully elucidated, accumulating evidence has provided a hypothesis as illustrated in Fig. 1. (Fujimura et al., 2008). UL-VWFMs are produced exclusively in vascular ECs and stored in an intracellular organelle termed Weidel-pallade bodies (WPBs) and then released into the circulation upon stimulation. Under physiological conditions, epinephrine acts as an endogenous stimulus, but under non-physiological conditions, DDAVP (1-deamino-8-D-arginine vasopressin), hypoxia, and several cytokines such as interleukin IL-2, IL-6, IL-8 and tumor necrosis factor (TNFα) act as stimuli that up-regulate VWF release. Once ECs are stimulated, UL-VWFMs and P-selectin, both stored in WPBs, move to the membrane surface of ECs, where P-selectin anchors UL-VWFMs on the ECs surface (Padilla et al., 2004). Under these circumstances, high shear stress generated in the microvasculature induces a change in the UL-VWFM from a globular to an extended form (Siedlecki et al., 1996). The ADAMTS13 protease efficiently cleaves the active extended form of UL-VWFM between the Tyr1605 and Met1606 residues in the A2 domain (Dent et al., 1990). In this context, it has been postulated that multiple exocites within the disintegrin-like/TSP1/cysteine-rich/spacer (DTCS) domains of ADAMTS13 play an important role in the interaction with the unfolded VWF-A2 domain (Akiyama et al., 2009). ADAMTS13 may more efficiently cleave newly released UL-VWFMs that exist as solid-phase enzymes anchored to the vascular EC surface by binding to CD36, because CD36 is a receptor for TSP1, which is a repeated domain within the ADAMTS13 molecule (Davis et al., 2009). When ADAMTS13 activity is reduced, UL-VWFM interacts more intensively with platelet GPIb and generates signals that further accelerate platelet activation (Fujimura et al., 2002; Moake, 2002) . A series of these reactions leads to platelet microaggregates and thrombocytopenia. However, little information has been available on the cleavage of the UL-VWFMs by ADAMTS13 in the sinusoidal microcirculation in ALD.

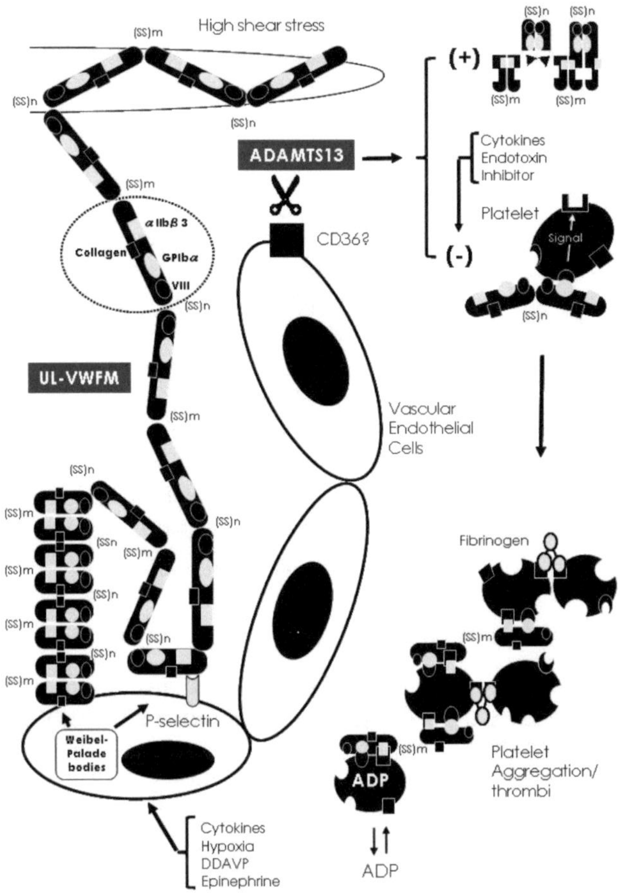

Fig. 1. Proposed mechanism of platelet thrombi formation under high shear stress in the absence of ADAMTS13:AC.

Unusually large von Willebrand factor multimers (UL-VWFMs) are produced in vascular endothelial cells (ECs) and stored in Weidel-pallade bodies (WPBs). UL-VWFMs are released from WPBs into the circulation upon stimulation by cytokines, hypoxia, DDAVP and epinephrine. P-selectin that co-migrates from WPBs anchors UL-VWFMs on the vascular EC surface. Under these circumstances, high shear stress changes the molecular conformation of UL-VWFMs from a globular to an extended form, allowing ADAMTS13 to access this molecule. In the absence of ADAMTS13:AC, UL-VWFMs remain uncleaved, allowing them to excessively interact with platelet glycoprotein (GP)Ibα and activate platelets via intra-platelet signaling, which result in the formation of platelet thrombi. Cytokines, endotoxin, and/or the inhibitor against ADAMTS13 may be candidates to decrease ADAMTS13 activity. (The dotted circle indicates a VWF subunit, which contains a set of binding domains with factor VIII, subendothelial collagen, platelet GPIbα, and integrin αIIbβ3.) (Partially modified from Fujimura et al, 2008).

5. Assays for plasma ADAMTS13:AC and ADAMTS13:INH

ADAMTS13:AC was determined with a classic VWFM assay in the presence of 1.5 mol/L urea using purified plasma derived VWF as a substrate, according to the method described by Furlan et al. (Furlan et al., 1996); the detection limit of this assay was 3% of the normal control in our laboratory (Kinoshita et al., 2001). In 2005, we developed a novel chromogenic ADAMTS13-act-ELISA using both an N- and C-terminal tagged recombinant VWF substrate (termed GST-VWF73-His). This assay was highly sensitive, and the detection limit was 0.5% of the normal control (Kato et al., 2006). Plasma ADAMTS13:AC levels highly correlated between VWFM assay and ADAMTS13-act-ELISA (Mean±SD, 102±23% vs. 99.1±21.5%, $r^2=0.72$, $p<0.01$) (Kato et al., 2006) . No interference of the ADAMTS13-act-ELISA occurred even in the presence of hemoglobin, bilirubin or chylomicrons in the samples, thus enabling distinction from the FRETS-VWF73 assay (Kokame et., 2005; Meyer et al., 2007). Because of its high sensitivity, easy handling, and lack of interference from plasma components, the ADAMTS13-act-ELISA is recommended for routine laboratory use.

The ADAMTS13:INH has also been evaluated with the chromogenic act-ELISA by means of the Bethesda method (Kasper et al., 1975). Prior to the assay, the test samples were heat-treated at 56°C for 60 min to eliminate endogenous enzyme activity, mixed with an equal volume of intact normal pooled plasma, and incubated for 2 hours at 37°C. The residual enzyme activity is measured after incubation. One Bethesda unit is defined as the amount of inhibitor that reduces activity by 50% of the control value, and values greater than 0.5 U/ml are significant.

6. ADAMTS13 activity and its related parameters in AH

Plasma ADAMTS13:AC was assayed according to the method of Furlan et al. (Furlan et al., 1996) with slight modifications (Mori et al., 2002). ADAMTS13:AC was markedly decreased in fatal SAH cases with multiorgan failure, in contrast to a mild-to-moderate decrease in SAH and AH survivors (Fig. 2a) (Uemura et al., 2005b; Matsuyama et al., 2007). Interestingly, ADAMTS13:AC in fatal SAH cases with multiorgan failure was extremely low, which is consistent with typical TTP. The VWF:AG level was remarkably increased in AH, especially in fatal SAH cases (Fig. 2b). Accordingly, VWF:AG relative to ADAMTS13:AC was extremely high in fatal SAH cases compared to AH and SAH survivors (Fig. 2c).

During recovery, ADAMTS13:AC returned to a normal range, and both VWF:AG levels and levels of VWF:AG relative to ADAMTS13:AC decreased in AH and SAH survivors; however, in fatal SAH cases, the activity remained extremely low while the VWF:AG levels were still high, resulting in an extremely high ratio of VWF:AG to ADAMTS13:AC (Matsuyama et al., 2007; Uemura et al., 2005b). These results suggest that plasma ADAMTS13:AC and its substrate, VWF:AG, are closely correlated with the severity of liver disturbance and may be useful markers for predicting the clinical outcome of AH, especially in SAH with multiorgan failure. Indeed, the prognosis was very poor in three SAH patients with extremely low ADAMTS13:AC and markedly high VWF:Ag. Furthermore, cirrhotic patients with superimposed AH showed higher levels of VWF:Ag (576% vs. 303%, $p<0.005$) and VWF:Ag relative to ADAMTS13:AC (14.0 vs. 5.3, $p<0.01$) than those with AH without LC, indicating that cirrhotic patients with superimposed AH may be a high risk for hepatic

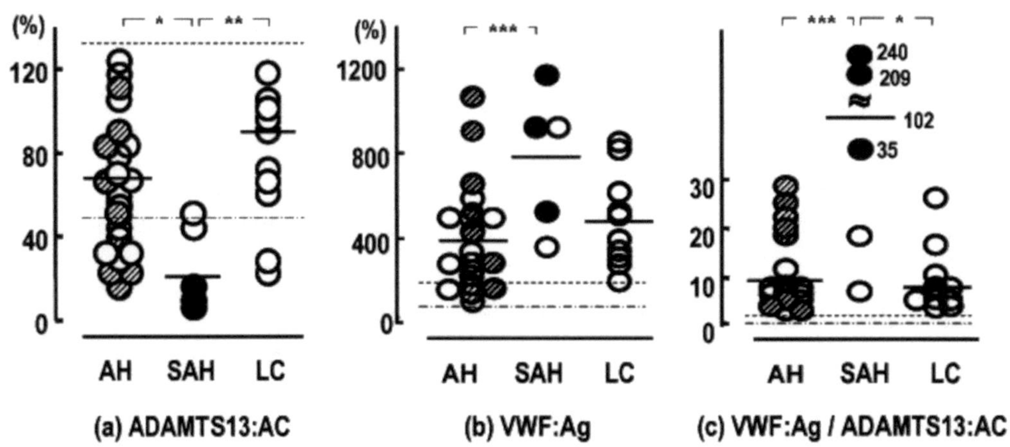

Fig. 2. Plasma values of ADAMTS13:AC, VWF:Ag, and the ratio of VWF:Ag to ADAMTS13:AC in the patients with AH, SAH, and alcoholic LC.
ADAMTS13:AC was significantly lower in AH, SAH and LC patients than in healthy subjects (a). The activity further decreased in the patients with SAH compared to those with AH and LC. In three fatal SAH cases, ADAMTS13:AC was extremely low. VWF:Ag was significantly higher in AH, SAH and LC patients than in healthy subjects (b). The antigen further increased in SAH patients compared to AH patients. In the three fatal SAH patients, VWF:Ag was extremely high. VWF:Ag relative to ADAMTS13 activity was markedly higher in AH, SAH and LC patients than in healthy subjects (c). It further increased in patients with SAH compared to those with AH and LC. In the three fatal SAH cases, it was extremely high. The dotted lines show the upper limit of the normal range, and dot-dashed lines the lower limit of the normal range. The normal range was 102±23% (mean±2SD, n=60) in ADAMTS13:AC, 100±53% in VWF:Ag, and 1.0 ± 0.4 for the ratio of VWF:Ag to ADAMTS13:AC, respectively. Open and shaded circles indicate survivors and the closed circles indicate non-survivors. The shaded circles show alcoholic LC with superimposed AH. AH=alcoholic hepatitis, SAH=severe alcoholic hepatitis, LC=alcoholic liver cirrhosis, ADAMTS13:AC=ADAMTS13 activity, VWF:Ag=von Willebrand factor antigen, VWF:Ag/ADAMTS13:AC=the ratio of VWF antigen to ADAMTS13 activity. *p<0.05, **p<0.01, and ***p<0.005 significantly different between the two groups. (Partially modified from Uemura et al., 2005b and Matsuyama et al., 2007).

failure (Matsuyama et al., 2007; Uemura et al., 2005b). In addition, in LC patients, ADAMTS13:AC tended to be lower as the cirrhotic stage progressed, suggesting that decreased ADAMTS13:AC is related to the functional liver capacity. Similar findings that ADAMTS13:AC decreases with increasing cirrhosis severity was recently reported (Feys et al., 2007; Uemura et al., 2008a).

In an univariate analysis ADAMTS13:AC was significantly correlated with 10 clinical variables, including functional liver capacity, inflammation signs, renal function, and platelet counts (Uemura et al., 2005b, 2008b) . VWF:Ag was significantly correlated with nine clinical variables, including functional liver capacity, anemia, inflammation signs, and platelet counts (Matsuyama et al., 2007; Uemura et al., 2008b). The factors associated with decreased ADAMTS13:AC and increased VWF:Ag, reduced functional liver capacity, augmented inflammation, and thrombocytopenia are consistent with the clinical characteristics that frequently appear in AH and SAH (Fujimoto et al., 1999; Haber et al., 2003; Ishii et al., 1993; Maddrey et al., 1978; McClain et al., 1999; Mookerjee et al., 2003). Remarkably, the imbalance between the ADAMTS13:AC and VWF:Ag levels might provide another mechanism for thrombocytopenia that usually occurs in AH even in the absence of signs of apparent disseminated intravascular coagulation (DIC).

On admission, UL-VWFM was detected in 4 (80.0%) of 5 SAH patients and in 5 (55.6%) of 9 AH patients, whose ADAMTS13:AC was less than 50% of normal control plasma levels (Fig. 3a) (Matsuyama et al., 2007). UL-VWFM-positive patients showed lower ADAMTS13:AC, higher plasma VWF:Ag, and a higher ratio of VWF:Ag to ADAMTS13:AC than UL-VWFM-negative patients (mean ADAMTS13:AC = 22% vs. 43%, $p<0.02$; VWF:Ag = 724% vs. 372 %, $p<0.05$; the ratio of VWF:Ag to ADAMTS13:AC = 66.0 vs. 8.2, $p<0.01$, respectively). In particular, UL-VWFM was detected in three fatal SAH patients with multiorgan failure (cases 1, 2, and 3, Fig. 3a) (Matsuyama et al., 2007). These findings of enhanced UL-VWFM production with deficient ADAMTS13 activity may, in part, contribute not only to the development of multiorgan failure but also to the progression of liver injury through microcirculatory disturbances in AH. Our results suggest an additional mechanism to explain multiorgan failure with liver disturbance, particularly in SAH patients. In order to confirm a TTP-like phenomenon as described above, it will be necessary to confirm the presence or absence of the platelet thrombi using samples obtained from liver and other organs in SAH patients.

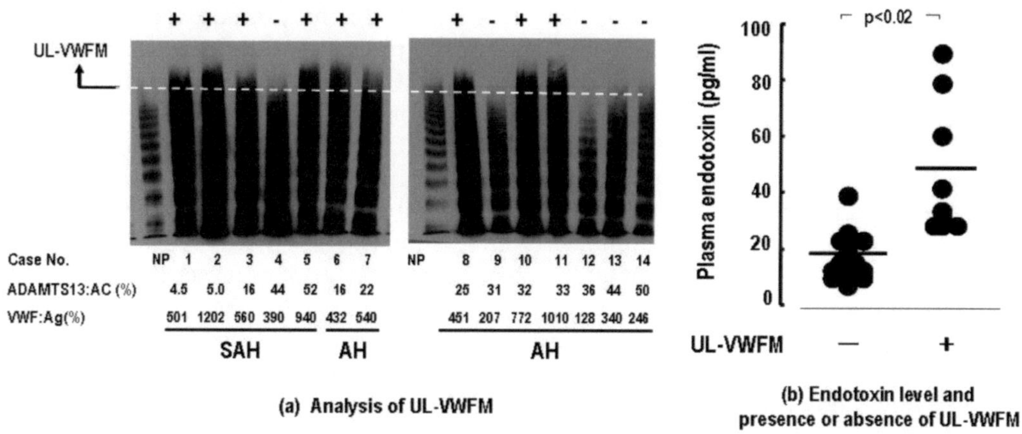

Fig. 3. The VWF multimer analysis and the difference in endotoxin level between UL-VWFM positive and negative patients in AH and SAH patients on admission.

UL-VWFM was detected in 4 of 5 SAH patients (80.0%, cases 1, 2, 3, and 5), and 3 of these patients died of hepatic failure with multiorgan failure (cases 1, 2 and 3) (a). In addition, UL-

VWFM was detected in 5 of 9 AH patients (55.6%, cases 6, 7, 8, 10, and 11), who had a moderate ADAMTS13 deficiency together with markedly high VWF:AG values (a). Plasma endotoxin concentrations were higher in UL-VWFM positive patients than UL-VWFM negative ones (b). AH=alcoholic hepatitis, SAH=severe alcoholic hepatitis, ADAMTS13: AC=ADAMTS13 activity, VWF:Ag=von Willebrand factor antigen, UL-VWFM= unusually large VWF multimer, NP shows the normal control plasma. (Partially modified from Matsuyama et al., 2007 and Ishikawa et al., 2010).

Hepatic microcirculatory disturbances are considered to play an important pathogenic role in ALD. VWF immunostaining was positive in sinusoidal lining cells and the scar-parenchyma interface even at the early stages of ALD (Urashima et al., 1993). Deficiencies in plasma ADAMTS13:AC and augmented VWF production in transformed vascular ESc might play an important role in sinusoidal microcirculatory disturbances and subsequent liver injury in AH patients. Furthermore, in SAH patients mild to severe hepatic veno-occlusive disease (VOD) was frequently observed (Goodman & Ishak, 1982; Kishi et al., 2000). After stem cell transplantation (SCT), plasma ADAMTS13:AC was significantly lower in patients with hepatic VOD than those without (Park et al., 2002). Prophylactic infusion of fresh frozen plasma (FFP) as a source of ADAMTS13 may be useful in preventing the development of hepatic VOD after SCT (Matsumoto et al., 2007), indicating a causative role of increased VWF production relative to decreased ADAMTS13:AC. Our present findings of markedly decreased ADAMTS13:AC and markedly increased VWF:AG may be involved in the pathogenesis of VOD in SAH patients.

7. Potential role of decreased ADAMTS13:AC in AH

The reason why ADAMTS13:AC decreases in AH and SAH patients remains to be clarified, but potential mechanisms may include: enhanced consumption due to the degradation of large quantities of UL-VWFM (Mannucci et al., 2001); cytokinemia- and/or endotoxemia-induced deficiency of ADAMTS13 (Ishikawa et al., 2010); the presence of inhibitors as detected in the majority of patients with "idiopathic" pregnancy- or drug-associated TTP (Fujimura & Matsumoto, 2010; Ishikawa et al., 2010); the decreased production of ADAMTS13 in HSCs (Kume et al., 2007); and the direct inhibition of the protease by ethanol and/or its metabolites. It is controversial whether ADAMTS13 deficiency is caused by decreased production in the liver. Kume et al. reported that HSC apoptosis plays an essential role in decreased ADAMTS13:AC using dimethylnitrosamine-treated rats, but not carbon tetrachloride (CCl_4)-treated animals (Kume et al., 2007), whereas Niiya et al. found upregulation of ADAMTS13 antigen and proteolytic activity in liver tissue using rats with CCl_4-induced liver fibrosis (Niiya et al., 2006). In our study, the ADAMTS13:AC gradually decreased (Fig. 4, upper panels), and the VWF:Ag progressively elevated with concomitant increase in concentrations of IL-6, IL-8, and TNFα from normal range to over 100 g/mL on admission (Fig. 4, lower panels) (Ishikawa et al., 2010).

The incidence of UL-VWFM detected in plasma became higher as concentrations of IL-6, IL-8, and TNFα increased (Ishikawa et al., 2010). At the recovery stage in survivors with AH and SAH, the ADAMTS13:AC increased to normal range, the VWF:Ag decreased, and the UL-VWFM disappeared with the decrease in the concentration of IL-6 and IL-8, whereas in a non-survivor with SAH, the ADAMTS13:AC remained at extremely low levels, the VWF:Ag was still high, and the UL-VWFM was persistently present with the increase in

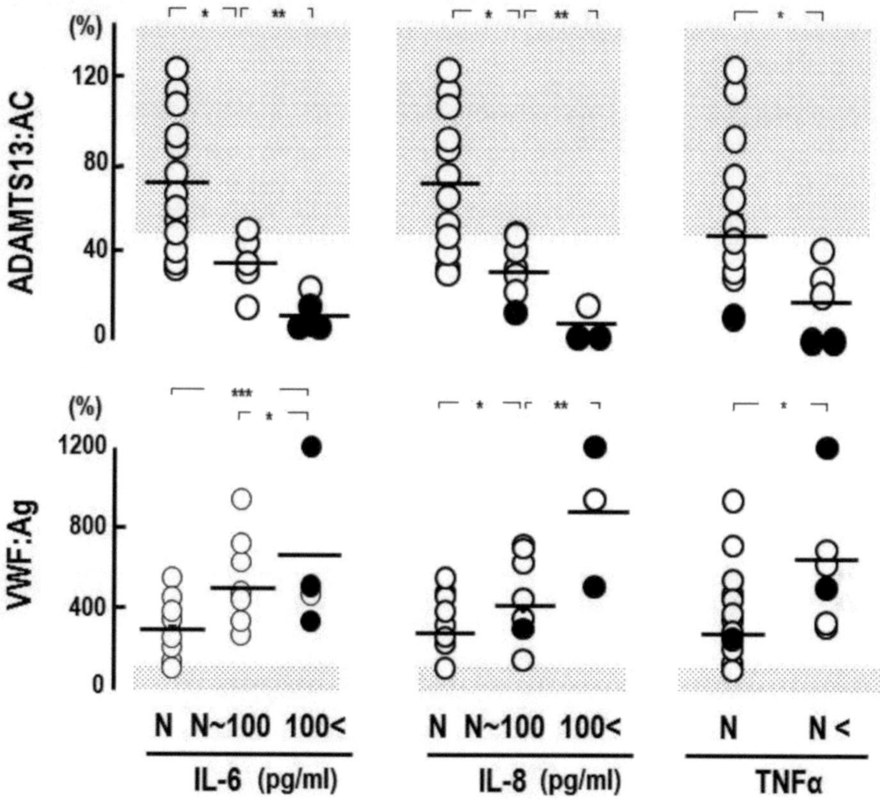

Fig. 4. Relation of plasma cytokine levels to ADAMTS13:AC and VWF:Ag in AH and SAH patients on admissionin.
ADAMTS13:AC concomitantly decreased with increasing concentrations of plasma IL-6 and IL-8, and the activity decreased in patients with TNFα concentrations higher than the normal range compared to those without (upper panels). On the other hand, VWF:Ag concomitantly increased with increasing concentrations of plasma IL-6 and IL-8, and the values increased in patients with TNFα concentration higher than the normal range compared to those without (lower panels). Shaded area shows normal ranges. IL-6= interleukin 6, IL-8=interleukin 8, TNFα=tumor necrosis factor α, N=normal range. $^{*}p<0.05$, $^{**}p<0.005$, and $^{***}p<0.001$ significantly different between the two groups. ADAMTS13:AC=ADAMTS13 activity, VWF:Ag=von Willebrand factor antigen. (Partially modified from Ishikawa et al., 2010).

concentrations of these cytokines (Ishikawa et al., 2010). These results indicate that the decrease in the ADAMTS13:AC and the increase in VWF:Ag in addition to UL-VWFM may be closely associated with increased proinflammatory cytokines including IL-6, IL-8, and TNFα. Recently, it was demonstrated that IL-6 inhibited the action of ADAMTS13 under flow condition, and both IL-8 and TNFα stimulated the release of UL-VWFM using human umbilical vein ECs (Bernardo et al., 2004). IFN-γ, IL-4, and TNFα also inhibit ADAMTS13 synthesis and activity in rat primary HSCs (Cao et al., 2008). Additionally, inflammation-associated ADAMTS13 deficiency promotes formation of UL-VWFM (Bockmeyer et al.,

2008; Claus et al., 2010). However, it is unknown whether IL-6 directly hampers the cleavage of UL-VWFM or if IL-6 down-regulates gene expression of ADAMTS13 whereby modifying the promoter activity.

Our study shows that plasma endotoxin concentration determined by a chromogenic substrate assay (Obayashi et al., 1984; Obayashi et al., 1985) was higher in patients with SAH and AH than in healthy subjects, and was markedly higher in patients with SAH than in AH (Fig. 5a) (Ishikawa et al., 2010). Our results are consistent with data previously reported (Fujimoto et al., 2000; Fukui et al., 1991; Fukui, 2005) most likely due to hepatic reticuloendothelial dysfunction and increased intestinal permeability caused by the opening of intestinal tight junctions by alcohol and its metabolite (Purohit et al., 2008). Upon admission, the endotoxin concentration correlated inversely with ADAMTS13 activity (Fig. 5b, upper panel), and positively with VWF:Ag (Fig. 5b, lower panel), and was higher in patients with UL-VWFM than those without (Fig. 3b). At the recovery stage, the endotoxin concentration decreased with the increase in ADAMTS13:AC and the decrease in VWF:Ag, and the disappearance of UL-VWFM together with the reduction of IL-6 and IL-8 concentrations (Ishikawa et al., 2010). These results indicate that enhanced endotoxemia

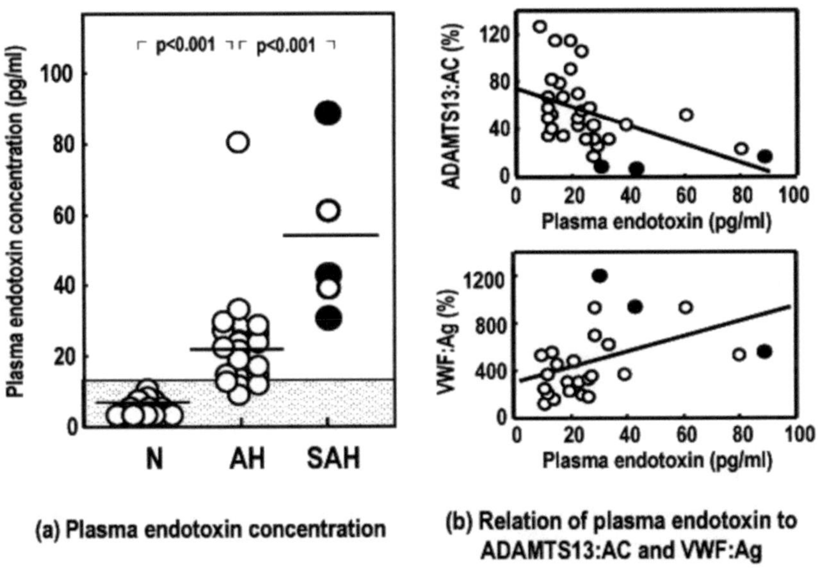

Fig. 5. Plasma endotoxin concentration and relation of endotoxin to ADAMTS13:AC and VWF:Ag in patients with alcoholic hepatitis.

Upon admission, plasma endotoxin concentrations were higher in patients with AH and SAH than in normal subjects, and the values were higher in SAH patients compared to AH (a). In addition, the endotoxin concentration correlated inversely with ADAMTS13:AC (r= - 0.474, p<0.01) (b, upper panel), and positively with VWF:Ag (r= - 0.406, p<0.05) (b, lower panel). N=normal healthy control, AH=alcoholic hepatitis, SAH=severe alcoholic hepatitis, ADAMTS13:AC=ADAMTS13 activity, VWF:Ag=von Willebrand factor antigen. Open circles indicate survivors, and closed circles nonsurvivors. Shaded area shows normal range. (Partially modified from Ishikawa et al., 2010).

may be closely related to the decrease in the ADAMTS13:AC and the appearance of UL-VWFM through the enhanced cytokinemia, leading to systemic microcirculatory disturbances and multiorgan failure, particularly in SAH patients. Intravenous infusion of endotoxin to healthy volunteers caused a decrease in plasma ADAMTS13:AC together with the appearance of UL-VWFM (Reiter et al., 2005). Severe secondary ADAMTS13 deficiency can be associated with sepsis-induced DIC and may contribute to the development of renal failure (Ono et al., 2006). These observations may support our data and hypothesis.

In response to alcohol intake, innate immune cells initiate and maintain hepatic inflammation via pattern recognition receptors, toll-like receptor 4 (TLR4) (Akira et al., 2006; Szabo, 1999). The TLR4 involves the co-receptors CD14 and myeloid differentiation (MD) protein 2 (MD2), and the LPS binding protein (LBP) (Chow et al., 1999; Visintin et al., 2001), which directly binds LPS and facilitates the association between LPS and CD14 (Wright et al., 1989). The activation of TLR4 in Kupffer cells by LPS is a key pathogenic mediator of ALD through production of inflammatory cytokines (TNFα and IL-6) and reactive oxygen species (Byun & Jeong, 2010; Soares et al., 2010). More recently, the disruption of interferon regulatory factor 3 in liver parenchymal cells has been shown to increase liver injury due to the deregulated expression of pro- and anti-inflammatory cytokines via Myd88-independent pathways (Hritz et al., 2008; Petrasek et al., 2011). It will be of particular interest to clarify the relation of ADAMTS13 to endotoxin-induced cytokinemia via the TLR4 signaling cascade in ALD.

Alternatively, another mechanism to reduce the activity of ADAMTS13 is the action of the plasma inhibitor against ADAMTS13. In our study, the inhibitor was detected in 80% of SAH patients and 21.4% of AH patients upon admission, and its inhibitory activity averaged 1.5 BU/ml in SAH and 1.0 BU/ml in AH (Ishikawa et al., 2010). Patients with the inhibitor showed lower ADAMTS13:AC and higher VWF:Ag than those without. At the recovery stage, the inhibitor was detected in 5 patients but disappeared with increased ADAMTS13:AC and decreased VWF:Ag, together with the decrease in concentrations of cytokines and endotoxin. Interestingly, patients with AH and SAH who had the inhibitor showed higher levels of serum total bilirubin, polymorphonuclear neutrophil count, plasma C-reactive protein, and plasma endotoxin concentration, and lower serum albumin levels than those with AH who had no inhibitor (Ishikawa et al., 2010). These results indicate that the decrease in the ADAMTS13:AC may be caused by the presence of its inhibitor, which is closely related to lower functional liver capacity, marked inflammation, and enhanced endotoxemia in patients with AH and SAH. Intravenous infusion of endotoxin to healthy volunteers induced the decrease in plasma ADAMTS13:AC together with the increase in VWF:Ag and the appearance of UL-VWFM during acute systemic inflammation (Reiter et al., 2005). From our results and previously reported findings (Reiter et al., 2005), endotoxemia itself might be a candidate to reduce plasma ADAMTS13:AC together with inflammatory cytokines in AH patients. It will be necessary to clarify what kinds of inhibitor is involved in association with inflammatory cytokines and endotoxin. Recently, we encountered two patient who developed TTP; one occurred in the course of hepatitis C virus (HCV)-related advanced LC (Yagita et al., 2005) and another occurred a month after pegylated-interferon alpha-2a therapy in a HCV-related case of chronic hepatitis (Kitano et al, 2006). In both cases, plasma ADAMTS13:AC was extremely low, and the inhibitor against ADAMTS13 was detected in the patient's heated plasma (2.0 BU/ml, 1.6 BU/ml, respectively) and purified IgG (0.19 BU/mg IgG, 0.4 BU/mg IgG, respectively).

Furthermore, we could detect IgG-inhibitor by western blot in 4 patients with advanced LC, who showed extremely lower ADAMTS13 activity (<3% of controls), but had no apparent clinical features of TTP, indicating the existence of "subclinical TTP" (Uemura et al., 2008a). Of 108 patients with idiopathic TTP whose plasma samples were sent to our department of Blood Transfusion Medicine, the inhibitor was detected in 54 (79.4%) of 68 patients analyzed, and its inhibitor activity was 0.5 to 2.0 BU/ml in 33 cases (61.1%), and more than 2.0 BU/ml in the remaining 21 cases (38.9%) (Matsumoto et al., 2004). Taken together, these observations suggest that the inhibitor activity detected in our patients with SAH and AH would be enough to reduce the activity of plasma ADAMTS13.

8. Clinical significance of plasma ADAMTS13:AC determination and future perspective in severe liver diseases

The introduction of ADAMTS13 to the field of hepatology not only enabled us to confirm the diagnosis of TTP early, but also provided novel insight into the pathophysiology of liver diseases. Some diseases were shown to be TTP itself, but others did not show any apparent clinical features of TTP, even in the presence of markedly decreased ADAMTS13:AC and increased UL-VWFM that correlate with TTP. Such TTP-like states, but not DIC, may indicate "subclinical TTP" as seen in advanced LC (Uemura et al., 2008a, Uemura et al., 2010) and SAH patients (Matsuyama et al., 2007; Uemura et al., 2005b; Uemura et al., 2008b), or "local TTP" as shown in patients with hepatic VOD after SCT (Matsumoto et al., 2007; Park et al., 2002) and patients with adverse events after living-donor liver transplantation (Ko et al., 2006). One would be unable to detect such TTP-like phenomena without the determination of ADAMTS13:AC, because the interaction of ADAMTS13 and UL-VWFM is the initial step in hemostasis, and their abnormalities do occur even in the absence of apparent imbalance in other conventional hemostatic factors. One could, then, notice that the origin of VWF, the substrate of ADAMS13, is indeed transformed hepatic sinusoidal and/or extrahepatic ECs, but not hepatocytes. The procoagulant and anticoagulant proteins synthesized in hepatocytes decrease as liver disease progresses, whereas VWF markedly increases. Under such circumstances, ADAMTS13 deficiency may lead to microcirculatory disturbances not only in the liver, but also in the systemic circulation. The determination of ADAMTS13 and its related parameters will thus be quite useful for better understanding the pathophysiology and for providing appropriate treatments especially in severe liver disease patients.

Regarding FFP infusion as a unique source of ADAMTS13, we clearly showed that pre-existing UL-VWFMs in the plasma of USS patients began to disappear within 1 hour and completely disappeared 24 hours after ADAMTS13 was replenished with infusions of FFP (Yagi et al., 2001), indicating that exogenous ADAMTS13 could efficiently cleave both UL-VWFMs pre-existing in the circulation and the newly produced molecules at the ECs' surface. Furthermore, prophylactic FFP infusion may be instrumental in preventing the development of hepatic VOD after SCT (Matsumoto et al., 2007). Our five patients with SAH were treated with FFP infusion together with supportive care, and two of them survived, but the remaining three did not (Ishikawa et al., 2010). One of the non-survivors showed a transient increase in ADAMTS13:AC during FFP infusion, which ultimately decreased. The other two patients died of hepatic failure (Ishikawa et al., 2010). The administration of FFP may be useful, in part, as a supplementation of ADAMTS13, but the effects might depend on the severity of the liver disturbance, or the degree of liver regeneration and multiorgan failure in SAH patients. Additionally, it is extremely important to monitor plasma ADAMTS13:AC in the treatment of thrombocytopenia associated with allograft dysfunction after liver transplantation. This is because the infusions of a platelet concentrate, but not FFP, under an imbalance of decreased ADAMTS13:AC to enhanced UL-VWFM production, may further exacerbate the formation of platelet aggregates mediated by uncleaved UL-VWFM, leading to graft failure via the "local TTP" mechanism (Ko et al., 2006). FFP infusion as ADAMTS13 replacement therapy may improve both liver dysfunction and thrombocytopenia in liver transplant patients.

From our point of view, it will be indispensable to measure ADAMTS13:AC when patients are encountered with unexplained thrombocytopenia in the course of liver disease. We are particularly interested in the conduct of clinical trials with recombinant ADAMTS13 preparations in severe liver diseases, including SAH, advanced LC, hepatic VOD and liver transplant patients. Further investigations will be necessary to define candidates for ADAMTS13 supplementation therapy, and to evaluate its potential therapeutic efficacy in severe liver diseases.

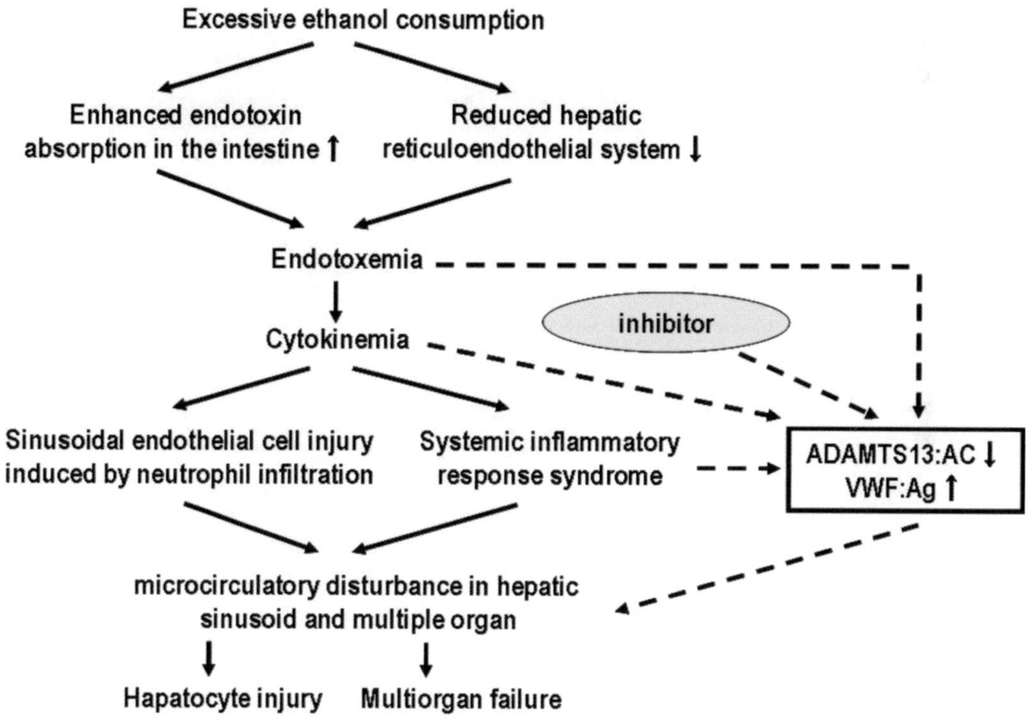

Fig. 6. A working hypothesis of ADAMTS13 and its related parameters in the progression of alcoholic hepatitis.

9. Conclusion

Enhanced gut-derived endotoxemia via hepatic reticuloendothelial dysfunction and increased intestinal permeability and subsequent cytokinemia may result in SECs injury and systemic inflammatory response syndrome, leading to microcirculatory disturbance in hepatic sinusoid and multiple organs, and finally, to the necrosis of hapatocytes and multiorgan failure in patients with AH, and particularly in patients with SAH (Fig. 6.). The imbalance between the enhanced production of UL-VWFM and the deficient activity of ADAMTS13 may, in part, contribute to not only sinusoidal microcirculatory disturbances and subsequent liver injury in AH, but also to the development of multiorgan failure through impaired organ microcirculation in SAH. Decreased ADAMTS13:AC and increased VWF:Ag could be induced by pro-inflammatory cytokinemia and the plasma inhibitor against ADAMTS13, both of which may be closely related to enhanced endotoxemia (Fig. 6.). The determination of ADAMTS13:AC and its substrate will give us new insights into the pathophysiology of acute ALD and help to elucidate additional therapeutic strategies including ADAMTS13 supplementation for this disease.

10. Acknowledgements

This work was supported in part by research grants from the Japanese Ministry of Education, Culture, and Science (to M.U., Y.F., SK., and M.M.), from the Research Program of Intractable Disease provided by the Ministry of Health, Labor, and Welfare of Japan (to H. F.), and from the Ministry of Health, Labour and Welfare of Japan for Blood Coagulation Abnormalities (to Y.F.). The authors sincerely thank Ayami Isonishi, Hiromichi Ishizashi, Seiji Kato, and Masatoshi Ishikawa for their extensive help in the assay of ADAMTS13 activity, VWF antigen, and UL-VWFM.

11. References

Akira, S.; Uematsu, S. & Takeuchi, O. (2006). Pathogen recognition and innate immunity. *Cell,* Vol. 124, No. 4, pp. 783-801, 0092-8674

Akiyama, M.; Takeda, S,; Kokame, K,; Takagi, J. & Miyata, T. (2009). Crystal structures of the noncatalytic domains of ADAMTS13 reveal multiple discontinuous exosites for von Willebrand factor. *Proc Natl Acad Sci U S A,* vol. 106, No. 46, pp. 19274-19279, 0027-8424

Albornoz, L.; Alvarez, D.; Otaso, JC.; Gadano, A.; Salviú, J.; Gerona, S.; Sorroche, P.; Villamil, A. & Mastai, R. (1999). Von Willebrand factor could be an index of endothelial dysfunction in patients with cirrhosis: relationship to degree of liver failure and nitric oxide levels. *J Hepatol,* Vol. 30, No. 3, pp. 451-455, 0168-8278

Amitrano, L.; Guardascione, MA.; Brancaccio, V.; Margaglione, M.; Manguso, F.; Iannaccone L.; Grandone, E. & Balzano, A. (2004). Risk factors and clinical presentation of portal vein thrombosis in patients with liver cirrhosis. *J Hepatol,* Vol. 40, No. 5, pp. 736-741, 0168-8278

Amorosi, EL. & Ultmann JE. (1966). Thrombotic thrombocytopenic purpura: report of 16 cases and review of the literature. *Medicine,* Vol. 45, pp. 139-159.

Arai, M.; Okuno, F.; Nagata, S.; Shigeta, Y.; Takagi, S.; Ebihara, Y.; Kobayashi, T.; Ishii, H. & Tsuchiya, M. (1986). Platelet dysfunction and alteration of prostaglandin metabolism after chronic alcohol consumption. *Scand J Gastroenterol,* Vol 21. No. 9, pp. 1091-1097, 0036-5521

Bernardo, A.; Ball, C.; Nolasco, L.; Moake, JF. & Dong, J. (2004). Effects of inflammatory cytokines on the release and cleavage of the endothelial cell-derived ultralarge von

Willebrand factor multimers under flow. *Blood*, Vol. 104, No. 1, pp. 100-106, 0006-4971

Bockmeyer, CL.; Claus, RA.; Budde, U.; Kentouche, K.; Schneppenheim, R.; Losche, W.; Reinhart, K. & Brunkhorst, FM. (2008). Inflammation-associated ADAMTS13 deficiency promotes formation of ultra-large von Willebrand factor. *Haematologica*, Vol. 93, No. 1, pp. 137-140, 0390-6078

Bode, C. & Bode, JC. (2005). Activation of the innate immune system and alcoholic liver disease: effects of ethanol per se or enhanced intestinal translocation of bacterial toxins induced by ethanol? *Alcohol Clin Exp Res*, Vol. 29, No. 11 Suppl, pp. 166S-171S, 0145-6008

Byun, JS. & Jeong, WI. (2010). Involvement of hepatic innate immunity in alcoholic liver disease. *Immune Netw*, Vol 10, No. 6, pp. 181-187, 1598-2629

Camargo, CA Jr.; Stampfer, MJ.; Glynn, RJ.; Gaziano, JM.; Manson, JE.; Goldhaber, SZ. & Hennekens, CH. (1997). Prospective study of moderate alcohol consumption and risk of peripheral arterial disease in US male physicians. *Circulation*, Vol 95, No. 3, pp. 577-580, 0009-7322

Cao, WJ.; Niiya, M.; Zheng, XW.; Shang, DZ. & Zheng, XL. (2008). Inflammatory cytokines inhibit ADAMTS13 synthesis in hepatic stellate cells and endothelial cells. *J Thromb Haemost*, Vol 6 、No. 7, pp. 1233-1255, 1538-7933

Chow, JC.; Young, DW.; Golenbock, DT.; Christ, WJ. & Gusovsky, F. (1999). Toll-like receptor-4 mediates lipopolysaccharide-induced signal transduction. *J Biol Chem*, Vol 274, No. 16, pp. 10689-10692, 0021-9258

Claus, RA.; Bockmeyer, CL.; Sossdorf, M. & Lösche, W. (2010). The balance between von-Willebrand factor and its cleaving protease ADAMTS13: biomarker in systemic inflammation and development of organ failure? *Curr Mol Med*, Vol. 10, No. 2, pp. 236-248, 1566-5240

Cowan, DH. & Hines, JD. (1971). Thrombocytopenia of severe alcoholism. *Ann Intern Med*, Vol. 74, No. 1, pp. 37-43, 0003-4819

Cowan, DH. (1980). Effect of alcoholism on hemostasis. *Semin Hematol*, Vol. 17, No. 2, pp. 137-147, 0037-1963

Davis, AK.; Makar, RS.; Stowell, CP.; Kuter, DJ. & Dzik, WH. (2009). ADAMTS13 binds to CD36: a potential mechanism for platelet and endothelial localization of ADAMTS13. *Transfusion*, Vol. 49, No. 2, pp. 206-213, 0041-1132

Dent, JA.; Berkowitz, SD.; Ware, J.; Kasper, CK. & Ruggeri, ZM. (1990). Identification of a cleavage site directing the immunochemical detection of molecular abnormalities in type IIA von Willebrand factor. *Proc Natl Acad Sci USA*, Vol. 87, No. 16, pp. 6306-6310, 0027-8424

Enomoto, N.; Takase, S.; Takada, N. & Takada, A. (1991). Alcohloic liver disease in heterozygotes of mutant and normal aldehyde dehydrogenase-2 gene. *Hepatology*, Vol. 13, No. 6, pp. 1071-1076, 0270-9139

Ferro, D.; Quintarelli, C.; Lattuada, A.; Leo, R.; Alessandroni, M.; Mannucci, PM. & Violi, F. (1996). High plasma levels of von Willebrand factor as a marker of endothelial perturbation in cirrhosis: relationship to endotoxemia. *Hepatology*, Vol. 23, No. 6, pp. 1377-1383, 0270-9139

Feys, HB.; Canciani, MT.; Peyvandi, F.; Deckmyn, H.; Vanhoorelbeke, K. & Mannucci, PM. (2007). ADAMTS13 activity to antigen ratio in physiological and pathological conditions associated with an increased risk of thrombosis. *Br J Haematol,* Vol. 138, No. 4, pp. 534-540, 0007-1048

French, SW.; Benson, NC. & Sun, PS. (1984). Centrilobular liver necrosis induced by hypoxia in chronic ethanol-fed rats. *Hepatology,* Vol. 4, No. 5, pp. 912-917, 0270-9139

Fujimoto, M.; Uemura, M.; Kojima, H.; Ishii, Y.; Ann T.; Sakurai, S.; Okuda, K.; Noguchi, R.; Adachi, S,; Kitano, H.; Hoppo, K.; Higashino, T.; Takaya, A. & Fukui, H. Prognostic factors in severe alcoholic liver injury. Nara Liver Study Group. (1999). *Alcohol Clin Exp Res,* Vol. 23, No. 4 Suppl, pp. 33S-38S, 0145-6008

Fujimoto, M.; Uemura, M.; Nakatani, Y.; Tsujita, S.; Hoppo, K.; Tamagawa, T.; Kitano, H.; Kikukawa, M.; Ann, T.; Ishii, Y.; Kojima, H.; Sakura,i S.; Tanaka, R.; Namisaki, T.; Noguchi, R.; Higashino, T.; Kikuchi, E.; Nishimura, K.; Takaya, A. & Fukui, H. (2000). Plasma endotoxin and serum cytokine levels in patients with alcoholic hepatitis: Relation to severity of liver diseases. *Alcohol Clin Exp Res,* Vol. 24, No. 4 Suppl, pp. 48S-54S, 0145-6008

Fujimura, Y.; Matsumoto, M.; Yagi, H.; Yoshioka, A.; Matsui, T. & Titani, K. (2002). von-Willebrand-factor-cleaving protease and Upshaw-Schulman syndrome. *Int J Hematol,* Vol. 75, No. 1, pp. 25-34, 0925-5710

Fujimura, Y.; Matsumoto, M. & Yagi, H. (2008). Thrombotic microangiopathy. Springer, Tokyo, pp. 625-639.

Fujimura, Y. & Matsumoto, M. (2010). Registry of 919 patients with thrombotic microangiopathies across Japan: database of Nara Medical University during 1998-2008. *Intern Med,* Vol. 49, No. 1, pp. 7-15, 0918-2918

Fujiwara, K.; Ogata, I.; Ohta, Y.; Hirata, K.; Oka, Y.; Yamada, S.; Sato, Y.; Masak,i N. & Oka, H. (1988). Intravascular coagulation in acute liver failure in rats and its treatment with antithrombin III. *Gut,* Vol. 29, No. 8, pp. 1103-1108, 0017-5749

Fukui, H.; Brauner, B.; Bode, JC. & Bode, C. (1991). Plasma endotoxin concentrations in patients with alcoholic and non-alcoholic liver disease: reevaluation with an improved chromogenic assay. *J Hepatol,* Vol. 12, No. 2, pp. 162-169, 0168-8278

Fukui, H. (2005). Relation of endotoxin, endotoxin binding proteins and macrophages to severe alcoholic liver injury and multiple organ failure. *Alcohol Clin Exp Res,* Vol. 29, No. 11 Suppl, pp. 172S-179S, 0145-6008

Furlan, M.; Robles, R. & Lämmle, B. (1996). Partial purification and characterization of a protease from human plasma cleaving von Willebrand factor to fragments produced by in vivo proteolysis. *Blood,* Vol. 87, No. 10, pp. 4223-4234, 0006-4971

Furlan, M.; Robles, R.; Galbusera, M.; Remuzzi, G.; Kyrle, PA.; Brenner, B.; Krause, M.; Scharrer, I.; Aumann, V.; Mittler, U.; Solenthaler, M. & Lämmle, B. (1998). von Willebrand factor-cleaving protease in thrombotic thrombocytopenic purpura and the hemolytic-uremic syndrome. *N Engl J Med,* Vol. 339, No. 22, pp. 1578-1584, 0028-4793

Goodman, ZD. & Ishak, KG. (1982). Occlusive venous lesions in alcoholic liver disease. A study of 200 cases. *Gastroenterology,* Vol. 83, No. 4, pp. 786-796, 0016-5085

Haber, PS.; Warner, Seth D.; Gorrell, MD. & McCaughan, GW. (2003). Pathogenesis and management of alcoholic hepatitis. *J Gastroenterol Hepatol,* Vol. 18, No. 12, pp. 1332-1344, 0815-9319

Haselager, EM. & Vreeken, J. (1977). Rebound thrombocytosis after alcohol abuse: a possible factor in the pathogenesis of thromboembolic disease. *Lancet,* Vol. 1, No. 8015, pp. 774-775, 0140-6736

Hattori, M.; Fukuda, Y.; Imoto, M,; Koyama, Y.; Nakano, I. & Urano, F. (1991). Histochemical properties of vascular and sinusoidal endothelial cells in liver diseases. *Gastroenterol Jpn,* Vol. 26, No. 3, pp. 336-343, 0435-1339

Haut, MJ. & Cowan, DH. (1974). The effect of ethanol on hemostatic properties of human blood platelets. *Am J Med,* Vol. 56, No. 1, pp. 22-33, 0002-9343

Hillbom, M. & Kaste, M. (1982). Alcohol intoxication: a risk factor for primary subarachnoid hemorrahage. *Neulology,* Vol. 32, No. 7, pp. 706-711, 0028-3878

Hillbom, M. & Kaste, M. (1983). Ethanol intoxication: a risk factor for ischemic brain infarction. *Stroke,* Vol. 14, No. 5, pp. 694-699, 0039-2499

Hillbom, M.; Muuronen, A.; Löwbeer, C.; Anggård, E.; Beving, H. & Kangasaho, M. (1985). Platelet thromboxane formation and bleeding time is influenced by ethanol withdrawal but not by cigarette smoking. *Thromb Haemost,* Vol. 53, No. 3, pp. 419-422, 0340-6245

Horn, T.; Christoffersen, P. & Henriksen, JH. (1987). Alcoholic liver injury: defenestration in noncirrhotic livers - a scanning electron microscopic study. *Hepatology,* Vol. 7, No. 1, pp. 77-82, 0270-9139

Hritz, I.; Mandrekar, P.; Velayudham, A.; Catalano, D.; Dolganiuc, A.; Kodys, K.; Kurt-Jones, E. & Szabo, G. (2008). The critical role of toll-like receptor (TLR) 4 in alcoholic liver disease is independent of the common TLR adapter MyD88. *Hepatology,* Vol. 48, No. 4, pp. 1224-1231, 0270-9139

Ishii, K.; Furudera, S.; Kumashiro, R.; Koga, Y.; Hamada, T.; Sata, M.; Abe, H. & Tanikawa, K. (1993). Clinical and pathological features, and the mechanism of development in severe alcoholic hepatitis, especially in comparison with acute type fulminant hepatitis. *Alcohol Alcohol Suppl,* Vol.1B, pp. 97-103, 1358-6173

Ishikawa, M.; Uemura, M.; Matsuyama, T.; Matsumoto, M.; Ishizashi, H.; Kato, S.; Morioka, C.; Fujimoto, M.; Kojima, H.; Yoshiji, H.; Tsujimoto, T.; Takimura, C.; Fujimura, Y. & Fukui, H. (2010). Potential role of enhanced cytokinemia and plasma inhibitor on the decreased activity of plasma ADAMTS13 in patients with alcoholic hepatitis: relationship to endotoxemia. *Alcohol Clin Exp Res,* Vol. 34, No. Suppl 1, pp. S25-33, 0145-6008

Itatsu, T.; Oide, H.; Watanabe, S.; Tateyama, M.; Ochi, R. & Sato, N. (1988). Alcohol stimulates the expression of L-type voltage-operated Ca^{2+} channels in hepatic stellate cells. *Biochem Biophys Res Commun,* Vol. 251, No. 2, pp. 533-537, 0006-291X

Kasper, CK.; Aledort, L.:, Aronson, D.; Counts, R.; Edson, JR.; van Eys J, Fratantoni J.; Green, D.; Hampton, J.; Hilgartner, M.; Levine, P.; Lazerson, J.; McMillan, C.; Penner, J.; Shapiro, S. & Shulman, NR. (1975). A more uniform measurement of factor VIII inhibitors. *Thromb Diath Haemorrh,* Vol. 34, No. 2, pp. 612. 0340-5338

Kasuda, S.; Nishiguchi, M.; Yoshida, S.; Ohtsu, N.; Adachi, N.; Sakurai, Y.; Shima, M.; Takahashi, M.; Hatake, K. & Kinoshita, H. (2009). Enhancement effect of ethanol on lipopolysaccharide-induced procoagulant status in human umbilical endothelial cells. *Soud Lek,* Vol. 54, No. 4, pp. 44-48, 0371-1854

Kato, S.; Matsumoto, M.; Matsuyama, T.; Isonishi, A.; Hiura, H. & Fujimura, Y. (2006). Novel monoclonal antibody-based enzyme immunoassay for determining plasma levels of ADAMTS13 activity. *Transfusion*, Vol. 46, No. 8, pp. 1444-1452, 0041-1132

Kinoshita, S.; Yoshioka, A.; Park, YD.; Ishizashi, H.; Konno, M.; Funato, M.; Matsui, T.; Titani, K.; Yagi, H.; Matsumoto, M. & Fujimura, Y. (2001). Upshaw-Schulman syndrome revisited: a concept of congenital thrombotic thrombocytopenic purpura. *Int J Hematol*, Vol. 74, No. 1, pp. 101-108, 0925-5710

Kishi, M.; Maeyama, S.; Iwaba, A.; Ogata, S.; Koike, J. & Uchikoshi, T. (2000). Hepatic veno-occlusive lesions and other histopathological changes of the liver in severe alcoholic hepatitis--a comparative clinicohistopathological study of autopsy cases. *Alcohol Clin Exp Res*, Vol. 24, No. 4 Suppl, pp. 74S-80S, 0145-6008

Kitano, K.; Gibo, Y.; Kamijo, A.; Furuta, K.; Oguchi, S.; Joshita, S.; Takahashi.; Ishida, F.; Matsumoto, M.; Uemura, M. & Fujimura, Y. (2006). Thrombotic thrombocytopenic purpura associated with pegylated-interferon alpha-2a by an ADAMTS13 inhibitor in a patient with chronic hepatitis C. *Haematologica*, Vol. 91, No. 8 Suppl, ECR34, 1592-8721

Kmieć, Z. Cooperation of liver cells in health and disease. (2001). *Adv Anat Embryol Cell Biol*, Vol. 161, No. III-XIII, pp. 1-151, 0301-5556

Knittel, T.; Neubauer, K.; Armbrust, T. & Ramadori, G. (1995). Expression of von Willebrand factor in normal and diseased rat livers and in cultivated liver cells. *Hepatology*, Vol. 21, No. 2, pp. 470-476, 0270-9139

Ko, S.; Okano, E.; Kanehiro, H.; Matsumoto, M.; Ishizashi, H.; Uemura, M.; Fujimura, Y.; Tanaka, K. & Nakajima, Y. (2006). Plasma ADAMTS13 activity may predict early adverse events in living donor liver transplantation: observations in 3 cases. *Liver Transpl*, Vol. 12, No. 5, pp. 859-869, 1527-6465

Kokame, K.; Matsumoto, M.; Soejima, K.; Yagi, H.; Ishizashi, H.; Funao, M.; Tamai, H.; Konno, M.; Kamide, K.; Kawano, Y.; Miyata, T. & Fujimura, Y. (2002). Mutations and common polymorphisms in *ADAMTS13* gene responsible for von Willebrand factor-cleaving protease activity. *Proc Natl Acad Sci USA*, Vol. 99, No. 18, pp. 11902-11907, 0027-8424

Kokame, K.; Nobe, Y.; Kokubo, Y.; Okayama, A. & Miyata, T. (2005). FRETS-VWF73, a first fluorogenic substrate for ADAMTS13 assay. *Br J Haematol*, Vol. 129, No. 1, pp. 93-100, 0007-1048

Kobayashi, T.; Wada, H.; Usui, M.; Sakura,i H.; Matsumoto, T.; Nobori, T.; Katayam, N.; Uemoto, S.; Ishizashi, H.; Matsumoto, M.; Fujimura, Y. & Isaji, S. (2009). Decreased ADAMTS13 levels in patients after living donor liver transplantation. Thromb Res, Vol. 124, No. 5, pp. 541-545, 0049-3848

Kume, Y.; Ikeda, H.; Inoue, M.; Tejima, K.; Tomiya, T.; Nishikawa, T.; Watanabe, N.; Ichikawa, T.; Kaneko, M.; Okubo, S.; Yokota, H.; Omata, M.; Fujiwara, K. & Yatomi, Y. (2007). Hepatic stellate cell damage may lead to decreased plasma ADAMTS13 activity in rats. *FEBS Lett*, Vol. 581, No. 8, pp. 1631-1634, 0014-5793

Langley, PG.; Hughes, RD. & Williams, R. Increased factor VIII complex in fulminant hepatic failure. (1985). *Thromb Haemostasis*, Vol. 54. No. 4, pp. 693-696 0340-6245

Levy, GG.; Nichols, WC.; Lian, EC.; Foroud, T.; McClintick, JN.; McGee, BM.; Yang, AY.; Siemieniak, DR.; Stark, KR.; Gruppo, R.; Sarode, R.; Shurin, SB.; Chandrasekaran, V.; Stabler, SP.; Sabio, H.; Bouhassira, EE.; Upshaw, JD.; Ginsburg, D. & Tsai, HM.

(2001). Mutations in a member of the ADAMTS13 gene family cause thrombotic thrombocytopenic purpura. *Nature,* Vol.413, No.6865, pp. 488-494, 0028-0836

Lindenbaum, J. & Hargrove, RL. (1968). Thrombocytopenia in alcoholics. *Ann Intern Med,* Vol. 68, No. 3, pp. 526-532, 0003-4819

Lippi, G.; Franchini, M.; Favaloro, EJ. & Targher, G. (2010). Moderate red wine consumption and cardiovascular disease risk: beyond the "French paradox". *Semin Thromb Hemost,* Vol. 36, No. 1, pp. 59-70, 0094-6176

Lisman, T.; Bongers, TN.; Adelmeijer, J.; Janssen, HL.; de Maat, MP.; de Groot, PG. & Leebeek, FW. (2006). Elevated levels of von Willebrand Factor in cirrhosis support platelet adhesion despite reduced functional capacity. *Hepatology,* Vol. 44, No. 1, pp. 53-61, 0270-9139

Maddrey, WC.; Boitnott, JK.; Bedine, MS.; Weber, FL Jr.; Mezey, E. & White, RI Jr. (1978). Corticosteroid therapy of alcoholic hepatitis. *Gastroenterology,* Vol. 75, No. 2, pp. 193-199, 0016-5085

Mak, KM. & Lieber, CS. (1984). Alterations in endothelial fenestrations in liver sinusoids of baboons fed alcohol: a scanning electron microscopic study. *Hepatology,* Vol. 4, No. 3, pp. 386-491, 0270-9139

Mandayam, S.; Jamal, MM. & Morgan, TR. (2004). Epidemiology of alcoholic liver disease. *Semin Liver Dis,* Vol. 24, No. 3, pp. 217-32, 0272-8087

Mandrekar, P. & Szabo, G. (2009). Signalling pathways in alcohol-induced liver inflammation. *J Hepatol,* Vol. 50, No. 6, pp. 1258-1266, 0168-8278

Manea, M.; Kristoffersson, A.; Schneppenheim, R.; Saleem, MA.; Mathieson, PW.; Mörgelin, M.; Björk, P.; Holmberg, L. & Karpman, D. (2007). Podocytes express ADAMTS13 in normal renal cortex and in patients with thrombotic thrombocytopenic purpura. *Br J Haematol,* Vol. 138, No. 5, pp. 651-662, 0007-1048

Mannucci, PM.; Canciani, MT.; Forza, I.; Lussana, F.; Lattuada, A. & Rossi, E. (2001). Changes in health and disease of the metalloproteinase that cleaves von Willebrand factor. *Blood,* Vol. 98, No. 9, pp. 2730-2735, 0006-4971

Matsumoto, M.; Chisuwa, H.; Nakazawa, Y.; Ikegami, T.; Hashikura, Y.; Kawasaki, S.; Yagi, H,; Ishizashi, H.; Matsui, T.; Titani K. & Fujimura, Y. (2000). Living-related liver transplantation rescues reduced vWF-cleaving protease activity in patients with cirrhotic biliary atresia. *Blood,* Vol. 96, 636a (abstr.), 0006-4971

Matsumoto, M.; Yagi, H.; Ishizashi, H.; Wada, H. & Fujimura, Y. (2004). The Japanese experience with thrombotic thrombocytopenic purpura-hemolytic uremic syndrome. *Semin Hematol,* Vol. 41, No. 1, pp. 68-74, 0037-1963

Matsumoto, M.; Kawa, K.; Uemura, M.; Kato, S; Ishizashi, H.; Isonishi, A.; Yagi, H.; Park, YD.; Takeshima, Y.; Kosaka, Y.; Hara, H.; Kai, S.; Kanamaru, A.; Fukuhara, S.; Hino, M.; Sako, M.; Hiraoka, A.; Ogawa, H.; Hara, J. & Fujimura, Y. (2007). Prophylactic fresh frozen plasma may prevent development of hepatic VOD after stem cell transplantation via ADAMTS13-mediated restoration of von Willebrand factor plasma levels. *Bone Marrow Transplant, Vol.* 40, No. 3, pp. 251-259, 0268-3369

Matsuyama, T.; Uemura, M.; Ishikawa, M.; Matsumoto, M.; Ishizashi, H.; Kato, S.; Morioka, C.; Fujimoto, M.; Kojima, H.; Yoshiji, H.; Takimura, C.; Fujimura, Y. & Fukui, H. (2007). Increased von Willebrand factor over decreased ADAMTS13 activity may contribute to the development of liver disturbance and multiorgan failure in patients with alcoholic hepatitis. *Alcohol Clin Exp Res,* Vo. 31, No. 1 Suppl 1, pp. 27S-35S, 0145-6008

McClain, CJ.; Barve, S.; Deaciuc, I.; Kugelmas, M. & Hill, D. (1999). Cytokines in alcoholic liver disease. *Semin Liver Dis,* Vol. 19, No. 2, pp. 205-219, 0272-8087

McClain, C.; Barve, S.; Joshi-Barve, S.; Song, Z.; Deaciuc, I.; Chen, T. & Hill D. (2005). Dysregulated cytokine metabolism, altered hepatic methionine metabolism and proteasome dysfunction in alcoholic liver disease. *Alcohol Clin Exp Res,* Vo. 29, No. 11 Suppl, pp. 180S-188S, 0145-6008

Menon, KV.; Gores, GJ. & Shah, VH. (2001). Pathogenesis, diagnosis, and treatment of alcoholic liver disease. *Mayo Clin Proc,* Vol. 76, no. 10, pp. 1021-1029, 0025-6196

Meyer, SC.; Sulzer, I.; Lämmle, B. & Kremer Hovinga, JA (2007). Hyperbilirubinemia interferes with ADAMTS-13 activity measurement by FRETS-VWF73 assay: diagnostic relevance in patients suffering from acute thrombotic microangiopathies. *J Thromb Haemost,* Vol. 5, No. 4, pp. 866-867, 1538-7933

Moake, JL. (2002). Thrombotic microangiopathies. *N Engl J Med,* Vol. 347, No. 8, pp. 589-599, 0028-4793

Mookerjee, RP.; Sen, S.; Davies, NA.; Hodges, SJ.; Williams, R. & Jalan, R. (2003). Tumor necrosis factor alpha is an important mediator of portal and systemic haemodynamic derangements in alcoholic hepatitis. *Gut,* Vol. 52, No. 8, pp. 1182-1187, 0017-5749

Mori, Y.; Wada, H.; Gabazza, EC.; Minami, N.; Nobori, T.; Shiku, H.; Yagi, H.; Ishizashi, H.; Matsumoto, M. & Fujimura, Y. (2002). Predicting response to plasma exchange in patients with thrombotic thrombocytopenic purpura with measurement of vWF-cleaving protease activity. *Transfusion,* Vol. 42, No. 5, pp. 572-580, 0041-1132

Moschcowitz, E. (1924). Hyaline thrombosis of the terminal arterioles and capillaries: a hitherto undescribed disease. *Proc NY Pathol Soc,* Vol. 24, pp. 21-24.

Mukamal, KJ.; Jadhav, PP.; D'Agostino, RB.; Massaro, JM.; Mittleman, MA.; Lipinska, I.; Sutherland, PA.; Matheney, T.; Levy, D.; Wilson, PW.; Ellison, RC.; Silbershatz, H.; Muller, JE. & Tofler, GH. (2001). Alcohol consumption and hemostatic factors: analysis of the Framingham Offspring cohort. *Circulation,* Vol. 104, No. 12, pp. 1367-1373, 0009-7322

Nath, B. & Szabo, G. (2009). Alcohol-induced modulation of signaling pathways in liver parenchymal and nonparenchymal cells: implications for immunity. *Semin Liver Dis,* Vol. 29, No. 2, pp. 166-177, 0272-8087

Neiman, J.; Rand, ML.; Jakowec, DM. & Packham, MA. (1989). Platelet responses to platelet-activating factor are inhibited in alcoholics undergoing alcohol withdrawal. *Thromb Res,* Vol. 56, No. 3, pp. 399-405, 0049-3848

Niiya, M.; Uemura, M.; Zheng, XW.; Pollak, ES.; Dockal, M.; Scheiflinger, F.; Wells, RG. & Zheng, XL. (2006). Increased ADAMTS-13 proteolytic activity in rat hepatic stellate cells upon activation in vitro and in vivo. *J Thromb Haemost,* Vol. 4, No. 5, pp. 1063-1070, 1538-7933

Nolan, JP. The role of intestinal endotoxin in liver injury: a long and evolving history. (2010). *Hepatology,* Vol. 52, No. 5, pp. 1829-1835, 0270-9139

Northup, PG.; Sundaram, V.; Fallon, MB.; Reddy, KR.; Balogun, RA.; Sanyal, AJ.; Anstee, QM.; Hoffma, MR.; Ikura, Y. & Caldwell, SH: Coagulation in Liver Disease Group.

(2008). Hypercoagulation and thrombophilia in liver disease. *J Thromb Haemost,* Vol. 6, No. *1,* pp. 2-9, 1538-7933

Numminen, H.; Syrjälä, M.; Benthin, G.; Kaste, M. & Hillbom, M. (2000). The effect of acute ingestion of a large dose of alcohol on the hemostatic system and its circadian variation. *Stroke,* Vol. 31, No. 6, pp. 1269-1273, 0039-2499

Obayashi, T. (1984). Addition of perchloric acid to blood samples for colorimetric limulus test using chromogenic substrate: Comparison with conventional procedures and clinical applications. *J Lab Clin Med,* Vol. 104, No. 3, pp. 321-330, 0022-2143

Obayashi, T.; Tamura, H.; Tanaka, S.; Ohki, M.; Takahashi, S.; Arai, M.; Masuda, M.& Kawai, T. (1985). A new chromogenic endotoxin-specific assay using recombined limulus coagulation enzymes and its clinical applications. *Clinica Climica Acta,* Vol. 149, No. 1, pp. 55-65, 0009-8981

Oka, K. & Tanaka, K. (1979). Intravascular coagulation in autopsy cases with liver diseases. *Thromb Haemost,* Vol. 42, No. 2, pp. 564-570, 0340-6245

Okano, E.; Ko, S.; Kanehiro, H.; Matsumoto, M.; Fujimura, Y. & Nakajima, Y. (2010). ADAMTS13 activity decreases after hepatectomy, reflecting a postoperative liver dysfunction. *Hepatogastroenterology,* Vol. 57, No. 98, pp. 316-320, 0172-6390

Ono, T.; Mimuro, J.; Madoiwa, S.; Soejima, K.; Kashiwakura, Y.; Ishiwata, A.; Takano, K.; Ohmori, T. & Sakata, Y. (2006). Severe secondary deficiency of von Willebrand factor-cleaving protease (ADAMTS13) in patients with sepsis-induced disseminated intravascular coagulation: its correlation with development of renal failure. *Blood,* Vol. 107, No. 2, pp. 528-534, 0006-4971

Oshita, M.; Takei. Y.; Kawano, S.; Yoshihara, H.; Hijioka, T.; Fukui, H.; Goto, M.; Masuda, E.; Nishimura, Y. & Fusamoto, H. (1993). Roles of endothelin-1 and nitric oxide in the mechanism for ethanol-induced vasoconstriction in rat liver. *J Clin Invest,* Vo. 91, No. 4, pp. 1337-1342, 0021-9738

Padilla, A.; Moake, JL.; Bernardo, A.; Ball, C.; Wang, Y.; Arya, M.; Nolasco, L.; Turner, N.; Berndt, MC.; Anvari, B.; López, JA. & Dong, JF. (2004). P-selectin anchors newly released ultralarge von Willebrand factor multimers to the endothelial cell surface. *Blood,* Vol. 103, No. 6, pp. 2150-2156, 0006-4971

Paintal, IS.; Minina, RJ. & Ramchandani, IK. (1975). Thrombccytopenia related to the severity of alcoholism. *Indian J Physiol Pharmacol,* Vol. 19, No. 4, pp. 199-202, 0019-5499

Park, YD.; Yoshioka, A.; Kawa, K.; Ishizashi, H.; Yagi, H.; Yamamoto, Y.; Matsumoto, M. & Fujimura, Y. (2002). Impaired activity of plasma von Willebrand factor-cleaving protease may predict the occurrence of hepatic veno-occlusive disease after stem cell transplantation. *Bone Marrow Transplant,* Vol. 29, No. 9, pp. 789-794, 0268-3369

Pereboom, ITA.; Adelmeijer, J.; van Leeuwen, Y.; Hendriks, HGD.; Porte, RJ. & Lisman, T. (2009). Development of a severe von Willebrand factor/ADAMTS13 dysbalance during orthotopic liver transplantation. *Am J Transpl,* Vol. 9, No. 5, pp. 1189-1196, 1600-6135

Petrasek, J.; Dolganiuc, A.; Csak, T.; Nath, B.; Hritz, I.; Kodys, K.; Catalano, D.; Kurt-Jones, E.; Mandrekar, P. & Szabo, G. (2011). Interferon regulatory factor 3 and type I interferons are protective in alcoholic liver injury in mice by way of crosstalk of parenchymal and myeloid cells. *Hepatology,* Vol. 53, No. 2, pp. 649-660, 0270-9139

Pluta, A.; Gutkowski, K. & Hartleb, M. (2010). Coagulopathy in liver diseases. *Adv Med Sci,* Vol. 55, No. 1, pp. 16-21, 1896-1126

Post, RM. & Desforges, JF. (1968a). Thrombocytopenia and alcoholism. *Ann Intern Med,* Vol. 68, No. 6, pp. 1230-1236, 0003-4819

Post, RM & Desforges, JF. (1968b). Thrombocytopenic effect of ethanol infusion. *Blood,* Vol. 31, No. 3, pp. 344-347, 0006-4971

Purohit, V.; Bode, JC.; Bode, C.; Brenner, DA.; Choudhry, MA.; Hamilton, F.; Kang, YJ.; Keshavarzian, A.; Rao, R.; Sartor, RB.; Swanson, C. & Turner, JR. (2008). Alcohol, intestinal bacterial growth, intestinal permeability to endotoxin, and medical consequences: summary of a symposium. *Alcohol,* Vol. 42, No. 5, pp. 349-361, 0741-8329

Rake, MO.; Flute, PT.; Shilkin, KB.; Lewis, ML.; Winch, J. & Williams, R. (1971). Early and intensive therapy of intravascular coagulation in acute liver failure. *Lancet,* Vol. 2, No. 7736, pp. 1215-1218, 0140-6736

Reiter, RA.; Varadi, K.; Turecek, PL.; Jilma, B. & Knöbl, P. (2005). Change in ADAMTS13 (von-Willebrand-factor-cleaving protease) activity after induced release of von Willebrand factor during acute systemic inflammation. *Thromb Haemost,* Vol. 93, No. 3, pp. 554-558, 0340-6245

Rimm, EB.; Klatsky,A.; Grobbee, D. & Stampfer, MJ. (1996). Review of moderate alcohol consumption and reduced risk of coronary heart disease: is the effect due to beer, wine, or spirits ? *BMJ,* Vol. 312, No. 7033, pp. 731-736, 0959-8138

Rockey, DC. (2001). Hepatic blood flow regulation by stellate cells in normal and injured liver. *Semin Liver Dis,* Vol. 21, No. 3, pp. 337-348, 0272-8087

Rubin, R & Rand, ML. (1994). Alcohol and platelet function. *Alcohol Clin Exp Res,* Vol. 18, No. 1, pp. 105-110, 0145-6008

Rubin, R. (1999). Effect of ethanol on platelet function. *Alcohol Clin Exp Res,* Vol. 23, No. 6, pp. 1114-1118, 0145-6008

Sakaguchi, S.; Takahashi, S.; Sasaki, T.; Kumagai, T. & Nagata, K. (2011). Progression of alcoholic and non-alcoholic steatohepatitis: common metabolic aspects of innate immune system and oxidative stress. *Drug Metab Pharmacokinet,* Vol. 26, No. 1, pp. 30-46, 1347-4367

Schaffner, F & Popper, H. (1963). Capillarization of hepatic sinusoids in man. *Gastroenterology,* Vol. 44, pp. 239-242, 0016-5085

Siedlecki, CA.; Lestini, BJ.; Kottke-Marchant, KK.; Eppell, SJ.; Wilson, DL. & Marchant, RE. (1996). Shear-dependent changes in the three-dimensional structure of human von Willebrand factor. *Blood,* Vol. 88, No. 8, pp. 2939-2950, 0006-4971

Siegel-Axel, DI & Gawaz, M. (2007). Platelets and endothelial cells. *Semin Thromb Hemost,* Vol. 33, No. 2, pp. 128-135, 0094-6176

Soares, JB.; Pimentel-Nunes, P.; Roncon-Albuquerque, R. & Leite-Moreira, A. (2010). The role of lipopolysaccharide/toll-like receptor 4 signaling in chronic liver diseases. *Hepatol Int,* Vol. 4, No. 4, pp. 659-972, 1936-0533

Soejima, K.; Mimura, N.; Hirashima, M.; Maeda, H.; Takayoshi, H.; Nakazaki, T. & Nozaki C. (2001). A novel human metalloproteinase synthesized in the liver and secreted into the blood: Possibly, the von Willebrand factor-cleaving protease? *J Biochem,* Vol. 130, No. 4, pp. 475-480, 0021-924X

Sougioultzis, S.; Dalakas, E.; Hayes, PC. & Plevris, JN. (2005). Alcoholic hepatitis: from pathogenesis to treatment. *Curr Med Res Opin,* Vol. 21, No. 9, pp. 1337-1346, 0300-7995

Sullivan, LW. & Herbert, V. (1964). Suppression hematopoiesis by ethanol. *J Clin Invest,* Vol. 43, No. 11, pp. 2048-2062, 0021-9738

Suzuki, M.; Murata, M.; Matsubara, Y.; Uchida, T.; Ishihara, H.; Shibano, T.; Ashida, S.; Soejima, K.; Okada, Y. & Ikeda Y. (2004). von Willebrand factor-cleaving protease (ADAMTS-13) in human platelets. *Biochem Biophys Res Commun,* Vl. 313, No. 1, pp. 212-216, 0006-291X

Szabo, G. (1999). Consequences of alcohol consumption on host defence. *Alcohol Alcohol,* Vol. 34, No. 6, pp. 830-841, 735-0414

Tsai, HM. & Lian, EC. (1998). Antibodies to von Willebrand factor-cleaving protease in acute thrombotic thrombocytopenic purpura. *N Engl J Med,* Vol. 339, No. 22, pp. 1585-1594, 0028-4793

Tsukamoto, H.; Machida, K.; Dynnyk, A. & Mkrtchyan, H. (2009). "Second hit" models of alcoholic liver disease. *Semin Liver Dis,* Vol. 29, No. 2, pp. 178-187, 0272-8087

Turner, N.; Nolasco, L.; Tao, Z.; Dong, JF. & Moake, J. (2006). Human endothelial cells synthesize and release ADAMTS-13. *J Thromb Haemost,* Vol. 4, No. 6, pp. 1396-1404, 1538-7933

Uemura, M.; Tatsumi, K.; Matsumoto, M.; Fujimoto, M.; Matsuyama, T.; Ishikawa, M.; Iwamoto, T.; Mori, T.; Wanaka, A.; Fukui, H. & Fujimura, Y. (2005a). Localization of ADAMTS13 to the stellate cells of human liver. *Blood,* Vol. 106, No. 3, pp. 922-924, 0006-4971

Uemura, M.; Matsuyama, T.; Ishikawa, M.; Fujimoto, M.; Kojima, H.; Sakurai, S.; Ishii, I.; Toyohara, M.; Yamazaki, M.; Yoshiji, H.; Yamao, Y.; Matsumoto, M.; Ishizashi, H.; Fujimura, F. & Fukui, H. (2005b). Decreased activity of plasma ADAMTS13 may contribute to the development of liver disturbance and multiorgan failure in patients with alcoholic hepatitis. *Alcohol Clin Exp Res,* Vol. 29, No. 12 Suppl, pp. 264S-271S, 0145-6008

Uemura, M.; Fujimura, Y.; Matsumoto, M.; Ishizashi, H.; Kato, S.; Matsuyama, T.; Isonishi, A.; Ishikawa, M.; Yagita, M.; Morioka, C.; Yoshiji, H.; Tsujimoto, T.; Kurumatani, N. & Fukui, H. (2008a). Comprehensive analysis of ADAMTS13 in patients with liver cirrhosis. *Thromb Haemost,* Vol. 99, No. 6, pp. 1019-1029, 0340-6245

Uemura, M.; Fujimura, Y.; Matsuyama, T.; Matsumoto, M.; Ishikawa, M.; Ishizashi, H.; Kato, S.; Tsujimoto, T.; Fujimoto, M.; Yoshiji, H.; Morioka, C. & Fukui, H. (2008b). Potential role of ADAMTS13 in the progression of alcoholic hepatitis. *Curr Drug Abuse Rev,* Vol. 1, No. 2, pp. 188-196, 1874-4737

Uemura, M.; Fujimura, Y.; Ko, S.; Matsumoto, M.; Nakajima, Y. & Fukui, H. (2010). Pivotal role of ADAMTS13 function in liver diseases. *Int J Hematol,* Vol. 91, No. 1, pp. 20-29, 0925-5710

Urashima, S.; Tsutsumi, M.; Nakase, K.; Wang, JS. & Takada, A. (1993). Studies on capillarization of the hepatic sinusoids in alcoholic liver disease. *Alcohol Alcohol,* Vol. 1B Suppl, pp. 77-84, 1358-6173

Vidali, M.; Hietala, J.; Occhino, G.; Ivaldi, A.; Sutti, S.; Niemelä, O. & Albano, E. (2008). Immune responses against oxidative stress-derived antigens are associated with increased circulating tumor necrosis factor-alpha in heavy drinkers. *Free Radic Biol Med,* Vol. 45, No. 3, pp. 306-311, 0891-5849

Visintin, A.; Mazzoni, A.; Spitzer, JA. & Segal, DM. (2001). Secreted MD-2 is a large polymeric protein that efficiently confers lipopolysaccharide sensitivity to Toll-like receptor 4. *Proc Natl Acad Sci U S A,* Vol. 98, No. 21, pp. 12156-12161, 0027-8424

Walbran, BB.; Nelson, JS. & Taylor, JR. (1981). Association of cerebral infarction and chronic alcoholism: an autopsy study. *Alcohol Clin Exp Res,* Vol. 5, No. 4, pp. 531-535, 0145-6008

Wanless, IR.; Wong, F.; Blendis, LM.; Greig, P.; Heathcote, EJ. & Levy, G. (1995). Hepatic and portal vein thrombosis in cirrhosis: possible role in development of parenchymal extinction and portal hypertension. *Hepatology,* Vol. 21, No. 5, pp. 1238-1247, 0270-9139

Wright, SD.; Tobias, PS.; Ulevitch, RJ. & Ramos, RA. (1989). Lipopolysaccharide (LPS) binding protein opsonizes LPS-bearing particles for recognition by a novel receptor on macrophages. *J Exp Med,* Vol. 170, No. 4, pp. 1231-1241, 0022-1007

Wu, D. & Cederbaum, AI. (2009). Oxidative stress and alcoholic liver disease. *Semin Liver Dis,* Vol. 29, No. 2, pp. 141-154, 0272-8087

Yagi, H.; Konno, M.; Kinoshita, S.; Matsumoto, M.; Ishizashi, H.; Matsui, T.; Titani, K. & Fujimura, Y. (2001). Plasma of patients with Upshaw-Schulman syndrome, a congenital deficiency of von Willebrand factor-cleaving protease activity, enhances the aggregation of normal platelets under high shear stress. *Br J Haematol,* Vol. 115, No. 4, pp. 991-997, 0007-1048

Yagita, M.; Uemura, M.; Nakamura, T.; Kunitomi, A.; Matsumoto, M. & Fujimura, Y. (2005). Development of ADAMTS13 inhibitor in a patient with hepatitis C virus-related liver cirrhosis causes thrombotic thrombocytopenic purpura. *J Hepatol,* Vol. 42, No. 3, pp. 420-421, 0168-8278

Zheng, X.; Chung, D.; Takayama, TK.; Majerus, EM.; Sadler, JE. & Fujikawa, K. (2001). Structure of von Willebrand factor-cleaving protease (ADAMTS 13), metalloproteinase involved in thrombotic thrombocytopenic purpura. *J Biol Chem,* Vol. 276, No. 44, pp. 41089-41163, 0021-9258

11

The Role of Liver Transplantation in the Treatment of Alcoholic Liver Disease

Georgios Tsoulfas and Polyxeni Agorastou
Aristotle University of Thessaloniki
Greece

1. Introduction

In 1988 Starzl challenged the consensus view from 1983 that only a small percentage of patients with alcoholic liver disease (ALD) would be expected to meet the criteria for transplantation (National Institute of Health [NIH], 1984). Starzl and his team reported the successful liver transplantation (LT) of patients with ALD, and suggested that few patients returned to alcohol after liver transplantation (Starzl et al., 1988). Since then ALD has become one of the most common indications for LT in adults. However, despite this success, there remains significant debate and controversy regarding the indication, as several studies over time have shown that the public may not be supportive of the idea of allocating a limited resource, such as the liver graft, to patients with ALD. This chapter will discuss the pre-transplant evaluation of patients with ALD, the debate over the treatment of acute alcoholic hepatitis, and the outcome of LT for ALD, including the issue of relapse. Finally, certain ethical concerns such as the use of living donors and future challenges will be analyzed.

2. Pre-transplant evaluation of patients with ALD

Patients with ALD, as part of their pre-transplant evaluation, are assessed by a multi-disciplinary team consisting of hepatologists, surgeons, social workers and psychiatrists. The decision to list the patient depends on the status of the liver disease, which is expressed in most centers by the Model for End-stage Liver Disease (MELD) score. This is a relatively objective measurement of the patients' degree of liver disease by using the patient's bilirubin, creatinine and INR serum values to calculate the MELD score. The latter is empirically capped at 40 and represents a continuous variable ranging from 6 to 40 and it has proven to be highly accurate in assessing 3 month mortality once a cirrhotic patient is on the waiting list (Kamath et al., 2001). There is however the assertion that ALD patients may be under-referred for LT in the United States (Kotlyar et al. 2008). This may be because ALD may represent a negative determinant for many physicians to refer patients for LT, or there may be a lack of recognition of the contribution of excessive alcohol consumption to liver failure in the community. One study identified patients with liver failure in whom alcohol consumption was not recognized or acknowledged by the referring physicians (Day et al., 2008). It is not clear whether this was a purposeful omission or a genuine lack of recognition, but it does underscore the need for careful attention to the presence of alcoholic disorders in patients with liver failure.

2.1 Abstinence prior to LT for ALD

Patients with ALD undergo the standard pre-transplant evaluation, whose goal is to determine the suitability of the potential candidate to undergo the LT, as well as the urgency with which this has to be performed, based on the severity of the liver disease. Specifically for patients with ALD the issue of abstinence is critical in making these determinations. The apprehension that candidates for LT with ALD are likely to relapse and cause damage to the graft, makes it important to select those patients with the lower risk of relapse. To ensure this formal pretransplant substance misuse evaluations are required, including a broad psychosocial and substance abuse assessment. Factors analyzed include the pattern of previous alcohol use, diagnosis of alcohol use disorder, length of abstinence and features that would indicate a higher risk of future return to alcohol consumption (Dobbels et al., 2009; Gedaly et al., 2008). People judged suitable for LT are patients with severe end-stage liver disease, a clear understanding of the risks and benefits involved in the procedure, and a favorable psychiatric profile including acceptance of their alcoholism and factors in their family and social network that would ensure post-transplant sobriety.

Pretransplant abstinence offers the advantages of allowing the liver disease an opportunity to stabilize, as well as testing the patient's commitment and resolve to proceed with this treatment. The transplant team with the support of the psychiatrists and the abuse specialists has the ability during that period to evaluate the patient and the presence of a support network, as well as monitor their resolve through frequent visits, as well as unannounced testing. There remains significant debate regarding the extent of the required abstinence period. Specifically, the vast majority of transplant centers (85%) in the United States require 6 months of abstinence prior to transplantation, with a significant number expecting the patients to sign a formal contract (Everhart & Beresford, 1997). This view was changed in 2005, following the UNOS and French Consensus Conference on LT, as there was not an agreement in the literature regarding the 6 month sobriety period (Mathurin, 2005).

People in favor of the 6 month abstinence period cite 3 main advantages. First, the period of pretransplantation abstinence may allow liver recovery, even to the extent of a LT becoming unnecessary, with one study showing significant improvement within 3 months (Veldt et al., 2002). Second, it can help identify those patients unable to abstain, and thus more likely to relapse after the LT. This cannot happen reliably when a patient presents with decompensated liver disease, as "death-bed repentance", no matter how genuine, may not accurately reflect future intentions. Finally, the time of abstinence can and should be used for intensive rehabilitation and treatment for the alcohol dependence, as relapse is more frequent within the first year after quitting alcohol. Others have questioned the need for an arbitrary period of abstinence pre-LT. All agree that the 6 month period is not based on prospectively gathered data, but rather on custom and practice (Neuberger et al., 2002). The main argument against the enforced time period of abstinence has been that it may be more of a selection method favored by insurance companies, rather than an effective predictor for post-transplant abstinence. Some of the key studies in the field have advocated that full psychosocial assessment as part of the pretransplant evaluation of the ALD patient may be more important than a universal application of a 6 month abstinence rule (Pfitzmann et al., 2007). Additionally, these studies have shown that the frequency of both minor and harmful drinking is frequent in the first 5 years after LT, despite careful pre-transplant assessment, although it is equally useful to distinguish between harmful drinking and "slips" (DiMartini et al., 2006; Pfitzmann et al., 2007). Setting a fixed time period for pre-LT abstinence as a rigid rule, fails to take into account the multiple clinical and psychosocial variables of ALD patients. Patients with ALD are not immune from hepatocellular carcinoma (HCC), and as such cannot have an arbitrary waiting time period placed on them, as in that case there is the real danger of the HCC getting outside Milan criteria, and thereby precluding any chance of a LT. This is not to say that there should not be a proper evaluation of the severity of the alcohol dependence in these patients, or measures taken to achieve sustained abstinence and prevent relapse; however, in order to reach a consensus on a period of abstinence prior to the LT, large, multicentric, randomized longitudinal prospective studies are needed to analyze the decision making methods carefully and completely (Beresford & Everson, 2000).

The question of the 6 month abstinence period prior to a LT is only part of the effort to identify predictors of post-LT relapse. In addition to the studies supporting that the length of sobriety is a strong predictor of recidivism, there are others reporting that patients with a DSM-IV diagnosis of abuse had a lower relapse probability than those with alcohol dependence (DiMartini et al., 2006; Karim et al., 2010). DiMartini et al. showed that variables such as alcohol dependence, short length of sobriety, family history of alcohol consumption and the use of other substances identified patients with a major risk of relapse (DiMartini et al., 2010). Despite that there are studies showing that pre-LT behavior is a poor predictor of relapse, or that other variables such as demographic, family and social ones come into play (De Gottardi et al., 2007; Foster et al., 1997; Kelly et al., 2006; Pfitzmann et al., 2007). Overall, this multitude of often competing possible predictors of recidivism, further stresses the need for an accurate stratification of potential candidates to identify those most likely to remain abstinent, and thus benefit the most from a LT.

2.2 Comorbidities associated with ALD

There is a significant number of comorbidities among patients with ALD which ultimately may limit their suitability for LT, unless properly addressed. Some of these comorbidities may be a direct effect of alcoholism, or they may be medical conditions commonly occurring in alcoholics. Patients with alcoholic cirrhosis may have alcohol related heart disease, such as alcoholic cardiomyopathy, in addition to the cirrhotic cardiomyopathy that is attributed to cirrhosis itself, and this may be related to the total lifetime use of alcohol (Urbano-Marquez et al., 1989). Alcoholic cardiomyopathy has specific diagnostic criteria and is associated with active alcohol intake. For that reason interventions that would lead to alcohol cessation would also prevent progression to cardiac failure. Additional medical comorbidities include neurologic disease ranging from myopathy to fixed deficits, with the latter being at times hard to differentiate from the hepatic encephalopathy that is associated with cirrhosis and can be reversible following LT (Keefe, 1997). Chronic pancreatitis and malnutrition are other problems commonly seen in these patients, whereas one cannot ignore the coexistence of other liver disease, such as chronic hepatitis C virus (HCV) infection or hepatocellular carcinoma (HCC), which can affect the urgency of LT, and especially the overall prognosis.

2.3 Acute alcoholic hepatitis

Acute alcoholic hepatitis (AH) represents a treatment dilemma for the medical team, as it may occur in patients with previously normal liver or with established cirrhosis. Patients with a previously normal liver present an opportunity, from a technical standpoint, as the liver transplantation is significantly easier with the absence of the trademarks of end-stage liver disease, such as portal hypertension (Figure 1 a, b).

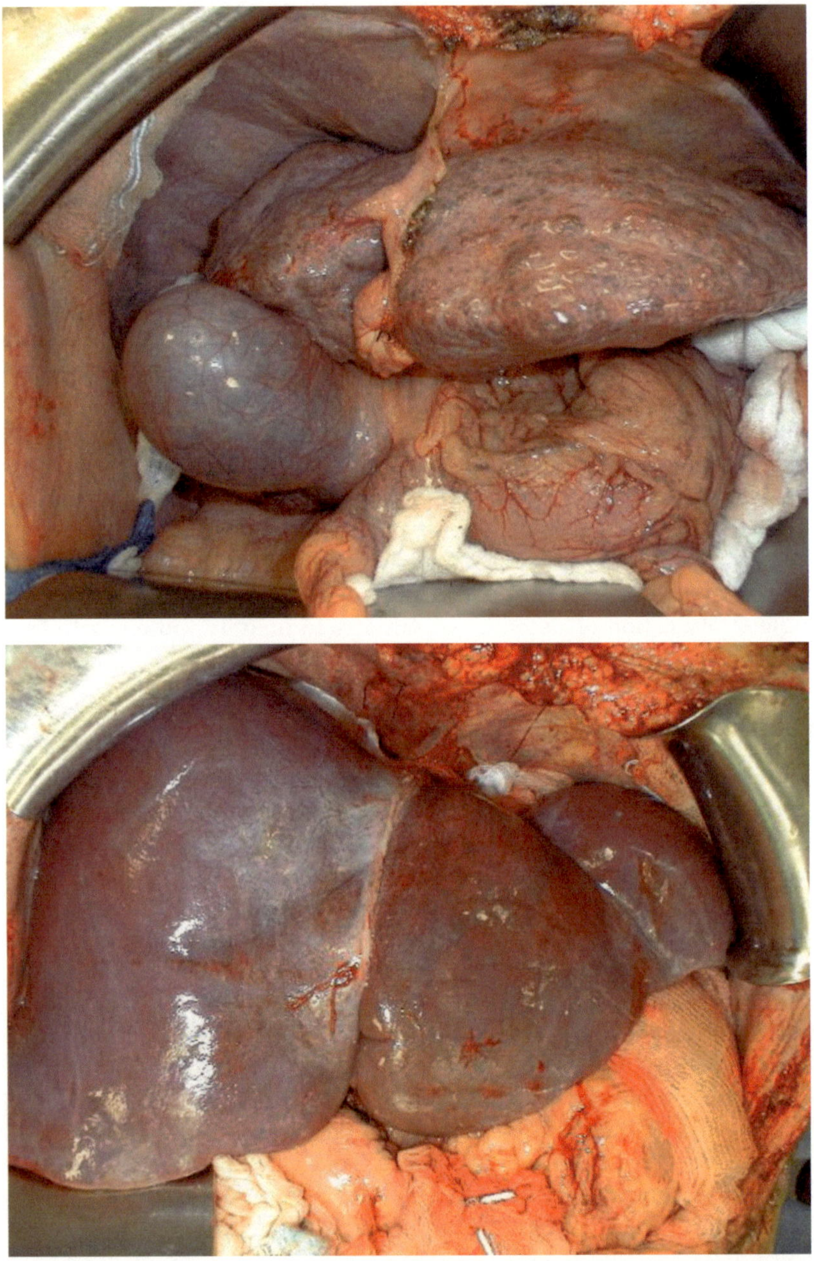

Fig. 1. a, b: Different types of livers encountered in patients with alcoholic liver disease. (a) This patient has acute alcoholic hepatitis on top of previously established cirrhosis. The hepatectomy stage of the LT is much more challenging in this patient. (b) This patient has acute alcoholic hepatitis without any previous evidence of cirrhosis, with the liver revealing some edema, but no cirrhosis.

Unfortunately, in the severe form, even with maximal medical treatment, there is a 40-50% mortality within 1 month after diagnosis (Dureja & Lucey, 2010). This very high mortality, despite the organ shortage, has led to many advocating LT for that subset of patients who have failed medical treatment. To date, only corticosteroids and pentoxifylline are considered to potentially improve short-term survival, although the results of meta-analysis remain controversial (Imperiale et al., 1990; Mathurin et al., 2011). Currently, the majority of transplant centers are reluctant to offer LT for patients with acute AH, although there is an effort to identify that subset of patients that will fail medical treatment with corticosteroids and likely benefit the most from LT. Experience has been mixed regarding transplantation for these patients, although there are some encouraging new studies, where strict selection can lead to favorable results, both in terms of survival, as well as in terms of relapse (Castel et al., 2009; Tome & Lucey, 2003). One of these studies was a European multicenter study about a carefully selected group of patients suffering from their first episode of severe AH and for whom medical treatment had failed. They had received a favorable psychosocial assessment and had excellent intermediate survival and low frequency of significant drinking after LT (Castel et al., 2009). Based on these results, transplant groups on both sides of the Atlantic have argued in favor of placement on the LT waiting list of patients with life-threatening AH who meet criteria.

3. Outcome of LT for ALD and ethical issues

3.1 Outcome of LT for ALD

The overall survival of patients who underwent LT for ALD is statistically comparable to that of patients who underwent LT for other indications. Data from the European Liver Transplant Registry 2008 revealed 1-, 5-, and 10-year patient survival rates for ALD of 96%, 88% and 76% respectively, as compared to 97%, 80% and 72% for patients with other indications (European Liver Transplantation Registry [ELTR], 2008). Similar survival rates have been reported for ALD patients in the US after LT: 92% at 1 year, 86% at 3 and 5 years and 76% at 9 years (Bhagat et al., 2009). It has been shown that patients with ALD had similar patient and graft survival rates, if not better in some cases, compared to those of patients undergoing LT for other indications (Dumortier et al., 2007; Mutimer et al., 2006; Romano et al., 1999). In a "perfect" world patients would have a single aetiology for their end-stage liver disease, unfortunately in the real world patients may undergo LT for ALD in the presence of other comorbidities, which can significantly affect the result. The most common is HCV, where there have been data of a more rapid progression of the liver disease in immunocompetent patients with the combination of ALD and HCV (Cromie et al., 1996; Pessione et al., 1998). However, other, more recent studies have shown that patients transplanted for ALD plus HCV had a better survival than patients with HCV alone and similar survival to those with ALD alone (Aguilera et al., 2009). This could be partly explained by the greater use of antiviral treatment in patients with HCV and ALD, as they were younger than the HCV alone patients. Furthermore, data from the European Liver Transplantation Registry have shown similar post-LT survival rates between patients with ALD and ALD plus a viral etiology (HCV and HBV), although patients with ALD plus HCV had a significantly shorter survival compared to those with ALD plus HBV infection (Burra et al., 2010). These data support the notion that ALD represents a good indication for LT, even in the presence of hepatitis virus infection.

Regarding long-term morbidity and survival in patients with ALD, there appears to be an effect from a high prevalence of medical comorbidities, including de novo cancers. In one study of a group of patients undergoing LT for ALD, 5 year graft and patient survival were significantly lower than non-alcoholics undergoing LT, mainly due to cardiorespiratory, cerebrovascular and neoplastic problems (Jain et al., 2000). When compared to patients receiving LT for other indications, those transplanted for ALD are at a greater risk of de novo malignancy, and especially aerodigestive cancers possibly due to the chronic alcohol use (Oo et al., 2005; Watt et al., 2009). These comorbidities are associated with worse survival (Bellamy et al., 2001; Duvoux et al., 1999). These studies do not show an association between new-onset cancers and alcoholic relapse. An important factor may be the high prevalence of chronic heavy tobacco use in this population, in combination with the immunosuppression. This presents the question of whether patients with ALD require specific surveillance programs for de novo tumours after LT. Also, if the link between tobacco use and death from either cancer or cardiovascular disease holds true, then an obvious way to improve post-transplant health is through the promotion of smoking cessation, especially in LT recipients with alcoholism.

3.2 Impact of recidivism on survival after LT for ALD

Not unexpectedly, better survival rates were observed for patients that remained abstinent after LT than those who returned to alcohol use. Still in trying to identify the impact of recidivism on survival after LT, first we have to overcome the problem of a lack of a commonly accepted definition and the fact that the reported rates of recidivism vary widely at different follow-up periods post-LT. In one of the better prospective studies, DiMartini et al., showed that 22% of patients had used some alcohol by the first year after LT and 42% had a drink by 5 years (DiMartini et al., 2006). By 5 years, 26% drank at a heavier use pattern and 20% in a frequent pattern. In another prospective study by DiMartini et al., there were five different patterns of alcohol consumption identified, based on the time of relapse and the subsequent pattern (DiMartini et al., 2010). Approximately 80% of the patients either did not drink or consumed only small amounts rarely. Among the remaining 20%, there were 3 patterns of harmful drinking, varied according to the time of relapse and the consumption of alcohol (sustained, heavy use or subsequently modified drinking). These data were similar to the retrospective data from Tang et al., who found harmful drinking in 16% of the patients (Tang et al., 1998). The problem of identifying a commonly-accepted definition for recidivism and the prevailing rates is made more difficult by the fact that most of these studies are based on data obtained through self-report questionnaires, interviews with patients and/or family members, or even retrospective analysis of routine screening tests. In all of this there is an apparent risk of underestimation.

However, there is disagreement on the impact of recidivism on post-transplant survival. Specifically, there have been studies showing no significant impact on survival rates (Burra et al., 2003; Gerhardt et al., 1996). These have been contradicted by other studies reporting 5- and 10-year survivals of 69% and 20% respectively in patients with alcohol relapse following LT, and the argument that attention needs to be paid to the different patterns of relapse, rather than the overall rate (DiMartini et al., 2006). It does appear that the long-term survival of patients who resume heavy drinking is lower compared to those who remain abstinent or have minor slips (Cuadrado et al., 2005; Pfitzmann et al., 2007). Interestingly enough, a significant factor for the decreased survival appears to be an association with developing malignancies, rather than recurrent end-stage liver disease. The influence of slips on LT outcome remains unclear, but there is the general perception that, although a slip should be considered an adverse event, it is unlikely to cause harm if it does not lead to a full-blown relapse (Cuadrado et al., 2005; Pfitzmann et al., 2007). One area where clinicians should pay particular attention to alcohol recidivism is when it is combined with concomitant HCV infection, since it may exacerbate the liver damage with rapid progression to cirrhosis and graft loss (Bellamy et al., 2001; Neuberger et al., 2002; Tome & Lucey, 2003). This can often lead to a late onset of acute or chronic rejection, whose management can be a nightmare in the patient with HCV recurrence (which is the vast majority of patients).

A question closely related to the effect of recidivism on survival after LT for ALD, is that of the quality of life after the LT. In a study in the UK of patients undergoing LT for ALD over a 10-year period, it was seen that overall in the long term at least 50% of the patients will drink again at some time post-LT, although at lower levels of alcohol intake than before the transplant (Perreira et al., 2000). The group at greatest risk for harmful drinking appears to be the patients with the most predictive factors for relapse, and thus the group that would benefit the most from professional counselling. Even so, the overall quality of life after LT for ALD, based on three different questionnaires, is high and in general similar to the level expected in the general population. When everything is put together regarding the issue of recidivism after LT for ALD, the challenge is the need for improved methodology and tools in monitoring post-transplantation abstinence, in order to better evaluate the effect of relapse. Ultimately, the question is critical, as it raises the issue of proper stewardship of a limited resource for society.

3.3 Cost-effectiveness of LT for ALD

As liver transplantation has not really been the subject of a randomized controlled trial, there is some uncertainty regarding the magnitude of the benefit and cost-effectiveness for specific patient groups. In an attempt to answer this question a study from England and Wales attempted an economic evaluation of liver transplantation in that area (Longworth et al., 2003). Cost-effectiveness was measured using incremental cost per quality-adjusted life years (QALY; commonly referred to as cost-utility analysis). The results of a comparison group, representing experience in the absence of LT, are estimated using a combination of observed data from patients waiting for transplant and published prognostic models. The analysis was limited to three disease groups for which prognostic models were available at the beginning of the study, one of which was the group of patients with ALD. Overall, a higher proportion of patients with ALD were assessed for a transplant but not placed on the waiting list. The estimated gain in quality-adjusted life-years from transplantation was positive for each of the disease groups. The mean incremental cost per quality-adjusted life-year from time of listing to 27 months was €54,000 (€13,500 to €93,500). The study showed that LT increases survival and health-related quality of life of ALD patients, although the cost-effectiveness estimates within that 27 month period were poorer for patients with ALD than for patients with PBC or

PSC. The authors suggested that this may reflect the cost of the higher number of ALD patients assessed for each transplant.

3.4 Ethical issues

The indication of ALD for LT is unlike many of the others as it involves the proper use of a scarce resource for patients with a potentially "self-inflicted" disease. Some have argued that since alcohol dependence as an "addiction" carries a neurobiological and a genetic component, then it may be more appropriate to treat it more as a medical condition. This does not answer the problem fully, as what matters is the outcome and if we accept that self-control has no role in the management of alcoholism then relapse would be all but a certainty. Others have challenged the ethics of the "6-month abstinence" rule, based on lack of evidence making it an arbitrary decision (Everhart & Beresford, 1997). Studies have found that although neither the presence of histological alcoholic hepatitis in the explant, nor any history of drinking within 6 months correlated with subsequent relapses (Tome et al., 2002; Wells et al., 2007). Against this background of conflicting data, there is a lack of consensus from country to country regarding the timing and suitability of patients with ALD for LT. One has to consider whether rules such as the "6-month" one represent an attempt towards an ethical approach to patient selection for LT, or whether they are a matter of practicality. For example, in the United States, the evaluation process usually results in the presentation of a comprehensive clinical and psychosocial assessment to the transplant program's selection committee. When the selection committee decides to recommend transplantation, the approval of the third party payer is necessary before the patient is placed on the waiting list. The 6-month rule has been widely adopted by the US insurance industry, without adequate data, leading to anecdotal reports of the difficult decisions involved (Boren, 1994). There are certain lessons that can be drawn regarding sobriety and prognosis after LT for ALD, which may have more validity than simply following the 6-month rule. Specifically, no single measure is a reliable prognosticator for future relapses into harmful drinking after transplantation, and although the duration of abstinence has been associated with subsequent drinking, it is an imprecise prognostic tool. Furthermore, there is more value in a careful evaluation by a trained addiction specialist with a special interest in transplant medicine, with such a psychosocial assessment helping determine the risk of relapse into significant alcohol abuse, but not with an absolute certainty. Finally, when all is said and done, the severely ill patient who has been drinking recently, but has other favorable prognostic indicators with respect to post-transplant behavior, represents a very difficult question for any transplant program.

Another issue is that since the need to restrict access to LT for patients with ALD is based on the donor shortage, then it could be argued that these recipients should be held to different standards when there is the possibility of a living donor. The answer to this question should still relate to the outcome and long-term results of LT for this group of patients, as no matter how willing the living donor may be, it must be made certain that the benefit to the recipient is worth the risk to the donor. Consideration of ALD patients as recipients for Living Donor Liver Transplantation (LDLT) has raised similar issues as those seen with cadaveric donation for these patients. Since most living donors are closely related to the recipient, they have watched the progression of ALD in the recipients over time and many may not regard the pathogenesis of ALD as totally unavoidable. This would result to donors seeing recipient relapses with alcohol, no matter how frequent or clinically significant, as ingratitude. Thus, for every patient with ALD being considered for LDLT there are individual conditions and relationships, which dictate significant less tolerance with alcohol relapse in LDLT compared to cadaveric donation.

The answer to many of these concerns has been the utilization of the 6 month abstinence rule by most programs. Notwithstanding the shortcomings of this rule regarding its predictive capacity that have been described elsewhere in this chapter, there are also certain issues unique to LDLT that may limit its use. Specifically, with a cadaveric LT there is the "luxury" of waiting given the organ shortage, and so that period can be used to test the abstinence and intervene; in LDLT the biggest advantage is the short preparative period and waiting time needed, something which would be negated by the strict use of the 6 month rule. Additionally, there are several Asian countries where, because of religious considerations, LDLT is the main type of LT, as cadaveric donation is limited or nonexistent. Thus, in these countries patients with ALD may have limited options. These two points are not meant to suggest that patients with ALD should be able to proceed with LDLT without addressing the issue of alcohol abuse and the possibility of recidivism, as that would be a disservice to the gift of the donor. A study by Hwang et al. from the Asan Medical Center in Korea of patients with ALD undergoing LDLT concluded that the pretransplant abstinence seemed to be beneficial and that for ethical reasons the 6 month abstinence rule should be strictly observed in LDLT (Hwang et al., 2006). When considering the ethical aspects of living organ donation, it is certainly reasonable to exclude recipients with significant factors for relapse. Also, we need to consider the unique aspects of the donor-recipient relationship, similar to those seen in the case of LDLT for patients with HCC. Along these lines a factor that may help is that a very close relationship between the donor and the recipient may be critical in preventing alcohol relapse or at least an escalation to significant alcohol abuse. The same study from South Korea found 3- and 5-year relapse rates of 20% in these patients undergoing LDLT for ALD, lower than many of the studies with cadaveric LT (Hwang et al., 2006). This issue cannot be simply ignored as in Korea, for example, at the Asan Medical Center 134 LDLTs had been performed by 2003, of which only four were for ALD (Moon & Lee, 2004). Although the actual prevalence of ALD in S. Korea may not be known, it is thought that 6% of patients with cirrhosis have ALD. This means that the trends are changing, as the 20-year vaccination program for Hepatitis B virus has reduced the incidence of the disease in the population, there is a gradual increase in alcohol consumption which will eventually lead to a higher need for LDLT for patients with ALD.

4. Future challenges

4.1 Psychosocial assessment

Evaluating the role of LT in the treatment of patients with ALD is a work in progress as significant challenges remain. Chief among them is the need for improved psychometric tools and assessments that would be able to predict with greater accuracy the pattern of alcohol use after transplant and the effect of that on the liver graft. This could lead to more targeted interventions with higher likelihood of success. A number of predictive tools have been considered as part of the assessment. The University of Michigan Alcoholism Prognosis Scale examines a number of psychosocial domains with a higher score suggesting increased stability leading to improved prognosis and Lucey et al. have suggested this broad-based tool as a useful alternative to the fixed pre-LT abstinence period (Lucey et al., 1997). Other tools include the alcohol abstinence self-Efficacy Scale which rates an individual's ability to self-determine in the context of relapse precipitants (DiClemente et al., 1994). Although it has shown good reliability and validity in alcohol treatment settings, it has yet to be proven in the liver transplant setting. Beresford, an addiction psychiatrist from the University of Michigan, who introduced the concept of psychosocial assessment of ALD transplant candidates, alerted the transplant community to the clinical insights into the factors involved in maintaining sobriety reported in the addiction literature (Beresford, 1994). Based on the studies of Vaillant and of Strauss and Bacon, he constructed a panel of negative prognostic factors that he used to assess prospective ALD patients as candidates for LT (Strauss & Bacon, 1951; Vaillant, 1995). These included psychiatric comorbid conditions, such as uncontrolled polysubstance abuse or unstable character disorder, a history of many failed rehabilitation attempts, social isolation as shown by lack of a fixed employment and living alone without a spouse or companion.

All of this has led to psychosocial assessment becoming part of the norm in liver transplant centers, where the use of agreed clinical guidelines and candidate selection criteria offer the assessment team a framework upon which to base complex decisions and an opportunity to explain the assessment and decision to the patient. It also allows transplant centers the opportunity to audit their selections and outcomes against accepted listing criteria. These observations, together with those by DiMartini documenting the five patterns of alcohol use, need validation in a large prospective cohort, and if successful can help clinicians identify tailored monitoring and interventions. Behavioral and pharmacological therapies may be necessary and helpful, but it is essential that they are individualized and that the support required is discussed and agreed upon with the candidate and their support system (DiMartini et al., 2010).

4.2 Genetic element of ALD

Also, further data are needed to clarify the element of genetic predisposition in alcohol abuse, as this too could help identify people at greater risk. Recent high-throughput technologies, such as micro arrays, genomics and proteomics have led to novel concepts in our understanding of several liver pathologies (Decaciuc et al., 2004; Seth et al., 2006). Application of these technologies has identified novel pathways that could not have been discovered using traditional methods and opened up several lines of investigation for understanding the mechanism involved in alcohol-mediated liver injury. Hepatic gene profiling using DNA micro arrays are reported from animal models of ALD and human ALD (Decaciuc et al., 2004; Seth et al., 2006). The ALD transcriptome profile is dominated by alcohol metabolism and inflammation related molecules, thus differing from other liver diseases (Seth et al., 2003). Additionally, several functional groups of genes showed similar qualitative and quantitative changes also in rodents as a result of chronic alcohol exposure regardless of the type of array platform (Decaciuc et al., 2004). This finding shows the existence of common mechanisms of alcohol effect on the liver across species.

In the past, genetic studies in ALD have focused on genes involved in alcohol metabolism (ADH, ALDH, CYP2E1), oxidative stress (GST, superoxide dismutase), endotoxin (TNF-a, CD14, TLR4), cytokines (IL-10), immune (cytotoxic T-lymphocyte antigen-4) and fibrosis (collagen, MMPs, osteopontin, TGF-b) and have been extensively reviewed (Stickel & Osterreicher, 2006). All appear to have an effect, but to date the search for single nucleotide polymorphisms (SNPs) in a hypothesis-driven candidate gene approach has been rather disappointing in identifying risk factors for ALD. Some of the reasons have been that most of the studies involved have either lacked statistical power due to small sample size, or investigated polymorphisms in a single or a few candidate genes or were subject to population stratification, Type 1 and 2 errors, or have failed to account for factors such as obesity and the confounding effect of Non-alcoholic steatohepatitis (NASH). Susceptibility to ALD, like most other multifactorial complex diseases, is controlled by a number of genes, each of which makes its own contribution. Therefore, what is needed is a genome-wide approach, in carefully designed large studies in order to identify various degree of risk genetic variants associated with ALD. The lack of an a priori hypothesis has helped Genome Wide Association (GWA) technologies yield successful outcomes in a variety of several common liver diseases (Karlsen et al., 2010; Kolleritis et al., 2009; Romeo et al., 2008). Advantage should also be taken of the understanding gained from research in other liver diseases, such as NASH, that show increasing parallels with ALD development. Recent advances in newer technologies enabling genome wide search for millions of SNPs, whole genome sequencing, global epigenetic profiles, and non-coding regulatory elements (miRNA) are the future research areas to construct the architecture of ALD and identify ways to predict and intervene in its progression. In these times of financial turmoil, a global well-coordinated effort is required to invest in future research to provide answers for a problem common in all different countries.

5. Conclusion

Liver transplantation has become over the last few decades one of the main treatments for advanced ALD. However, in order to optimize the results of this treatment, as well as fully establish its societal acceptance, it is imperative that careful patient selection takes place and that attention is paid not only to the peri-operative but also to the pre- and post-transplant periods. We need to stratify ALD potential transplant candidates according to the risk of relapse. Unfortunately, as we have seen in this chapter, to date the results reported from different studies are mostly inconclusive regarding the evaluation of predictive factors for alcoholic relapse after LT. Also, a defined pre-LT abstinence period for ALD candidates for transplantation appears to be justified, both as a way to ensure compliance, as well as an opportunity to effect some interventions to possibly recover liver function to the extent that a LT might not be needed. Even so, there are no strong data supporting the 6 month abstinence rule, and that means that we need to reach a consensus on this specific issue by conducting longitudinal, prospective studies. Just as important is the need to avoid the ease that strict "yes or no" rules and regulations offer (such as the 6 month rule) and concentrate more on creating and using improved psychomotor tools and assessments that will allow us to better evaluate and help these patients. The question of the definition of alcohol relapse is another area where further studies are needed. The reason is that although a number of patients return to some degree of alcohol use after LT, recidivism leading to liver disease threatening the graft is uncommon. Additionally, post-LT surveillance programs for the early detection of cardiovascular problems and de novo malignancies are also needed, given the apparent higher prevalence in this population. To fully achieve this, patients with ALD need to be evaluated and followed by a team of professionals, including internists, surgeons, hepatologists, psychiatrists and social workers who will be able to fully address their complicated needs.

6. References

Aguilera V, Berenguer M, Rubin A, et al. (2009). Cirrhosis of mixed etiology (hepatitis C virus and alcohol): posttransplantation outcome - comparison with hepatitis C virus-related cirrhosis and alcoholic-related cirrhosis. *Liver Transpl*, Vol.15, No.1, pp.79-87

Bellamy CO, DiMartini AM, Ruppert K, et al. (2001). Liver transplantation for alcoholic cirrhosis: long-term follow-up and impact of disease recurrence. *Transplantation*, Vol.72, No.4, pp. 619-626

Beresford TP, Everson GT. (2000). Liver transplantation for alcoholic liver disease: bias, beliefs, 6-month rule, and relapse - but where are the data? *Liver Transpl*, Vol.6, No.6, pp. 777-778

Beresford TP. (1994). Psychiatric assessment of alcoholic candidates for liver transplantation, In: *Liver Transplantation and the alcoholic patient: medical, surgical and psychosocial issues,* Lucey MR, Merion RM, Beresford TP, pp.29-49, Cambridge, UK: Cambridge University Press

Bhagat V, Mindikoglu AL, Nudo CG, et al. (2009). Outcomes of liver transplantation in patients with cirrhosis due to non alcoholic steatohepatitis versus patients with cirrhosis due to alcoholic liver disease. *Liver Transpl*, Vol.15, No.12, pp. 1814-1820

Boren SD. (1994). I had a tough day today, Hillary. *N Engl J Med*, Vol.330, No.7, pp. 500-502

Burra P, Senzolo M, Adam R, et al. (2010). Liver transplantation for alcoholic liver disease in Europe: a study from the ELTR (European Liver Transplant Registry). *Am J Transplant*, Vol.10, No.1, pp. 138-148

Burra P, Mioni D, Cillo U, et al. (2003). Long-term medical and psycho-social evaluation of patients undergoing orthotopic liver transplantation for alcoholic liver disease. *Transpl Int*, Vol.13, No. S1, pp. S174-178

Castel H, Moreno C, Antonini T, et al. (2009). Early transplantation improves survival of non-responders to steroids in severe alcoholic hepatitis: a challenge to the 6 months rule of abstinence. *Hepatology*, Vol.4, No., pp. 307-8

Cromie SL, Jenkins PJ, Bowden DS, et al. (1996). Chronic hepatitis C: effect of alcohol on hepatitis activity and viral titre. *J Hepatol*, Vol.25, No.6, pp. 821-826

Cuadrado A, Fabrega E, Casafont F, et al. (2005). Alcohol recidivism impairs long-term patient survival after orthotopic liver transplantation for alcoholic liver disease. *Liver Transpl*, Vol.11, No.4, pp. 420-426

Day E, Best D, Sweeting R, et al. (2008). Detecting lifetime alcohol problems in individuals referred for liver transplantation for non-alcoholic liver failure. *Liver Transpl*, Vol.14, No.11, pp. 1609-1613

Deaciuc IV, Arteel GE, Peng X, et al. (2004). Gene expression in the liver of rats fed alcohol by means of intragastric infusion. *Alcohol*, Vol.33, No.1, pp. 17-30

DeGottardi A, Spahr L, Gelez P, et al. (2007). A simple score for predicting alcohol relapse after liver transplantation: results from 387 patients over 15 years. *Arch Intern Med*, Vol.167, No.11, pp.1183-1188

DiClemente CC, Carbonari JP, Montgomery RP, et al. (1994). The Alcohol Abstinence Self-Efficacy scale. *J Stud Alcohol*, Vol.55, No.2, pp. 141-148

DiMartini A, Dew MA, Day N, et al. (2010). Trajectories of alcohol consumption following liver transplantation. *Am J Transplant*, Vol.10, No.10, pp. 2305-2312

DiMartini A, Day N, Dew MA, et al. (2006). Alcohol consumption patterns and predictors of use following liver transplantation for alcoholic liver disease. *Liver Transpl*, Vol.12, No.5, pp. 813-820

Dobbels F, Vanhaecke J, Dupont L, et al. (2009). Pretransplant predictors of posttransplant adherence and clinical outcome: an evidence base for pretransplant psychosocial screening. *Transplantation*, Vol.87, No.10, pp. 1497-1504

Dumortier J, Guillaud O, Adham M, et al. (2007). Negative impact of de novo malignancies rather than alcohol relapse on survival after liver transplantation for alcoholic cirrhosis: a retrospective analysis of 305 patients in a single center. *Am J Gastroenterol*, Vol.102, No.5, pp. 1032-1041

Dureja P, Lucey MR. (2010). The place of liver transplantation in the treatment of severe alcoholic hepatitis. *J Hepatol*, Vol.52, No.5, pp. 759-764

Duvoux C, Delacroix I, Richardet JP, et al. (1999). Increased incidence of oropharyngeal squamous cell carcinoma after liver transplantation for alcoholic cirrhosis. *Transplantation*, Vol.67, No.3, pp. 418-421

Everhart JE, Beresford TP. (1997). Liver transplantation for alcoholic liver disease: a survey of transplantation programs in the United States. *Liver Transpl*, Vol.3, No.3, pp. 220-226

European Liver Transplantation Registry. (2008). Data. *ELTR website*. http://www.eltr.org.publi/results.php3

Foster PF, Fabrega F, Karademir S, et al. (1997). Prediction of abstinence from ethanol in alcoholic recipients following liver transplantation. *Hepatology*, Vol.25, No.6, pp. 1469-1477

Gedaly R, McHugh PP, Johnston TD, et al. (2008). Predictors of relapse to alcohol and illicit drugs after liver transplantation for alcoholic liver disease. *Transplantation*, Vol.86, No.8, pp. 1090-1095

Gerhardt TC, Goldstein RM, Urschel HC, et al. (1996). Alcohol use following liver transplantation for alcoholic cirrhosis. *Transplantation*, Vol.62, No.8, pp. 1060-1063

Hwang S, Lee SG, Kim KK, et al. (2006). Efficacy of 6-month pretransplant abstinence for patients with alcoholic liver disease undergoing living donor liver transplantation. *Transplant Proc*, Vol.38, No.9, pp. 2937-2940

Imperiale TF, McCullough AJ. (1990). Do corticosteroids reduce mortality from alcoholic hepatitis? A meta-analysis of the randomized trials. *Ann Intern Med*, Vol. 113, No.4, pp. 299-307

Jain A, DiMartini A, Kashyap R, et al. (2000). Long term follow-up after liver transplantation for alcoholic liver disease under tacrolimus. *Transplantation*, Vol.70, No.9, pp. 1135-1142

Kamath PS, Wiesner RH, Malinchoc M, et al. (2001). A model to predict survival in patients with end-stage liver disease. *Hepatology*, Vol.33, No.2, pp. 464-470

Karim Z, Intaraprasong P, Scudamore CH, et al. (2010). Predictors of relapse to significant alcohol drinking after liver transplantation. *Can J Gastroenterol*, Vol. 24, No.4, pp. 245-250

Karlsen TH, Franke A, Melum E, et al. (2010). Genome-wide association analysis in primary sclerosing cholangitis. *Gastroenterology*, Vol.138, No.3, pp. 1102-1111

Keefe EB. (1997). Comorbidities of alcoholic liver disease that affect outcome of orthotopic liver transplantation. *Liver Transpl Surg*, Vol.3, pp. 251-257

Kelly M, Chick J, Gribble R, et al. (2006). Predictors of relapse to harmful alcohol after orthotopic liver transplantation. *Alcohol Alcohol*, Vol.41, No.3, pp. 278-283

Kolleritis B, Coassin S, Kiechl S, et al. (2009). A common variant in the adiponutrin gene influences liver enzyme levels. *J Med Genet*, Vol.213, No.2, pp. 116-119

Kotlyar DS, Burke A, Campbell MS, et al. (2008). A critical review of candidacy for orthotopic liver transplantation in alcoholic liver disease. *Am J Gastroenterol*, Vol.103, No.3, pp. 734-743

Longworth L, Young T, Buxton MJ, et al. (2003). Midterm cost-effectiveness of the liver transplantation program of England and Wales for three disease groups. *Liver Transpl*, Vol.9, No.12, pp. 1295-1307

Lucey MR, Carr K, Beresford TP, et al. (1997). Alcohol use after liver transplantation in alcoholics: a clinical cohort follow-up study. *Hepatology*, Vol.25, No.5, pp. 1223-1227

Mathurin P, O'Grady J, Carithers RL, et al. (2011). Corticosteroids improve short-term survival in patients with severe alcoholic hepatitis: meta analysis of individual patient data. *Gut*, Vol.60, No.2, pp. 255-260

Mathurin P. (2005). Is alcoholic hepatitis an indication for transplantation? Current management and outcomes. *Liver Transpl*, Vol.11, No.S2, pp. S21-S24

Moon DB, Lee SG. (2004). Adult-to-adult living donor liver transplantation at the Asan Medical Center. *Yonsei Med J*, Vol.45, No.6, pp. 1162-1168

Mutimer DJ, Gunson B, Chen J, et al. (2006). Impact of donor age and year of transplantation on graft and patient survival following liver transplantation for hepatitis C virus. *Transplantation*, Vol.81, No.1, pp. 7-14

National Institute of Health. (1984). Consensus development conference statement: liver transplantation. *Hepatology*, Vol.4, No.S1, pp. S1075-S1105

Neuberger J, Schulz KH, Day K, et al. (2002). Transplantation for alcoholic liver disease. *J Hepatol*, Vol.36, No.1, pp. 130-137

Oo YH, Gunson BK, Lancashire RJ, et al. (2005). Incidence of cancers following orthotopic liver transplantation in a single center: comparison with national cancer incidence rates for England and Wales. *Transplantation*, Vol.80, No.6, pp. 759-764

Perreira SP, Howard LM, Muiesan P, et al. (2000). Quality of life after liver transplantation for alcoholic liver disease. *Liver Transpl*, Vol.6, No.6, pp. 762-768

Pessione F, Degos F, Marcellin P, et al. (1998). Effect of alcohol consumption on serum hepatitis C virus RNA and histological lesions in chronic hepatitis C. *Hepatology*, Vol.27, No.6, pp. 1717-1722

Pfitzmann R, Schwenzer J, Rayes N, et al. (2007). Long-term survival and predictors of relapse after orthotopic liver transplantation for alcoholic liver disease. *Liver Transpl*, Vol.13, No.2, pp. 197-205

Romano DR, Jimenez C, Rodriguez F, et al. (1999). Orthotopic liver transplantation in alcoholic liver cirrhosis. *Transplant Proc*, Vol.31, No.6, pp. 2491-2493

Romeo S, Kozlitina J, Xing C, et al. (2008). Genetic variation in PNPLA3 confers susceptibility to nonalcoholic fatty liver disease. *Nat Genet*, Vol.40, No.12, pp. 1461-1465

Starzl TE, Van Thiel D, Tzakis AG, et al. (1988). Orthotopic liver transplantation for alcoholic cirrhosis. *JAMA*, Vol.260, No.17, pp. 1542-2544

Seth D, Cordoba S, Gorrell MD, et al. (2006). Intrahepatic gene expression in human alcoholic hepatitis. *J Hepatol*, Vol.45, No.2, pp. 306-320

Seth D, Leo MA, McGuinness PH et al. (2003). Gene expression profiling of alcoholic liver disease in the baboon (Papio hamadryas) and human liver. *Am J Pathol*, Vol.163, No.6, pp. 2303-2317

Stickel F, Osterreicher CH. (2006). The role of genetic polymorphisms in alcoholic liver disease. *Alcohol Alcohol*, Vol.41, No.3, pp. 209-224

Strauss R, Bacon SD. (1951). Alcoholism and social stability. *Q J Stud Alcohol*, Vol.12, pp. 231-260

Tome S, Lucey MR. (2003). Timing of liver transplantation in alcoholic cirrhosis. *J Hepatol*, Vol.39, No.3, pp. 320-327

Tome S, Martinez-Rey C, Gonzalez-Quintela A, et al. (2002). Influence of superimposed alcoholic hepatitis on the outcome of liver transplantation for and-stage alcoholic liver disease. *J Hepatol*, Vol.36, No.6, pp. 793-798

Tang H, Boulton R, Gunson B, et al. (1998). Patterns of alcohol consumption after liver transplantation. *Gut*, Vol.43, No.1, pp. 140-145

Urbano-Marquez A, Estruch R, Navarro-Lopez F, et al. (1989). The effects of alcoholism on skeletal and cardiac muscle. *N Engl J Med*, Vol.320, No.7, pp. 409-415

Vaillant GE. (1995). *The natural history of alcoholism revisited*. Harvard University Press, Cambridge, MA.

Veldt BJ, Laine F, Guillygomarch A, et al. (2002). Indication of liver transplantation in severe alcoholic liver cirrhosis: qualitative evaluation and optimal timing. *J Hepatol*, Vol.36, No.1, pp. 93-98

Watt KDS, Pedersen RA, Kremers WK, et al. (2009). Long-term probability of and mortality from de novo malignancy after liver transplantation. *Gastroenterology*, Vol.137, No.6, pp. 2010-2017

Wells JT, Said A, Agni R, et al. (2007). The impact of acute alcoholic hepatitis in the explanted recipient liver on outcome after liver transplantation. *Liver Transpl*, Vol.13, No.12, pp. 1728-1735